Evidence-based Management of

STROKE

José Biller
José M. Ferro

tfm Publishing Limited, Castle Hill Barns, Harley, Nr Shrewsbury, SY5 6LX, UK.
Tel: +44 (0)1952 510061; Fax: +44 (0)1952 510192
E-mail: nikki@tfmpublishing.com; Web site: www.tfmpublishing.com

Design & Typesetting: Nikki Bramhill BSc Hons Dip Law
First Edition: © June 2011
ISBN: 978 1 903378 76 2

Cover image: © 2011 3d4medical, www.3d4medical.com

Printed by Gutenberg Press Ltd., Gudja Road, Tarxien, PLA 19, Malta.
Tel: +356 21897037; Fax: +356 21800069.

Contents

page

Foreword   v

Contributors   vi

Acknowledgements   ix

Using evidence-based medicine   x

Chapter 1   Thrombolysis in ischemic stroke   1
Lars Marquardt, Jens Regula, Christian Hametner,
Werner Hacke

Chapter 2   Management of stroke risk factors   19
Gustavo A. Ortiz, Ralph L. Sacco

Chapter 3   Antithrombotic therapies in stroke prevention   45
James F. Meschia

Chapter 4   Anticoagulant therapy in prevention of ischemic stroke   59
Harold P. Adams, Jr.

Chapter 5   Interventions for acute ischemic stroke   89
Gabriel A. Smith, Zakaria Hakma, Christopher M. Loftus

Chapter 6   Interventions for carotid artery   107
disease and intracranial stenosis
Gabriel A. Smith, Zakaria Hakma, Christopher M. Loftus

Chapter 7   Surgery for acute ischemic stroke   123
Katayoun Vahedi, Marie-Germaine Bousser

Chapter 8   Management of ruptured cerebral aneurysms and   135
aneurysmal subarachnoid hemorrhage
Stephen F. Shafizadeh, Rudy J. Rahme, Christopher S.
Eddleman, Bernard R. Bendok, H. Hunt Batjer

Chapter 9   Management of spontaneous intracerebral hemorrhage   175
Barbara Voetsch, Carlos S. Kase

Chapter 10   Cerebral venous sinus thrombosis   205
José M. Ferro, Patrícia Canhão

Chapter 11   Ischemic stroke in children   221
E. Steve Roach

Chapter 12   Stroke in pregnancy and puerperium   239
Rima M. Dafer

Chapter 13   Oral contraceptives, hormonal therapy and stroke   255
Kerstin Bettermann

Chapter 14   The management of cerebrovascular   279
complications in cardiac procedures
Sara Hocker, José Biller

Chapter 15   Central nervous system vascular malformations   301
A. Jess Schuette, C. Michael Cawley, Daniel L. Barrow

Index   317

Foreword

The World Health Organization estimates that worldwide approximately 15 million people will suffer a stroke each year. The burden of stroke is high and accounts for 5.54 million deaths worldwide, with two thirds of these deaths occurring in less developed countries. It is the prevalence of stroke and the resultant disability that resulted in the practice of vascular neurology to continue to evolve and incorporate those rapid changes in technology and the implementation of revolutionary advances in stroke management.

This book is designed to fill a growing need of clinicians who treat and care for stroke patients to have access to a state-of-the art, and user-friendly reference. Each chapter is a succinct compilation of basic research and clinical advances. It is hoped that this evidence-based book will provide an important, concise and robust management perspective of the clinical spectrum of cerebrovascular disorders, and thus improve patient care. To achieve this goal, we were fortunate to have the intellectual rigor and scientific excellence of many of our transcontinental medical and surgical colleagues who are experts in stroke care, management and research.

Finally, we are well aware that a caveat exists with all texts which provide recommendations so, we invite our readers to inform us of differences of opinion with our recommendations and of areas that were either overlooked or need further comment.

José Biller MD, FACP, FAAN, FAHA
Professor and Chairman
Department of Neurology
Loyola University Chicago
Stritch School of Medicine
2160 S. 1st Avenue
Bldg. 105, Room 2700
Maywood, IL 60153, USA
Phone: 708-216-2438
Fax: 708-216-5617
e-mail: jbiller@lumc.edu

José M. Ferro MD, PhD
Professor and Chairman
Department of Neurosciences
Neurology Service, 6th Floor
Hospital de Santa Maria
University of Lisbon
Lisbon, Portugal
1649-028 Lisbon
Phone/Fax: 00 351 21 7957474
e-mail: jmferro@fm.ul.pt

Contributors

Harold P. Adams, Jr., MD Professor of Neurology, Division of Cerebrovascular Diseases, Department of Neurology, Carver College of Medicine, University of Iowa Health Care Stroke Center, University of Iowa, Iowa City, Iowa, USA

Daniel L. Barrow MD MBNA/Bowman Professor and Chairman, Director, Emory Stroke Center, Department of Neurosurgery, Emory University School of Medicine, Atlanta, Georgia, USA

H. Hunt Batjer MD Michael J. Marchese Professor and Chair, Department of Neurosurgery, Feinberg School of Medicine, Northwestern University, Chicago, Illinois, USA

Bernard R. Bendok MD Associate Professor of Neurosurgery and Radiology, Department of Neurosurgery, Feinberg School of Medicine, Northwestern University, Chicago, Illinois, USA

Kerstin Bettermann MD PhD Assistant Professor of Neurology, Department of Neurology, Penn State College of Medicine, Hershey, Pennsylvania, USA

José Biller MD FACP FAAN FAHA Professor and Chairman, Department of Neurology, Loyola University Chicago, Stritch School of Medicine, Maywood, Illinois, USA

Marie-Germaine Bousser MD Professor in Neurology, Neurology Department, Lariboisière Hospital, Assistance Publique Hôpitaux de Paris, Paris, France

Patrícia Canhão MD PhD Assistant Professor and Consultant Neurologist, Department of Neurosciences, Hospital de Santa Maria, University of Lisbon, Lisboa, Portugal

C. Michael Cawley MD Associate Professor, Department of Neurosurgery, Emory University, Atlanta, Georgia, USA

Rima M. Dafer MD MPH FAHA Associate Professor of Neurology, Loyola University Chicago, Stritch School of Medicine, Maywood, Illinois, USA

Christopher S. Eddleman MD PhD Cerebrovascular Fellow, Department of Neurosurgery and Radiology, UT Southwestern Medical Center, Dallas, Texas, USA

José M. Ferro MD PhD Chairman and Full Professor, Department of Neurosciences, Hospital de Santa Maria, University of Lisbon, Lisboa, Portugal

Werner Hacke MD PhD Professor of Neurology, University of Heidelberg, Department of Neurology, Heidelberg, Germany

Zakaria Hakma MD Chief Neurosurgical Resident, Department of Neurosurgery, Temple University Hospital, Philadelphia, USA

Christian Hametner MD Neurology Registrar, University of Heidelberg, Department of Neurology, Heidelberg, Germany

Sara Hocker MD Fellow, Division of Critical Care Neurology, Mayo Clinic, Rochester, Minnesota, USA

Carlos S. Kase MD Professor of Neurology, Boston Medical Center, Boston University School of Medicine, Boston, Massachusetts, USA

Christopher M. Loftus MD Dr. h.c. FACS Professor and Chairman of the Department of Neurosurgery, Temple University Hospital; Chairman of the AANS International Outreach Committee; WFNS Assistant Treasurer; and Assistant Dean for International Affiliations, Temple University School of Medicine, Philadelphia, USA

Lars Marquardt MD DPhil Consultant Neurologist, University of Heidelberg, Department of Neurology, Heidelberg, Germany

James F. Meschia MD Professor of Neurology, and Chair of the Cerebrovascular Division, Mayo Clinic, Jacksonville, Florida, USA

Gustavo A. Ortiz MD Assistant Professor of Clinical Neurology, University of Miami, Miller School of Medicine, Miami, Florida, USA

Rudy J. Rahme MD Post-Doctoral Research Fellow, Department of Neurosurgery, Feinberg School of Medicine, Northwestern University, Chicago, Illinois, USA

Jens Regula MD Neurology Registrar, University of Heidelberg, Department of Neurology, Heidelberg, Germany

E. Steve Roach MD Professor and Chief, Division of Child Neurology, Ohio State University School of Medicine, Nationwide Children's Hospital, Columbus, Ohio, USA

Ralph L. Sacco MS MD FAAN FAHA Professor and Olemberg Family Chair in Neurological Disorders, Miller Professor of Neurology, Epidemiology, and Human Genetics, University of Miami, Miller School of Medicine, Miami, Florida, USA

A. Jess Schuette MD Resident, Department of Neurosurgery, Emory University, Atlanta, Georgia, USA

Stephen F. Shafizadeh MD PhD DC Resident Physician, PGY-6 and infolded Cerebrovascular and Skull Base Fellow, Department of Neurosurgery, Feinberg School of Medicine, Northwestern University, Chicago, Illinois, USA

Gabriel A. Smith BS Medical Student, Temple University School of Medicine, Philadelphia, USA

Katayoun Vahedi MD Consultant Neurologist, Neurology Department, Lariboisière Hospital, Assistance Publique Hôpitaux de Paris, Paris, France

Barbara Voetsch MD PhD Assistant Professor of Neurology, Lahey Clinic Medical Center, Tufts University School of Medicine, Burlington, Massachusetts, USA

Acknowledgements

We especially thank the contributing authors for their generosity in giving their time, effort, and expertise to the preparation of this book. The encouragement, dedication, and professionalism of Nikki Bramhill, Director, tfm Publishing Ltd., and Jonathan Gregory, Commissioning Editor, tfm Publishing Ltd, are gratefully acknowledged. Our gratitude also extends to Linda Turner and Luisa Mendonça for their wonderful secretarial and administrative support during this project.

Dedication

To the patients who suffer from the cerebrovascular diseases and their families, and to all "students of medicine", young and old, who appreciate the value of evidence-based medicine.

Using evidence-based medicine

The process of gathering evidence is a time-consuming task. One of the main reasons for supporting the use of evidence-based medicine, is the rate of change of new practices, and the increasing tendency for specialisation. Medical information is widely available from a variety of sources for clinicians but keeping up-to-date with current literature remains an almost impossible task for many with a busy clinical workload. *Evidence-based Management of Stroke* has been written to aid this process. The chapters in this book have been written by internationally renowned experts who have applied the principles of evidence-based medicine and taken relevant clinical questions and examined the current evidence for the answers. The authors were asked to quote levels and grades of evidence for each major point, and to provide a summary of key points and their respective evidence levels at the end of each chapter. The levels of evidence and grades of evidence used in this book are shown in Tables 1 and 2 and are widely used in evidence-based medicine.

Table 1. Levels of evidence.

Level	Type of evidence
Ia	Evidence obtained from systematic review or meta-analysis of randomised controlled trials
Ib	Evidence obtained from at least one randomised controlled trial
IIa	Evidence obtained from at least one well-designed controlled study without randomisation
IIb	Evidence obtained from at least one other type of well-designed quasi-experimental study
III	Evidence obtained from well-designed non-experimental descriptive studies, such as comparative studies, correlation studies and case studies
IV	Evidence obtained from expert committee reports or opinions and/or clinical experience of respected authorities

Table 2. Grades of evidence.

Grade of evidence	Evidence
A	At least one randomised controlled trial as part of a body of literature of overall good quality and consistency addressing the specific recommendation (evidence levels Ia and Ib)
B	Well-conducted clinical studies but no randomised clinical trials on the topic of recommendation (evidence levels IIa, IIb, III)
C	Expert committee reports or opinions and/or clinical experience of respected authorities. This grading indicates that directly applicable clinical studies of good quality are absent (evidence level IV)

Chapter 1

Thrombolysis in ischemic stroke

Lars Marquardt MD DPhil, Consultant Neurologist
Jens Regula MD, Neurology Registrar
Christian Hametner MD, Neurology Registrar
Werner Hacke MD PhD, Professor of Neurology
University of Heidelberg
Department of Neurology
Heidelberg, Germany

Introduction

The majority of strokes are due to a blockage of an artery in the brain by a blood clot of different origins. Prompt treatment with thrombolytic drugs can restore blood flow before major brain damage has occurred and could improve recovery after stroke. Thrombolytic drugs, however, can also cause serious bleeding in the brain, which can be fatal. Recombinant tissue plasminogen activator (rt-PA or alteplase) is licensed for use in selected stroke patients.

Thrombolytic therapy results in a significant net reduction in the proportion of patients dying or dependent in activities of daily living. This overall benefit seems to be apparent despite an increase in symptomatic intracranial haemorrhages [1]. Either way, revascularization is important to achieve a good outcome – the faster, the better [2] **(Ia/A)**. International guidelines (American Stroke Association and European Stroke Organisation) are recommended for additional frequently updated information.

Intravenous thrombolysis

Within 3 hours of symptom onset

In 1996, the US Food and Drug Administration (FDA) approved the use of intravenous rt-PA as treatment for acute ischemic stroke in a 3-hour time window after symptom onset. The European Medicines Evaluation Agency (EMEA) followed in 2002 by granting a restricted license for the use of rt-PA for treatment of ischemic stroke patients within 3 hours of symptom onset.

These decisions were substantially based on the results of the National Institute of Neurological Disorders and Stroke (NINDS) rt-PA Stroke Study, in which 624 patients with ischemic stroke were treated intravenously with either placebo or rt-PA (0.9mg/kg, maximum 90mg) within 3 hours of symptom onset [3] **(Ia/A)**. Favorable outcome (complete or nearly complete neurological recovery 3 months after stroke) was achieved in 31-50% of patients treated with rt-PA compared to 20-38% of patients given placebo. The number needed to treat with rt-PA for a favorable outcome after 3 months was 7. The benefit was similar 1 year after stroke [4] **(Ia/A)**. The major risk of treatment was symptomatic brain hemorrhage, which occurred in 6.4% of patients treated with rt-PA and 0.6% of patients given placebo. However, the death rate in the two treatment groups was similar at 3 months (17% vs. 20%) and 1 year (24% vs. 28%) [3-4] **(Ia/A)**.

In contrast, the ECASS (European Cooperative Acute Stroke Study) and ECASS II studies did not show statistically significant superiority of rt-PA for the primary endpoints when treatment was given within 6 hours [5-6] **(Ia/A)**. However, a post hoc analysis concluded that those patients treated within 3 hours appeared to benefit from rt-PA [7, 8] **(Ia/A)**. In ECASS II, 800 patients were assigned to treatment with either rt-PA (0.9mg/kg) or placebo. Another post hoc analysis of ECASS II showed that the likelihood of either death or dependency was lower among the patients treated with rt-PA compared to placebo [5]. Similarly to the NINDS results, the rate of symptomatic intracranial hemorrhage was increased with rt-PA treatment (8.8% vs. 3.4%).

The EMEA granted a license for rt-PA on condition of a prospective registry of patient treatment experience with rt-PA given within the 3-hour window from symptom onset (Safe Implementation of Thrombolysis in Stroke-Monitoring Study, SITS-MOST), which reported that the frequency of symptomatic intracerebral hemorrhage (per NINDS definition) at 24 hours after rt-PA was 7.3% (95% CI, 6.7-7.9%). For efficacy, the frequency of scores of 0, 1, and 2 on the combined modified Rankin Scale (mRS) at 90 days was 54.8% (95% CI, 53.5-56.0%) among rt-PA patients [9]. These findings appear to confirm the potential safety of rt-PA within the 3-hour window in European centers.

Furthermore, subsequent to the approval of rt-PA for treatment of patients with acute ischemic stroke, several groups reported on the utility of the treatment in a community setting sometimes reporting higher rates of intracranial bleeding associated with rt-PA treatment than described in NINDS or ECASS [10-16]. However, it is now clear that the risk of hemorrhage is proportional to the degree to which the NINDS protocol is not followed [10, 17-18].

There is strong evidence that there is a significant time effect for treatment with rt-PA even within the 3-hour time window (see Figure 1). A pooled data analysis of rt-PA trials showed that earlier treatment results in a better outcome. A similar finding has been described in a subgroup analysis based on NINDS data [19]. Treatment initiated within 90 minutes of symptom onset was associated with an odds ratio (OR) of 2.11 (95% CI, 1.33-3.55) for favorable outcome at 3 months compared to 1.69 (95% CI, 1.09-2.62) within 90 to 180 minutes after onset [20].

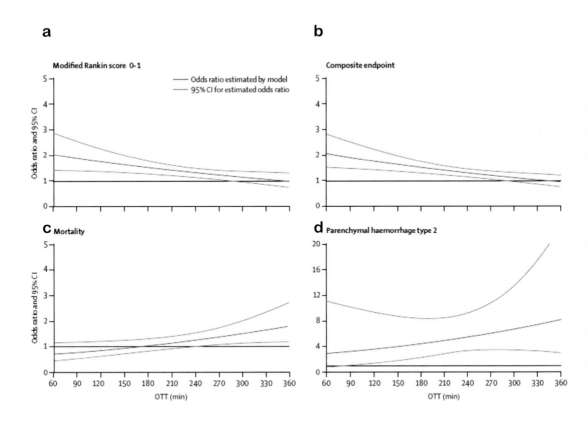

Figure 1. Relation of stroke onset to start of treatment (OTT) with treatment effect after adjustment for prognostic variables assessed by: a) day 90 modified Rankin score 0-1 versus 2-6 (interaction p=0.0269, n=3530 [excluding EPITHET data p=0.0116, n=3431]); b) global test that incorporates modified Rankin score 0-1 versus 2-6, Barthel Index score 95-100 versus 90 or lower and NIHSS score 0-1 versus 2 or more (interaction p=0.0111, n=3535 [excluding EPITHET data p=0.0049, n=3436]); c) mortality (interaction p=0.0444, n=3530 [excluding EPITHET7 data p=0.0582, n=3431]); and d) parenchymal haemorrhage type 2 (interaction p=0.4140, n=3531 [excluding EPITHET data p=0.4578, n=3431]). Thus, for parenchymal haemorrhage type 2, the fitted line is not statistically distinguishable from a horizontal line. For each graph, the adjusted odds ratio is shown with the 95% CIs. *Reproduced with permission from Lees KR, Bluhmki E, von Kummer R, et al* [2]. *Copyright © 2010, Elsevier.*

Patients with major strokes (National Institute of Health Stroke Scale [NIHSS] score >22) have a very poor prognosis, but some positive treatment effect with rt-PA has been documented [21]. However, the risk of hemorrhage is high in these patients; hence, the decision to treat with rt-PA should be made with caution.

Early ischemic changes on a baseline CT scan do not seem to be associated with adverse outcome, although these findings are associated with a higher risk of symptomatic intracranial haemorrhage [22-23].

Several factors associated with an increased risk of intracranial bleeding following rt-PA treatment for ischemic stroke have been identified in several post hoc analyses [24]. These include elevated serum glucose, a history of diabetes, baseline symptom severity, advanced age, increased time to treatment, previous aspirin use, a history of congestive heart failure, low plasminogen activator inhibitor activity, and NINDS protocol violations. However, none of these factors reversed the overall benefit of rt-PA.

Although rare, there are other complications besides intracranial hemorrhage one has to look out for by treating stroke patients with rt-PA, including systemic bleeding, myocardial rupture if the agent is given within a few days of acute myocardial infarction, and reactions such as anaphylaxis [25].

Expanded time window

Based on pooled analyses from the ATLANTIS, ECASS, and NINDS rt-PA stroke trials published in 2004, it has been suggested that there should be a benefit for systemic thrombolysis for acute stroke beyond a 3-hour time window [20]. Recently these data have been updated with new and up-to-date analyses, coming to the conclusion that patients benefit from intravenous rt-PA treatment at least up to 4.5 hours after onset [2]. In addition, a post hoc analysis of data acquired in the SITS-ISTR project between 2002 and 2007 compared close to 12,000 patients treated with rt-PA within 3 hours of stroke onset with 664 patients who received treatment within 3-4.5 hours [26] (Ia/A). It has been concluded that treatment with rt-PA remains safe when given at 3-4.5 hours after ischemic stroke, offering an opportunity for patients who cannot be treated within the standard 3-hour time window.

In 2008, the ECASS-3 study has provided new data on systemic thrombolysis with rt-PA in a time window of 3-4.5 hours after stroke onset [27] (Ia/A). This multicenter, randomized, placebo-controlled, prospective study enrolled over 800 patients to either systemic treatment with rt-PA or placebo within 3-4.5 hours after stroke symptom onset. Persons older than 80 years, those with a baseline NIHSS score >25, those taking oral anticoagulants, and those who had the combination of a previous stroke and diabetes mellitus were excluded from participation. Symptomatic intracranial hemorrhage, as defined by the criteria used in the NINDS study, was diagnosed in 7.9% of subjects treated with rt-PA and 3.5% when given placebo (OR 2.38; 95% CI, 1.25-4.52; $p<0.006$). However, this increased incidence of hemorrhage is consistent with other clinical rt-PA trials [3, 5, 6, 28-29]. The frequency of the primary efficacy outcome in ECASS-3 (defined as mRS score of 0 to 1 at 90 days after treatment) was significantly greater with rt-PA (52.4%) than with placebo (45.2%; OR 1.34; 95% CI, 1.02-1.76; risk ratio 1.16; 95% CI, 1.01-1.34; $p<0.04$). The number needed to treat to achieve the primary efficacy outcome was 14. Mortality in the two ECASS-3 treatment groups did not differ significantly, although it was nominally higher among the subjects treated with placebo [27] (Ia/A).

A recently published subgroup outcome analysis of ECASS-3 data has shown, that treatment with rt-PA is effective and safe in various subgroups, including older patients (<65 years: OR 1.61; 95% CI, 1.05-2.48; > or =65 years: 1.15; 0.80-1.64; p=0.230). The effectiveness was independent of the severity of stroke at baseline (NIHSS score 0-9: 1.28; 0.84-1.96; NIHSS score 10-19: 1.16; 0.73-1.84; NIHSS score > or = 20: 2.32; 0.61-8.90; p=0.631). The incidence of symptomatic intracranial hemorrhage seemed to be independent of previous antiplatelet drug use (no: 2.41; 1.09-5.33; yes: 2.33; 0.79-6.90; p=0.962) and time from onset of symptoms to treatment (181-210 min: 1.62; 0.26-10.25; 211-240 min: 1.97; 0.82-4.76; 241-270 min: 3.15; 1.01-9.79; p=0.761). However, patients older than 65 years had a higher risk of hemorrhage (<65 years: 0.74; 0.28-1.96; > or =65 years: 5.79; 2.18-15.39; p=0.004) [30] **(IIb/B)**.

Other agents

Intravenous streptokinase was associated with an unacceptable risk of hemorrhage and death [31-32] **(III/B)**. Thrombolytic agents like anistreplase, staphylokinase, reteplase or urokinase might be considered for treatment of acute ischemic stroke but none of these agents have been sufficiently used in clinical trials. Desmoteplase administered to patients selected on the basis of perfusion/diffusion mismatch was associated with a higher rate of reperfusion and better clinical outcome compared with placebo in two small randomized clinical trials [33-34] **(III/B)**. Although these findings were not confirmed in a phase III study, this agent will be evaluated further. There is preliminary evidence that the systemic administration of ancrod, a defibrogenating enzyme derived from snake venom, might be associated with improved outcomes after stroke [35-36] **(III/B)** and a favorable benefit-risk profile [37-38] **(III/B)**. Further studies are on their way to investigate the potential of this substance.

Intra-arterial thrombolysis

Besides intravenous thrombolysis, reperfusion strategies include intra-arterial thrombolysis and mechanical methods to aid reperfusion like the use of mechanical clot disruption, clot retrieval or stenting devices. There are not sufficient data to advise on the optimal reperfusion strategy. However, it seems likely that the important determinant of therapeutic efficacy is the speed and safety with which reperfusion can be achieved. It may also be that the time available to achieve reperfusion is longer in the posterior than in the anterior circulation [39].

Middle cerebral artery (MCA) occlusion

In patients suffering from thrombotic occlusion of the MCA, intra-arterial application of pro-urokinase within 6 hours has been shown to improve outcome in a randomized study [40]. A meta-analysis of three small randomized controlled trials (PROACT I, PROACT II, MELT) suggested a beneficial outcome effect of intra-arterial thrombolytic therapy in patients with proximal MCA occlusion [41] **(Ia/A)**. However, pro-urokinase is commercially not available and there are no randomized controlled trials using rt-PA for intra-arterial thrombolysis.

Basilar artery (BA) occlusion

In acute basilar occlusion, one trial included 16 patients but was underpowered [42]. A systematic review including 420 patients with BA occlusion compared intravenous to intra-arterial thrombolysis and found no significant difference between the two treatment options [43] (IIa/B).

A prospective registry (Basilar Artery International Cooperation Study, BASICS) investigated 592 patients with acute BA occlusion for differences regarding antithrombotic therapy, intravenous or intra-arterial thrombolysis. However, most patients received intra-arterial thrombolysis. No statistically significant superiority for intra-arterial over intravenous thrombolysis was found. Therefore, unequivocal superiority of intra-arterial over intravenous thrombolysis is not shown [44] (IIb/B).

The so called 'bridging concept' is currently preferred in most centers in cases of proven vessel occlusion. Therefore, rt-PA is given with 60% of the full recommended dosage as first-line treatment and – in case of non-response – either with local application of rt-PA at the thrombus site, with mechanical recanalization devices or with mechanical clot disruption, or a combination of mentioned techniques. Standard treatment of patients with BA occlusion in non-specialized centers or where neuroradiological intervention is not available, should be intravenous application of rt-PA, since there are no trials to support the superiority of intra-arterial thrombolysis in patients with BA occlusion [45] (IIb/B).

Although there is no evidence from relevant trials it seems obvious that rapid treatment for acute BA occlusion should improve efficacy and outcome. However, the time window for thrombolysis seems to be larger than in acute MCA occlusion.

Mechanical intra-arterial recanalization

An intra-arterial embolectomy device (Merci Retriever®) has been tested in patients with a large vessel stroke within 8 hours in a multicenter trial (MERCI). Recanalization was achieved in 46% (69/151) of patients on an intention to treat analysis. This rate was significantly higher than that expected using an historical control of 18% (p<0.0001). Clinically significant procedural complications occurred in 7.1% patients. Symptomatic intracranial hemorrhage was observed in 7.8% patients. Good neurological outcomes (modified Rankin score ≤2) were more frequent at 90 days in patients with successful recanalization compared with patients with unsuccessful recanalization (46% vs. 10%; p<0.0001), and mortality was less (32% vs. 54%; p=0.01) [46] (IIb/B).

A trial using a modified version of the Merci Retriever® (Multi MERCI) including 164 patients could not show a significantly higher recanalization rate associated with second-generation devices compared to the ones of first generation. A favorable outcome (mRS ≤2) occurred in 36% and death in 34% with both being significantly related to vascular recanalization. Patients with MCA occlusion whose recanalization failed with intravenous rt-PA, but had recanalization with the Merci Retriever®, tended to have a good outcome (47.1% vs. 15.4%). In a multivariate analysis, final revascularization was the strongest independent predictor of good outcome at 90 days. Symptomatic intracerebral hemorrhage and peri-procedural complication rates were similar in all groups [47] **(IIb/B)**.

The prospective RECANALISE study compared recanalisation rates, neurological improvement at 24 hours, and functional outcome at 3 months in patients (n=160) with acute artery occlusion who were treated with either intravenous rt-PA (n=107) or with a combined intravenous endovascular approach (and thrombectomy if necessary) (n=53). The recanalisation rate was 52% in patients treated only intravenously compared to 87% in patients treated with the intravenous endovascular approach (adjusted relative risk [RR] 1.49; 95% CI, 1.21-1.84; p=0.0002). Early neurological improvement (NIHSS score of 0 or 1 or an improvement of 4 points or more at 24 hours) occurred in 39% in the intravenous group compared to 60% in the intravenous endovascular group (adjusted RR 1.36; 0.97-1.91; p=0.07). However, favourable outcome at 90 days was not significantly different in the two groups. Mortality rate at 90 days and symptomatic intracranial hemorrhage after treatment was similar in both groups. Better clinical outcome was associated with recanalisation in both groups and with time to recanalisation in the intravenous endovascular group [48] **(IIb/B)**.

Other considerations

Angioedema

Orolingual angioedema with obstruction of the upper airways is a potentially life-threatening complication of rt-PA treatment in stroke patients, especially in those with previous intake of ACE inhibitors. The estimated incidence is about 5-10% [49] **(III/B)**.

Posterior circulation

Patients with ischemic stroke in the posterior circulation were included in several acute stroke studies with intravenous rt-PA, especially if they were CT-based and patients fulfilled the NIHSS criteria. Patients with stroke in the posterior circulation count rarely more than 4 points on the NIHSS, because the scale underrates brainstem and cerebellar symptoms. Although posterior circulation stroke is often disabling, it is not routinely treated as consequently as anterior circulation ischemia. International guidelines support thrombolysis within 4.5 hours, irrespective of the involved territory.

Stroke on awakening

Mostly multimodal imaging is used to diagnose patients with stroke on awakening. If time of falling asleep is set as stroke onset, patients are often not eligible for thrombolytic therapy anymore because of over-estimation of the time window.

In the AbESTT-II trial, patients were treated randomly with abciximab or placebo in different time windows (0-5 hours vs. 5-6 hours vs. wake-up cohort) based on CT imaging. The study was terminated early due to excessive bleeding risk in the abciximab-treated patients. Patients with stroke on awakening had an even higher bleeding risk up to 18% if treated with abciximab [50].

Using a 6-hour time window after awakening, as well as the MRI mismatch-concept, outcome was comparable in the rt-PA-treated and placebo-treated group. No symptomatic intracranial haemorrhage was observed. Feasibility of multimodal imaging to select patients with stroke on awakening for thrombolysis was shown [51]. Patients with stroke on awakening and with known stroke onset did not show any major differences regarding patient characteristics, etiology, clinical and radiological characteristics [52].

Age >80 years

The European license for rt-PA is restricted to patients between 18 years and 80 years of age. An increasing number of stroke patients are older than 80 years, mainly due to demographic development.

Three-month mortality was higher in patients aged >80 years compared to patients <80 years. Favorable outcome (mRS ≤1) and intracranial hemorrhage (asymptomatic, symptomatic, or fatal) were similarly frequent in both groups. Stroke severity, time to thrombolysis, glucose level, and history of coronary heart disease independently predicted outcome, whereas age did not [49] **(III/B)**.

The overall rate of hemorrhagic complications after rt-PA treatment for ischemic stroke in octogenarians was 6.9%, compared to 5.3% in younger patients (p=0.61). Baseline imaging method (CT or MRI) had no significant influence on intracranial haemorrhage, mortality or on favourable outcome on the mRS after 3 months [53].

Nonagenarians and octogenarians were identified in the CASES registry. Both groups were equally hypertensive and predominantly had severe strokes (NIHSS score >15; 58% and 52%). Rate of symptomatic intracranial haemorrhage (7% nonagenarians vs. 4% octogenarians), and 30-day favorable functional outcomes ([mRS ≤1] 30% vs. 26%) did not show a significant difference when comparing the two age groups. 90-day mortality (52% vs. 33%; p=0.087) was higher in the older group [54] **(III/B)**.

Cervical artery dissection (CAD)

A study from the Swiss intravenous thrombolysis databank analysed [55] rt-PA-treated patients with cervical artery dissection with regard to favorable 3-month outcome, intracranial cerebral hemorrhage and recurrent ischemic stroke. Patients with CAD had less favorable outcome (36% vs. 44%) compared to non-CAD patients. Intracranial hemorrhages were equally frequent (both 14%). Recurrent cerebral ischemia was less frequent in CAD patients (1.8% vs. 3.7%). rt-PA-treated patients with CAD did not recover as well as rt-PA-treated non-CAD patients. rt-PA treatment should not be excluded in patients who may have CAD. Hemodynamic factors or frequent tandem occlusions might explain less favorable outcome of CAD patients [55].

Insufficient data exist on the efficacy of rt-PA in CAD, but complication rates were not greater than thrombolysis for other ischemic stroke. In conclusion, thrombolysis in CAD appears safe but more data on efficacy are required [56] **(III/B)**.

There are no randomized trials specifically analyzing thrombolysis in CAD patients, but these patients were not excluded from the large randomized thrombolytic trials. In contrast, patients with CAD were excluded from intra-arterial thrombolysis trials [57].

Role of anticoagulation

Patients on oral anticoagulation were excluded from the large rt-PA trials because of the fear of an increased bleeding risk. Variations in INR values in patients on oral anticoagulation are common. Rapid diagnosis of the actual anticoagulation state is essential for the patient being eligible for thrombolysis or not. Measuring INR on admission by point of care testing in an emergency setting is sufficiently precise in patients on oral anticoagulation with acute stroke. This substantially reduces the time interval until INR values are available and therefore may hasten the initiation of thrombolysis [58] **(IIa/B)**.

Blood pressure

Blood pressure monitoring and treatment is controversial in acute stroke management. Patients with the highest and lowest levels of blood pressure in the first 24 hours after stroke are more likely to have early neurological decline and poorer outcomes [59]. A low or low-normal blood pressure at stroke onset is unusual [60], and may be the result of a large cerebral infarct, cardiac failure, ischemia, hypovolemia or sepsis.

High blood pressure was positively correlated with worse outcome after thrombolysis. Systolic blood pressure after rt-PA treatment was significantly higher in patients with hemorrhagic complications than in those without. No correlation between blood pressure levels and stroke severity at admission was found. This indicates that rt-PA-induced hemorrhage is influenced by post-thrombolytic systolic blood pressure. Arterial hypertension should be treated diligently after thrombolysis, especially within the first 32 hours [61].

The relationship between hemorrhage and acute diffusion-weighted imaging (DWI) lesion volumes and blood pressure was analyzed in the search for reliable predictors of hemorrhagic transformation (HT) and parenchymal hemorrhage (PH) after thrombolysis in stroke. Patients with PH had larger DWI lesion volumes (63.1+/-56.1ml) than those without HT (27.6+/-39.0ml). Weighted average systolic blood pressure (SBP) 24 hours after treatment was higher in patients with PH (159.4+/-18.8mm Hg) relative to those without HT (143.1+/-20.0mm Hg). Regression analysis strongly indicated that PH and HT was predicted by DWI lesion volume (OR=1.16 per 10ml), atrial fibrillation (OR=9.33), and post-thrombolysis (24-hour weighted average) SBP (OR=1.59 per 10mm Hg). Therefore, withholding rt-PA from patients with very large baseline DWI volumes and more stringent BP control after thrombolysis in stroke should be considered [62].

Pre-treatment blood pressure protocol violations (systolic blood pressure >185mm Hg and diastolic blood pressure >110mm Hg) in patients receiving rt-PA were independently associated with a higher likelihood of symptomatic intracranial hemorrhage (OR: 2.59) [63] **(IIa/B)**.

Multivariable analysis based on SITS registry data found high systolic blood pressure 2 to 24 hours after thrombolysis to be associated with worse outcome (p<0.001) and symptomatic hemorrhage. Withholding antihypertensive therapy for up to 7 days in patients with a history of arterial hypertension was associated with worse outcome, whereas initiation of antihypertensive therapy in newly recognized moderate hypertension was associated with a favorable outcome [64] **(IIa/B)**.

The impact of early blood pressure changes on DWI lesion evolution and clinical outcome was studied in stroke patients treated with rt-PA. Variability of SBP and diastolic blood pressure was associated with DWI lesion growth and worse 3-month outcome. SBP variability emerged as an independent predictor of DWI lesion growth and worse stroke outcome in rt-PA-treated patients without recanalization, but not in recanalized patients. Its impact varies depending on the occurrence of early recanalization after thrombolysis [65].

Lipid levels

The SPARCL study showed an increased risk of intracerebral hemorrhage with statin use [66]. After adjusting for covariates, low LDL cholesterol (OR 0.968 per 1mg/dL increase; 95% CI, 0.941-0.995), current smoking (OR 14.568; 95% CI, 1.590-133.493), and higher NIHSS score (OR 1.265 per 1-point increase; 95% CI, 1.047-1.529) were independently associated with hemorrhagic complications after recanalization therapy for ischemic stroke [67].

After multivariate analysis, the frequency of any intracranial haemorrhage remained independently associated with previous statin use (OR 3.1; 95% CI, 1.53 -6.39; p=0.004), atrial fibrillation (OR 2.5; CI, 1.35-4.75; p=0.004), NIHSS score (OR 1.1; CI, 1.00-1.10; p=0.037), and worse collateralization (OR 1.7; CI, 1.19-2.42; p=0.004). There was no association of outcome with prior statin use, total cholesterol level, or low-density lipoprotein cholesterol level. Prior statin use, but not cholesterol levels on admission, is associated with a higher frequency of any intracranial haemorrhage after intra-arterial thrombolysis without an impact on outcome [68] **(III/B)**.

High admission triglyceride levels were independently associated with a higher risk of intracranial haemorrhage, but were not associated with a reduced chance of a favorable functional outcome at 3 months. Total cholesterol levels, LDL levels and statin use had no influence on both the occurrence of intracranial haemorrhage or functional outcome after thrombolysis [69].

Blood glucose

Elevated serum glucose is associated with an increased risk for intracranial bleeding and hemorrhagic transformation when treated with rt-PA. Unfavorable outcome due to parenchymal hematoma after thrombolysis is correlated with a higher blood glucose level. A significant and linear increase in risk of hematoma related to an increase in blood glucose levels has been shown [70].

Admission hyperglycemia in rt-PA-treated patients seemed be independently associated with an increased risk of death (adjusted risk ratio 1.5), symptomatic intracranial haemorrhage (OR 1.69), and decreased probability of a favorable outcome at 90 days (OR 0.7), all of them increasing incrementally with admission glucose and independent of presence of diabetes [71] (IIa/B).

Hypoglycemia (<50mg/dL [2.8mmol/L]) may mimic acute ischemic infarction, and should be treated by an intravenous dextrose bolus or infusion of 10-20% glucose [72].

Body temperature

Elevated body temperature might worsen the outcome after thrombolysis. Patients with an unfavorable outcome had more prominent temperature elevation than patients who had a favorable outcome after treatment with rt-PA (+1°C vs. +0.6°C; p=0.02), despite similar baseline temperature resulting in a reduced odds (OR 0.34) of good outcome after thrombolysis [73] (IIb/B).

Relevance of microbleeds

Detection of microbleeds is usually done with MRI using T2*-sequences or susceptibility-weighted imaging. The role of microbleeds in rt-PA-treated patients is controversial. The BRASIL study (Bleeding Risk Analysis in Stroke Imaging before Thrombolysis) analyzed the relevance of cerebral microbleeds in patients treated with rt-PA. Patients with microbleeds (15.1%) had a slightly higher risk of symptomatic intracranial haemorrhage than those without (5.8% vs. 2.7%, p=0.170), resulting in a non-significant absolute risk increase of 3.1%. If there is any increased risk for symptomatic intracranial haemorrhage attributable to microbleeds, it is likely to be small and unlikely to exceed the benefits of thrombolysis [74] (IIa/B). Microbleeds may be associated with symptomatic intracranial haemorrhage but there is still no conclusive answer to this question [75-76].

Neuroprotection

No neuroprotection programme has shown improved outcome on its predefined primary endpoint (e.g. Selfotel, lubeluzole, gavestinel, repinotan). All these substances have failed to show their clinical effectiveness. NXY-059 was tested in the SAINT I & II trials showing its ineffectiveness [77]. A meta-analysis has suggested a mild benefit with citicoline [78]; a clinical trial with this agent is in progress. G-CSF, hypothermia, transcranial laser stimulation and other drugs and treatment options are actually being tested for their neuroprotective properties.

Conclusions

Time lost is brain lost in acute cerebral ischaemia. Thrombolytic therapy is of proven and substantial benefit for many patients with acute cerebral ischaemia. Successful treatment means the patient is more likely to make a good recovery from their stroke resulting in several positive effects for the individual, relatives/caregivers and society. However, besides this proven benefit, frequency of thrombolysis in acute stroke is still too low. Now and in the future, every effort must be made to treat all eligible patients with intravenous rt-PA as soon as possible. Expansion of the time window to 4.5 hours after symptom onset must not lead to a delay in the commencement of treatment. Furthermore, alternative methods such as intra-arterial thrombolysis and mechanical thrombectomy might be a promising treatment option for subgroups of patients and should be investigated further. To be able to tailor optimal treatment to the individual patient, further research is needed, especially from randomised controlled trials.

Key points	Evidence level
• rt-PA (0.9mg/kg of body weight, maximum dose 90mg) should be administered to eligible patients who can be treated within 3 hours of onset of ischemic stroke.	Ia/A
• Every effort must be made to treat patients with rt-PA as early as possible after stroke symptom onset, even within the 3-hour time window, because the efficacy declines rapidly over time.	Ia/A
• Intravenous administration of ancrod, tenecteplase, reteplase, desmoteplase, urokinase, or other thrombolytic agents outside the setting of a clinical trial is not recommended.	III/B
• rt-PA should be administered to eligible patients who can be treated in the time period of 3-4.5 hours after stroke.	Ia/A

Continued

Key points *continued*	Evidence level

- The efficacy of intravenous treatment with rt-PA within 3-4.5 hours after stroke in patients with the following characteristics is not well established: age >80 years, on oral anticoagulants, international normalized ratio (INR) >1.7, NIHSS score >25, a history of stroke plus diabetes. — **IIb/B**
- Intra-arterial administration of rt-PA might be a treatment option for patients with acute large vessel occlusion, but should be limited to specialized centers. — **IIa/B**
- Intra-arterial mechanical thrombectomy might be a therapeutic option for patients with large vessel occlusion. — **IIb/B**
- Intra-arterial mechanical thrombectomy appears to be a possible treatment option for patients who do not respond to an intravenous rt-PA application or in patients ineligible for systemic thrombolysis. — **IIb/B**
- In acute basilar occlusion, patients should be treated as early as possible for efficacy with either intravenous, intra-arterial thrombolysis or mechanical thrombectomy or in combination. — **IIb/B**
- Selected patients may profit from the so called 'bridging concept'. — **IV/C**
- In acute artery occlusion, a combined intravenous and intra-arterial thrombolysis-thrombectomy approach might be considered. — **IIb/B**
- Orolingual angioedema must be thought of as a life-threatening complication of rt-PA treatment. — **III/B**
- Patients with posterior circulation stroke should be considered for thrombolysis. — **IV/C**
- Multiparametric imaging might be useful in selecting patients with stroke on awakening in order to initiate thrombolysis. — **IIa/B**
- Intravenous rt-PA may be administered to selected patients over 80 years of age. — **III/B**
- Intravenous thrombolysis should not be withheld from patients with suspected cervical artery dissection. — **III/B**
- Patients on effective oral anticoagulation should not be treated with rt-PA. — **IV/C**
- Early point-of-care testing in patients on oral anticoagulation may improve the time to thrombolysis. — **IIa/B**
- Blood pressure of 185/110mm Hg or higher should be lowered before thrombolysis. — **IV/C**
- Elevated blood pressure is associated with hemorrhagic complications after rt-PA treatment and should therefore be treated consequently. — **IIa/B**
- Statin use does not seem to be a contraindication for rt-PA treatment, although statins can cause hemorrhagic complications. — **III/B**

Continued

Key points *continued*	Evidence level
◆ Cessation of statin therapy in rt-PA-associated bleeding might not be necessary, although the evidence is inconclusive.	IV/C
◆ Elevated blood glucose levels on admission exceeding 180mg/dL (10mmol/L) should be lowered.	IIa/B
◆ Elevated body temperature may worsen outcome after thrombolysis and should be treated.	IIb/B
◆ Patients with microbleedings or leukoaraiosis should be considered for thrombolysis, although the risk of hemorrhage might be elevated.	IIa/B
◆ Administration of neuroprotective substances is not recommended.	Ia/A
◆ Administration of glycoprotein IIb/IIIa inhibitors is not recommended.	Ia/A
◆ rt-PA may be used in patients with seizures at stroke onset, if the neurological deficit is related to acute cerebral ischemia.	IV/C

References

1. Wardlaw JM, Murray V, Berge E, Del Zoppo GJ. Thrombolysis for acute ischaemic stroke. *Cochrane Database Syst Rev* 2009; 4: CD000213.
2. Lees KR, Bluhmki E, von Kummer R, Brott TG, Toni D, Grotta JC, Albers GW, Kaste M, Marler JR, Hamilton SA, Tilley BC, Davis SM, Donnan GA, Hacke W; ECASS, ATLANTIS, NINDS and EPITHET rt-PA Study Group, Allen K, Mau J, Meier D, del Zoppo G, De Silva DA, Butcher KS, Parsons MW, Barber PA, Levi C, Bladin C, Byrnes G. Time to treatment with intravenous alteplase and outcome in stroke: an updated pooled analysis of ECASS, ATLANTIS, NINDS, and EPITHET trials. *Lancet* 2010; 375(9727): 1695-703.
3. The National Institute of Neurological Disorders and Stroke rt-PA Stroke Study Group. Tissue plasminogen activator for acute ischemic stroke. *N Engl J Med* 1995; 333: 1581-7.
4. Kwiatkowski TG, Libman RB, Frankel M, Tilley BC, Morgenstern LB, Lu M, Broderick JP, Lewandowski CA, Marler JR, Levine SR, Brott T; National Institute of Neurological Disorders and Stroke Recombinant Tissue Plasminogen Activator Stroke Study Group. Effects of tissue plasminogen activator for acute ischemic stroke at one year. *N Engl J Med* 1999; 340: 1781-7.
5. Hacke W, Kaste M, Fieschi C, von Kummer R, Dávalos A, Meier D, Larrue V, Bluhmki E, Davis S, Donnan G, Scheider D, Diez-Tejedor E, Trouilas P. Randomised double-blind placebo-controlled trial of thrombolytic therapy with intravenous alteplase in acute ischaemic stroke (ECASS II). *Lancet* 1998; 352: 1245-51.
6. Hacke W, Kaste M, Fieschi C, Toni D, Lesaffre E, von Kummer R, Boysen G, Bluhmki E, Höxter G, Mahagne MH, Hennerici M. Intravenous thrombolysis with recombinant tissue plasminogen activator for acute stroke. *JAMA* 1995; 274: 1017-25.
7. Steiner T, Bluhmki E, Kaste M, Toni D, Trouillas P, von Kummer R, Hacke W; ECASS Study Group. The ECASS 3-hour cohort: secondary analysis of ECASS data by time stratification: European Cooperative Acute Stroke Study. *Cerebrovasc Dis* 1998; 8: 198-203.
8. Hacke W, Bluhmki E, Steiner T, Tatlisumak T, Mahagne MH, Sacchetti ML, Meier D. Dichotomized efficacy end-points and global end-point analysis applied to the ECASS intention-to-treat data set: post hoc analysis of ECASS I. *Stroke* 1998; 29(10): 2073-5.

9. Wahlgren N, Ahmed N, Da'valos A, Ford GA, Grond M, Hacke W, Hennerici MG, Kaste M, Kuelkens S, Larrue V, Lees KR, Roine RO, Soinne L, Toni D, Vanhooren G; SITS-MOST Investigators. Thrombolysis with alteplase for acute ischaemic stroke in the Safe Implementation of Thrombolysis in Stroke Monitoring Study (SITS-MOST): an observational study [published correction appears in *Lancet* 2007; 369: 826]. *Lancet* 2007; 369: 275-82.

10. Katzan IL, Hammer MD, Furlan AJ, Hixson ED, Nadzam DM; Cleveland Clinic Health System Stroke Quality Improvement Team. Quality improvement and tissue-type plasminogen activator for acute ischemic stroke: a Cleveland update. *Stroke* 2003; 34: 799-800.

11. Albers GW, Bates VE, Clark WM, Bell R, Verro P, Hamilton SA. Intravenous tissue-type plasminogen activator for treatment of acute stroke: the Standard Treatment with Alteplase to Reverse Stroke (STARS) study. *JAMA* 2000; 283: 1145-50.

12. Grond M, Stenzel C, Schmulling S, Rudolf J, Neveling M, Lechleuthner A, Schneweis S, Heiss WD. Early intravenous thrombolysis for acute ischemic stroke in a community-based approach. *Stroke* 1998; 29: 1544-9.

13. Derex L, Hermier M, Adeleine P, Pialat JB, Wiart M, Berthezene Y, Phillippeau F, Honnorat J, Froment JC, Trouillas P, Nighoghossian N. Clinical and imaging predictors of intracerebral haemorrhage in stroke patients treated with intravenous tissue plasminogen activator. *J Neurol Neurosurg Psychiatry* 2005; 76: 70-5.

14. Trouillas P, Nighoghossian N, Getenet JC, Riche G, Neuschwander P, Froment JC, Turjman F, Jin JX, Malicier D, Fournier G, Gabry AL, Ledoux X, Derex L, Berthezene Y, Adeleine P, Xie J, Ffrench P, Dechavanne M. Open trial of intravenous tissue plasminogen activator in acute carotid territory stroke: correlations of outcome with clinical and radiological data. *Stroke* 1996; 27: 882-90.

15. Tanne D, Verro P, Mansbach H, *et al*. Overview and summary of phase IV data on use of t-PA for acute ischemic stroke. *Stroke Interventionalist* 1998; 1: 3.

16. Tanne D, Bates V, Verro P, Kasner SE, Binder JR, Patel SC, Mansbach HH, Daley S, Schultz LR, Karanjia PN, Scott P, Dayno JM, Vereczkey- Porter K, Benesch C, Book D, Coplin WM, Dulli D, Levine SR; t-PA Stroke Survey Group. Initial clinical experience with IV tissue plasminogen activator for acute ischemic stroke: a multicenter survey. *Neurology* 1999; 53: 424-7.

17. Katzan IL, Hammer MD, Hixson ED, Furlan AJ, Abou-Chebl A, Nadzam DM; Cleveland Clinic Health System Stroke Quality Improvement Team. Utilization of intravenous tissue plasminogen activator for acute ischemic stroke. *Arch Neurol* 2004; 61: 346-50.

18. Graham GD. Tissue plasminogen activator for acute ischemic stroke in clinical practice: a meta-analysis of safety data. *Stroke* 2003; 34: 2847-50.

19. Marler JR, Tilley BC, Lu M, Brott TG, Lyden PC, Grotta JC, Broderick JP, Levine SR, Frankel MP, Horowitz SH, Haley EC Jr, Lewandowski CA, Kwiatkowski TP. Early stroke treatment associated with better outcome: the NINDS rt-PA stroke study. *Neurology* 2000; 55: 1649-55.

20. Hacke W, Donnan G, Fieschi C, Kaste M, von Kummer R, Broderick JP, Brott T, Frankel M, Grotta JC, Haley EC, Jr., Kwiatkowski T, Levine SR, Lewandowski C, Lu M, Lyden P, Marler JR, Patel S, Tilley BC, Albers G. Association of outcome with early stroke treatment: pooled analysis of ATLANTIS, ECASS, and NINDS rt-PA stroke trials. *Lancet* 2004; 363: 768-74.

21. Qureshi AI, Kirmani JF, Sayed MA, Safdar A, Ahmed S, Ferguson R, Hershey LA, Qazi KJ; Buffalo Metropolitan Area and Erie County Stroke Study Group. Time to hospital arrival, use of thrombolytics, and in-hospital outcomes in ischemic stroke. *Neurology* 2005; 64: 2115-20.

22. Patel SC, Levine SR, Tilley BC, Grotta JC, Lu M, Frankel M, Haley EC Jr, Brott TG, Broderick JP, Horowitz S, Lyden PD, Lewandowski CA, Marler JR, Welch KM; National Institute of Neurological Disorders and Stroke rt-PA Stroke Study Group. Lack of clinical significance of early ischemic changes on computed tomography in acute stroke. *JAMA* 2001; 286: 2830-8.

23. The NINDS t-PA Stroke Study Group. Intracerebral hemorrhage after intravenous t-PA therapy for ischemic stroke. *Stroke* 1997; 28: 2109-18.

24. Lansberg MG, Thijs VN, Bammer R, Kemp S, Wijman CA, Marks MP, Albers GW. Risk factors of symptomatic intracerebral hemorrhage after tPA therapy for acute stroke. *Stroke* 2007; 38: 2275-8.

25. Lyden PD. *Thrombolytic Therapy for Acute Stroke*, 2nd ed. Totowa, NJ, USA: Humana Press, 2005.

26. Wahlgren N, Ahmed N, Da'valos A, Hacke W, Milla'n M, Muir K, Roine RO, Toni D, Lees KR; SITS Investigators. Thrombolysis with alteplase 3-4.5 h after acute ischaemic stroke (SITS-ISTR): an observational study. *Lancet* 2008; 372: 1303-9.

27. Hacke W, Kaste M, Bluhmki E, Brozman M, Da'valos A, Guidetti D, Larrue V, Lees KR, Medeghri Z, Machnig T, Schneider D, von Kummer R, Wahlgren N, Toni D; ECASS Investigators. Thrombolysis with alteplase 3 to 4.5 hours after acute ischemic stroke. *N Engl J Med* 2008; 359(13): 1317-29.

28. Clark WM, Albers GW, Madden KP, Hamilton S; Thrombolytic Therapy in Acute Ischemic Stroke Study Investigators. The rtPA (alteplase) 0- to 6-hour acute stroke trial, part A (A0276g): results of a double-blind, placebo-controlled, multicenter study. *Stroke* 2000; 31: 811-6.

29. Clark WM, Wissman S, Albers GW, Jhamandas JH, Madden KP, Hamilton S. Recombinant tissue-type plasminogen activator (Alteplase) for ischemic stroke 3 to 5 hours after symptom onset: the ATLANTIS Study: a randomized controlled trial: Alteplase Thrombolysis for Acute Noninterventional Therapy in Ischemic Stroke. *JAMA* 1999; 282: 2019-26.

30. Bluhmki E, Chamorro A, Dávalos A, Machnig T, Sauce C, Wahlgren N, Wardlaw J, Hacke W. Stroke treatment with alteplase given 3.0-4.5 h after onset of acute ischaemic stroke (ECASS III): additional outcomes and subgroup analysis of a randomised controlled trial. *Lancet Neurol* 2009; 8(12): 1095-102.

31. The Multicenter Acute Stroke Trial - Europe Study Group. Thrombolytic therapy with streptokinase in acute ischemic stroke. *N Engl J Med* 1996; 335: 145-50.

32. (MAST-I) Group. Randomised controlled trial of streptokinase, aspirin, and combination of both in treatment of acute ischaemic stroke. Multicentre Acute Stroke Trial-Italy. *Lancet* 1995; 346: 1509-14.

33. Hacke W, Albers G, Al-Rawi Y, Bogousslavsky J, Dávalos A, Eliasziw M, Fischer M, Furlan A, Kaste M, Lees KR, Soehngen M, Warach S. The Desmoteplase in Acute Ischemic Stroke Trial (DIAS): a phase II MRI-based 9-hour window acute stroke thrombolysis trial with intravenous desmoteplase. *Stroke* 2005; 36: 66-73.

34. Furlan AJ, Eyding D, Albers GW, Al-Rawi Y, Lees KR, Rowley HA, Sachara C, Soehngen M, Warach S, Hacke W. Dose Escalation of Desmoteplase for Acute Ischemic Stroke (DEDAS): evidence of safety and efficacy 3 to 9 hours after stroke onset. *Stroke* 2006; 37: 1227-31.

35. Sherman DG, Atkinson RP, Chippendale T, Levin KA, Ng K, Futrell N, Hsu CY, Levy DE. Intravenous ancrod for treatment for acute ischemic stroke; the STAT study: a randomized controlled trial. Stroke Treatment with Ancrod Trial. *JAMA* 2000; 283: 2395-403.

36. The Ancrod Stroke Study Investigators. Ancrod for the treatment of acute ischemic brain infarction. *Stroke* 1994; 25: 1755-9.

37. Liu M, Counsell C, Zhao XL, Wardlaw J. Fibrinogen depleting agents for acute ischaemic stroke. *Cochrane Database Syst Rev* 2003; 3: CD000091.

38. Sherman DG. Antithrombotic and hypofibrinogenetic therapy in acute ischemic stroke: what is the next step? *Cerebrovasc Dis* 2004; 17(suppl 1): 138-43.

39. Macleod M. Current issues in the treatment of acute posterior circulation stroke. *CNS Drugs* 2006; 20(8): 611-21.

40. Furlan A, Higashida R, Wechsler L, Gent M, Rowley H, Kase C, Pessin M, Ahuja A, Callahan F, Clark WM, Silver F, Rivera F. Intra-arterial prourokinase for acute ischemic stroke. The PROACT II study: a randomized controlled trial. Prolyse in Acute Cerebral Thromboembolism. *JAMA* 1999; 282(21): 2003-11.

41. Ogawa A, Mori E, Minematsu K, Taki W, Takahashi A, Nemoto S, Miyamoto S, Sasaki M, Inoue T; MELT Japan Study Group. Randomized trial of intra-arterial infusion of urokinase within 6 hours of middle cerebral artery stroke: the middle cerebral artery embolism local fibrinolytic intervention trial (MELT) Japan. *Stroke* 2007; 38(10): 2633-9.

42. Macleod MR, Davis SM, Mitchell PJ, Gerraty RP, Fitt G, Hankey GJ, Stewart-Wynne EG, Rosen D, McNeil JJ, Bladin CF, Chambers BR, Herkes GK, Young D, Donnan GA. Results of a multicentre, randomised controlled trial of intra-arterial urokinase in the treatment of acute posterior circulation ischaemic stroke. *Cerebrovasc Dis* 2005; 20(1): 12-7.

43. Lindsberg PJ, Mattle HP. Therapy of basilar artery occlusion: a systematic analysis comparing intra-arterial and intravenous thrombolysis. *Stroke* 2006; 37(3): 922-8.

44. Schonewille WJ, Wijman CA, Michel P, Rueckert CM, Weimar C, Mattle HP, Engelter ST, Tanne D, Muir KW, Molina CA, Thijs V, Audebert H, Pfefferkorn T, Szabo K, Lindsberg PJ, de Freitas G, Kappelle LJ, Algra A; BASICS study group. Treatment and outcomes of acute basilar artery occlusion in the Basilar Artery International Cooperation Study (BASICS): a prospective registry study. *Lancet Neurol* 2009; 8(8): 724-30.

45. Seifert M, Ahlbrecht A, Dohmen C, Spuentrup E, Moeller-Hartmann W. Combined interventional stroke therapy using intracranial stent and local intraarterial thrombolysis (LIT). *Neuroradiology* 2010; Epub ahead of print.

46. Smith WS, Sung G, Starkman S, Saver JL, Kidwell CS, Gobin YP, Lutsep HL, Nesbit GM, Grobelny T, Rymer MM, Silverman IE, Higashida RT, Budzik RF, Marks MP; MERCI Trial Investigators. Safety and efficacy of mechanical embolectomy in acute ischemic stroke: results of the MERCI trial. *Stroke* 2005; 36(7): 1432-8.

47. Smith WS, Sung G, Saver J, Budzik R, Duckwiler G, Liebeskind DS, Lutsep HL, Rymer MM, Higashida RT, Starkman S, Gobin YP; Multi MERCI Investigators, Frei D, Grobelny T, Hellinger F, Huddle D, Kidwell C, Koroshetz W, Marks M, Nesbit G, Silverman IE. Mechanical thrombectomy for acute ischemic stroke: final results of the Multi MERCI trial. *Stroke* 2008; 39(4): 1205-12.

48. Mazighi M, Serfaty JM, Labreuche J, Laissy JP, Meseguer E, Lavallée PC, Cabrejo L, Slaoui T, Guidoux C, Lapergue B, Klein IF, Olivot JM, Abboud H, Simon O, Niclot P, Nifle C, Touboul PJ, Raphaeli G, Gohin C, Claeys ES, Amarenco P; RECANALISE investigators. Comparison of intravenous alteplase with a combined intravenous-endovascular approach in patients with stroke and confirmed arterial occlusion (RECANALISE study): a prospective cohort study. *Lancet Neurol* 2009; 8(9): 802-9.

49. Engelter ST, Reichhart M, Sekoranja L, Georgiadis D, Baumann A, Weder B, Müller F, Lüthy R, Arnold M, Michel P, Mattle HP, Tettenborn B, Hungerbühler HJ, Baumgartner RW, Sztajzel R, Bogousslavsky J, Lyrer PA. Thrombolysis in stroke patients aged 80 years and older: Swiss survey of IV thrombolysis. *Neurology* 2005; 65(11): 1795-8.

50. Adams HP Jr, Leira EC, Torner JC, Barnathan E, Padgett L, Effron MB, Hacke W; AbESTT-II Investigators. Treating patients with 'wake-up' stroke: the experience of the AbESTT-II trial. *Stroke* 2008; 39(12): 3277-82.

51. Breuer L, Schellinger PD, Huttner HB, Halwachs R, Engelhorn T, Doerfler A, Köhrmann M. Feasibility and safety of magnetic resonance imaging-based thrombolysis in patients with stroke on awakening: initial single-centre experience. *Int J Stroke* 2010; 5(2): 68-73.

52. Breuer L, Huttner HB, Dörfler A, Schellinger PD, Köhrmann M. Wake up stroke: overview on diagnostic and therapeutic options for ischemic stroke on awakening. *Fortschr Neurol Psychiatr* 2010; 78(2): 101-6.

53. Ringleb PA, Schwark Ch, Köhrmann M, Külkens S, Jüttler E, Hacke W, Schellinger PD. Thrombolytic therapy for acute ischaemic stroke in octogenarians: selection by magnetic resonance imaging improves safety but does not improve outcome. *J Neurol Neurosurg Psychiatry* 2007; 78(7): 690-3.

54. Mateen FJ, Buchan AM, Hill MD; CASES Investigators. Outcomes of thrombolysis for acute ischemic stroke in octogenarians versus nonagenarians. *Stroke* 2010; 41(8): 1833-5.

55. Engelter ST, Rutgers MP, Hatz F, Georgiadis D, Fluri F, Sekoranja L, Schwegler G, Müller F, Weder B, Sarikaya H, Lüthy R, Arnold M, Nedeltchev K, Reichhart M, Mattle HP, Tettenborn B, Hungerbühler HJ, Sztajzel R, Baumgartner RW, Michel P, Lyrer PA. Intravenous thrombolysis in stroke attributable to cervical artery dissection. *Stroke* 2009; 40(12): 3772-6.

56. Menon R, Kerry S, Norris JW, Markus HS. Treatment of cervical artery dissection: a systematic review and meta-analysis. *J Neurol Neurosurg Psychiatry* 2008; 79(10): 1122-7.

57. Baumgartner RW. Management of spontaneous dissection of the cervical carotid artery. *Acta Neurochir Suppl* 2010; 107: 57-61.

58. Rizos T, Herweh C, Jenetzky E, Lichy C, Ringleb PA, Hacke W, Veltkamp R. Point-of-care International Normalized Ratio testing accelerates thrombolysis in patients with acute ischemic stroke using oral anticoagulants. *Stroke* 2009; 40(11): 3547-51.

59. Castillo J, Leira R, García MM, Serena J, Blanco M, Dávalos A. Blood pressure decrease during the acute phase of ischemic stroke is associated with brain injury and poor stroke outcome. *Stroke* 2004; 35(2): 520-6.

60. Leonardi-Bee J, Bath PM, Phillips SJ, Sandercock PA; IST Collaborative Group. Blood pressure and clinical outcomes in the International Stroke Trial. *Stroke* 2002; 33(5): 1315-20.

61. Perini F, De Boni A, Marcon M, Bolgan I, Pellizzari M, Dionisio LD. Systolic blood pressure contributes to intracerebral haemorrhage after thrombolysis for ischemic stroke. *J Neurol Sci* 2010; 297(1-2): 52-4.

62. Butcher K, Christensen S, Parsons M, De Silva DA, Ebinger M, Levi C, Jeerakathil T, Campbell BC, Barber PA, Bladin C, Fink J, Tress B, Donnan GA, Davis SM; EPITHET Investigators. Post-thrombolysis blood pressure elevation is associated with hemorrhagic transformation. *Stroke* 2010; 41(1): 72-7.

63. Tsivgoulis G, Frey JL, Flaster M, Sharma VK, Lao AY, Hoover SL, Liu W, Stamboulis E, Alexandrov AW, Malkoff MD, Alexandrov AV. Pre-tissue plasminogen activator blood pressure levels and risk of symptomatic intracerebral hemorrhage. *Stroke* 2009; 40(11): 3631-4.

64. Ahmed N, Wahlgren N, Brainin M, Castillo J, Ford GA, Kaste M, Lees KR, Toni D; SITS Investigators. Collaborators (11): Wahlgren N, Dávalos A, Ford GA, Grond M, Hacke W, Hennerici M, Kaste M, Larrue V, Lees KR, Roine R, Toni D. Relationship of blood pressure, antihypertensive therapy, and outcome in ischemic

stroke treated with intravenous thrombolysis: retrospective analysis from Safe Implementation of Thrombolysis in Stroke-International Stroke Thrombolysis Register (SITS-ISTR). *Stroke* 2009; 40(7): 2442-9.

65. Delgado-Mederos R, Ribo M, Rovira A, Rubiera M, Munuera J, Santamarina E, Delgado P, Maisterra O, Alvarez-Sabin J, Molina CA. Prognostic significance of blood pressure variability after thrombolysis in acute stroke. *Neurology* 2008; 71(8): 552-8.

66. Amarenco P, Benavente O, Goldstein LB, Callahan A 3rd, Sillesen H, Hennerici MG, Gilbert S, Rudolph AE, Simunovic L, Zivin JA, Welch KM; Stroke Prevention by Aggressive Reduction in Cholesterol Levels Investigators. Results of the Stroke Prevention by Aggressive Reduction in Cholesterol Levels (SPARCL) trial by stroke subtypes. *Stroke* 2009; 40(4): 1405-9.

67. Bang OY, Saver JL, Liebeskind DS, Starkman S, Villablanca P, Salamon N, Buck B, Ali L, Restrepo L, Vinuela F, Duckwiler G, Jahan R, Razinia T, Ovbiagele B. Cholesterol level and symptomatic hemorrhagic transformation after ischemic stroke thrombolysis. *Neurology* 2007; 68(10): 737-42.

68. Meier N, Nedeltchev K, Brekenfeld C, Galimanis A, Fischer U, Findling O, Remonda L, Schroth G, Mattle HP, Arnold M. Prior statin use, intracranial hemorrhage, and outcome after intra-arterial thrombolysis for acute ischemic stroke. *Stroke* 2009; 40(5): 1729-37.

69. Uyttenboogaart M, Koch MW, Koopman K, Vroomen PC, Luijckx GJ, De Keyser J. Lipid profile, statin use, and outcome after intravenous thrombolysis for acute ischaemic stroke. *J Neurol* 2008; 255(6): 875-80.

70. Paciaroni M, Agnelli G, Caso V, Corea F, Ageno W, Alberti A, Lanari A, Micheli S, Bertolani L, Venti M, Palmerini F, Billeci AM, Comi G, Previdi P, Silvestrelli G. Acute hyperglycemia and early hemorrhagic transformation in ischemic stroke. *Cerebrovasc Dis* 2009; 28(2): 119-23.

71. Poppe AY, Majumdar SR, Jeerakathil T, Ghali W, Buchan AM, Hill MD; Canadian Alteplase for Stroke Effectiveness Study Investigators. Admission hyperglycemia predicts a worse outcome in stroke patients treated with intravenous thrombolysis. *Diabetes Care* 2009; 32(4): 617-22.

72. Huff JS. Stroke mimics and chameleons. *Emerg Med Clin North Am* 2002; 20(3): 583-95.

73. Ernon L, Schrooten M, Thijs V. Body temperature and outcome after stroke thrombolysis. *Acta Neurol Scand* 2006; 114(1): 23-8.

74. Fiehler J, Albers GW, Boulanger JM, Derex L, Gass A, Hjort N, Kim JS, Liebeskind DS, Neumann-Haefelin T, Pedraza S, Rother J, Rothwell P, Rovira A, Schellinger PD, Trenkler J; MR STROKE Group. Bleeding Risk Analysis in Stroke Imaging before thromboLysis (BRASIL): pooled analysis of T2*-weighted magnetic resonance imaging data from 570 patients. *Stroke* 2007; 38(10): 2738-44.

75. Singer OC, Fiehler J, Berkefeld J, Neumann-Haefelin T. Stroke MRI for risk assessment of intracerebral hemorrhage associated with thrombolytic therapy. *Nervenarzt* 2009; 80(2): 130, 132-6.

76. Derex L, Nighoghossian N. Intracerebral haemorrhage after thrombolysis for acute ischaemic stroke: an update. *J Neurol Neurosurg Psychiatry* 2008; 79(10): 1093-9.

77. Diener HC, Lees KR, Lyden P, Grotta J, Dávalos A, Davis SM, Shuaib A, Ashwood T, Wasiewski W, Alderfer V, Hårdemark HG, Rodichok L; SAINT I and II Investigators. NXY-059 for the treatment of acute stroke: pooled analysis of the SAINT I and II Trials. *Stroke* 2008; 39(6): 1751-8.

78. Dávalos A, Castillo J, Alvarez-Sabín J, Secades JJ, Mercadal J, López S, Cobo E, Warach S, Sherman D, Clark WM, Lozano R. Oral citicoline in acute ischemic stroke: an individual patient data pooling analysis of clinical trials. *Stroke* 2002; 33(12): 2850-7.

Chapter 2

Management of stroke risk factors

Gustavo A. Ortiz MD, Assistant Professor of Clinical Neurology
Ralph L. Sacco MS MD FAAN FAHA, Professor and Olemberg Family
Chair in Neurological Disorders, Miller Professor of Neurology,
Epidemiology, and Human Genetics
University of Miami, Miller School of Medicine
Miami, Florida, USA

Introduction

Stroke is the leading cause of disability in the United States, with a devastating impact in the life of patients, families and communities. It is more often disabling than lethal, but nevertheless, is also the most common life-threatening neurological disorder, ranking third among all causes of death in the United States, after heart disease and cancer. In 2006, stroke accounted for approximately 1 out of every 18 deaths in the US. Every 4 minutes, someone dies of a stroke [1]. About 795,000 people experience a new or recurrent stroke every year. Approximately 610,000 of them are first attacks, and 185,000 are recurrent strokes [1]. In the population-based Northern Manhattan Study (NOMAS), the 30-day risk of recurrent stroke was more than twice that of cardiac events (including non-fatal MI) and the adjusted 5-year risk of non-fatal stroke was approximately twice as high as fatal cardiac events and four times higher than the risk of fatal stroke [2]. According to data from the National Center for Health Statistics (NCHS) and National Health and Nutrition Examination Survey (NHANES) from 2003 to 2006, an estimated 6,400,000 Americans ≥20 years of age have had a stroke and the overall stroke prevalence during this period is an estimated 2.9% [1]. The calculated direct and indirect cost of stroke for 2010 is $73.7 billion [1].

The use of intravenous recombinant tissue-type plasminogen activator (IV rt-PA) has been a major landmark in the treatment of acute ischemic stroke, since the publication of the National Institute of Neurological Disorders and Stroke trial in 1995 [3] and many other promising therapies for acute stroke are flourishing.

Stroke centers are continuing to increase and as of January 2009, there were over 541 primary stroke centers certified by The Joint Commission (TJC), 200 state-designated stroke centers and 1,330 hospitals participating in the "Get with the Guidelines – Stroke" program. It has been estimated that now more than 80% of the US population (250 million residents) lives within a 60-minute drive of a TJC certified stroke center or a state-designated stroke center, and 68.2% (211 million residents) lives within a 30-minute drive [4]. However, acute stroke treatment is only utilized among the minority of all strokes occurring in the US. Only 3-8.5% of patients with stroke receive IV rt-PA in the US [5]. Effective prevention is still the best approach for reducing the burden of stroke: it has been estimated that as many as 70-80% of strokes could be prevented by appropriate application of prevention measures [6].

Our goal in this chapter is to review the evidence-based recommendations for the management of stroke risk factors, and how this information can be applied in clinical practice. Management of carotid atherosclerotic disease, intracranial arterial stenosis and cardioembolic disease, including atrial fibrillation are not discussed, as they fall beyond the scope of this chapter. The definitions of class recommendations and levels of supportive evidence are shown in Table 1 based on the American Heart Association.

Table 1. American Heart Association/American Stroke Association (AHA/ASA) classification of recommendations and levels of evidence [105].

AHA/ASA classifications of recommendations

I: Evidence for or general agreement that treatment or procedure is useful and effective

II: Conflicting evidence or divergence of opinion about usefulness or effectiveness of treatment or procedure

IIa: Weight of evidence or opinion for treatment or procedure

IIb: Usefulness and effectiveness less well established

III: Evidence or general agreement that treatment or procedure is not useful or effective and may be harmful

AHA/ASA level of evidence

A: Based on multiple randomized clinical trials

B: Based on single randomized trial or non-randomized studies

C: Based on expert opinion or case studies

Non-modifiable risk factors

Stroke risk factors, similar to cardiovascular risk factors, may be classified as non-modifiable and modifiable. Most important non-modifiable risk factors are advanced age, gender, ethnicity and heredity, whereas the list of major modifiable factors includes hypertension (HTN), diabetes mellitus (DM), hypercholesterolemia, obesity, cigarette smoking and alcohol abuse. Non-modifiable risk factors are important to recognize, since they may be useful to identify those patients who are at highest risk of stroke and who may benefit from more rigorous prevention or treatment of other, modifiable risk factors.

Age

Age is the strongest non-modifiable stroke risk factor, doubling the risk for each successive decade after 55 years of age. This pattern was clearly shown in the Framingham Heart Study (55-year follow-up) for all cerebrovascular events combined, isolated transient ischemic attacks (TIAs), atherothrombotic strokes and combined ischemic and hemorrhagic strokes [7] (Figure 1). The increased risk with age reflects the cumulative effects of aging on

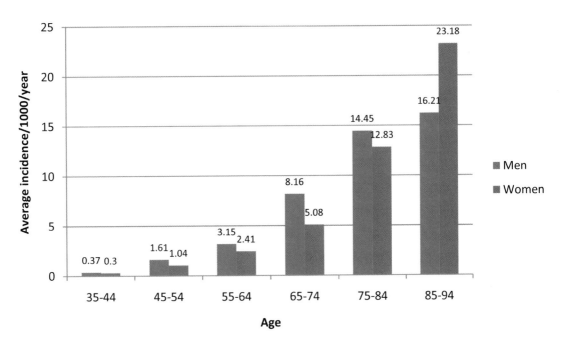

Figure 1. Incidence of completed strokes distributed by age. Data from the Framingham Heart Study: 55-year follow-up [7].

the cardiovascular system and the progressive nature of stroke risk factors [8]. As the proportion of our population living older than 80 increases, the estimated number of annual strokes will rise and lead to an increased public health problem.

Gender

Stroke has been considered to be overall more prevalent and generally have a higher age-specific incidence rate among men than in women [9], with the exceptions of ages between 35 to 44 years and >85 years of age, groups in which women have a slightly greater age-specific stroke incidence than men. Overall, more women have a stroke than men each year in the US largely due to their survival to older ages than men. Oral contraceptive use and pregnancy contribute to the increased risk of stroke in young women and the earlier cardiac-related deaths of men with cardiovascular disease may contribute to the relatively greater risk of stroke in older women [6]. However, an analysis of NHANES 1999 to 2004 data found that women 45 to 54 years of age are more than twice as likely as men to have suffered a stroke and have a >4-fold higher likelihood of having had a stroke, compared to women 35 to 44 years of age [10]. This raised the question of whether the increased incidence is due to aging alone or perhaps to hormone status and whether hormone therapy could affect the risk [1, 11]. However, randomized clinical trial data indicate that the use of postmenopausal hormone replacement therapy (estrogen plus progestin, or estrogen alone), increases stroke risk in overall healthy women and provided no protection for women with established heart disease or stroke [12-14]. A healthy lifestyle, with abstinence from smoking, low body mass index (BMI), moderate alcohol consumption, regular exercise and a healthy diet has been associated with a significantly reduced risk of stroke in an observational study of >37,000 women ≥45 years of age participating in the Women's Health Study [15].

Ethnicity

Greater stroke incidence and mortality rates have been found among African Americans and some Hispanic Americans. Studies such as the Atherosclerosis Risk in Communities (ARIC) study have shown a 38% higher incidence of stroke in African Americans, compared with European Americans. A higher prevalence of hypertension, obesity and diabetes within the black population may explain some, but not all the excess risk. Moreover, the impact of different stroke subtypes seems to be different across populations. According to data from NOMAS, the age-adjusted incidence of first ischemic stroke per 100,000 was 88 in whites, 191 in blacks and 149 in Hispanics. Compared with whites, the relative rates of intracranial atherosclerotic stroke among blacks was 5.85; extracranial atherosclerotic stroke, 3.18; lacunar stroke, 3.09; and cardioembolic stroke, 1.58. When comparing Hispanics (primarily from the Caribbean: Dominican, Cuban and Puerto Rican), with whites, the relative rates of intracranial atherosclerotic stroke was 5.00; extracranial atherosclerotic stroke, 1.71; lacunar stroke, 2.32; and cardioembolic stroke, 1.42 [16]. Regarding intracerebral hemorrhage, Mexican Americans, Latin Americans, African Americans, Native Americans, Japanese and Chinese people have higher incidences than do white Americans [17].

Genetic factors

The genetic hereditability of stroke risk factors, as well as the inheritance of susceptibility to the effects of such risk factors may mediate an increased stroke risk in cases of paternal and maternal history of stroke. But this may also be associated with familial sharing of cultural, environmental and lifestyle factors that may interact with the genetic factors [18]. Many of the established, modifiable stroke risk factors such as hypertension, diabetes and hyperlipidemia, have both a genetic and an environmental/behavioral component [18]. Familial inheritance of stroke risk has been strongly suggested in studies comparing incidence and prevalence of stroke in monozygotic and dizygotic twins [19, 20].

Single or multiple mutations have been involved in increased stroke risk. The methylene-tetrahydrofolate reductase gene mutation that leads to increased blood homocysteine levels is one single example [21-23]. Marfan syndrome (due to mutations in the fibrillin gene), neurofibromatosis types I and II, and cerebral autosomal dominant arteriopathy with subcortical infarcts and leukoencephalopathy (CADASIL) [24], are examples of multiple mutations. CADASIL, characterized by subcortical infarcts, dementia and migraine headaches, can be related to any of a series of mutations in the Notch3 gene.

Inheritance patterns may also include autosomal dominant traits, like some coagulopathies (protein C and S deficiencies, Factor V Leiden mutation), with increased risk of venous thrombosis [25-28]; or autosomal recessive traits, like in some disorders of clotting factors (e.g. Factors V, VII, X, XI and XIII), with increased risk of neonatal and childhood hemorrhage [6]. Other acquired coagulopathies, like the presence of anticardiolipin antibodies, or lupus anticoagulant can also be familial in up to 10% of cases [29, 30]. A genetic or familial component can be found in up to 10-20% of cases with arterial dissections, fibromuscular dysplasia and Moyamoya syndrome [31, 32].

In Fabry disease, a lysosomal storage disorder caused by α-galactosidase A deficiency, there is a progressive accumulation of globotriaosylceramide and related glycosphingolipids affecting mostly small vessels in the brain and other organs, leading to increased risk of stroke among other neurologic manifestations [33]. Human recombinant lysosomal α-galactosidase A has been found in two prospective randomized trials to reduce significantly microvascular deposits and plasma levels of globotriaosylceramide [34-36] **(Ib/A)**. No effects on stroke rates were found, but these studies had short follow-up periods. Specific gene therapy is not yet available, but Fabry disease is an example of available treatments for some of the risk factors that have a genetic predisposition or cause.

The American Heart Association/American Stroke Association (AHA/ASA) recommends to consider genetic counseling for patients with rare genetic causes of stroke (Class IIb, Level of evidence C), but there is still insufficient data to recommend genetic screening for the prevention of a first stroke.

Modifiable risk factors

Hypertension

Hypertension, a major risk factor for cerebral infarction and intracerebral hemorrhage, affects at least 65 million persons in the United States [37]. Blood pressure and the prevalence of hypertension increases with age [38] (Figure 2). The Framingham Study found that individuals with normal blood pressure at 55 years of age have a 90% lifetime risk for developing hypertension [39] and in the general population, over two thirds of persons >65 years of age are hypertensive [40]. Cardiovascular and stroke risk is linked continuously and consistently to blood pressure, independently of other risk factors [40].

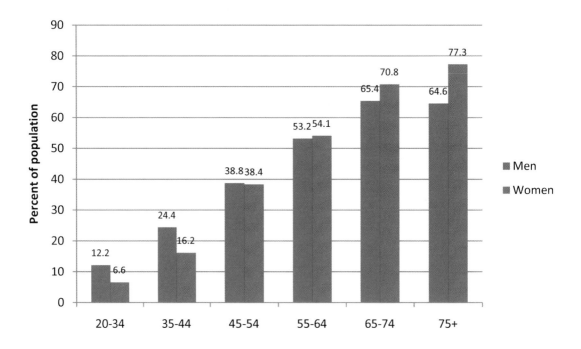

Figure 2. Prevalence of high blood pressure in adults ≥20 years of age by age and sex (NHANES: 2003-2006). Heart Disease and Stroke Statistics 2010 Update: A Report from the American Heart Association [1].

There is overwhelming evidence that control of blood pressure reduces stroke incidence and other target-organ damage, including renal failure and congestive heart failure [40]. Meta-analyses of randomized controlled trials have shown that antihypertensive treatment is associated with a 35-44% stroke risk reduction among hypertensive subjects [41, 42] **(Ia/A)**. With regards to isolated systolic hypertension in the elderly (systolic blood pressure >160mm Hg and diastolic blood pressure <90mm Hg), two large trials, the Systolic Hypertension in the Elderly Program (SHEP) and Systolic Hypertension in Europe (Syst-Eur) proved 36% and 42% risk reduction, respectively, in the actively treated groups [43, 44]. Hypertension, however, is still largely undiagnosed or inadequately treated. Only 70% of all hypertensive Americans are aware of having this condition, 60% are receiving treatment and 34% are well controlled. Minorities and the elderly are affected in larger proportions [40, 45].

Cardiovascular and stroke risk can be reduced in hypertensive patients by several categories of antihypertensive agents, such as thiazide diuretics, angiotensin-converting enzyme inhibitors (ACE-Is), angiotensin receptor blockers (ARBs), β-adrenergic receptor blockers (β-blockers) and calcium channel blockers (CCBs) [42, 46-49]. Hypertension can be controlled in most patients, but combination therapy with more than one agent is often required. There is a clear benefit of hypertension treatment for primary prevention of stroke. The choice of a particular regimen should be individualized, but blood pressure reduction seems to be the most important goal, independently of the specific agent used to achieve this goal. Programs to improve hypertension treatment compliance in the community need to be developed and supported [6]. Table 2 shows the recommendations from the American Heart Association/ American Stroke Association (AHA/ASA), regarding hypertension treatment and primary stroke prevention [6, 40].

Blood pressure control in the acute setting after an ischemic stroke is controversial, but specific guidelines need to be followed regarding blood pressure management before intravenous thrombolysis is considered [50]. Regarding secondary stroke prevention, only a few randomized studies have evaluated blood pressure control and recurrent stroke risk reduction. A meta-analysis of seven randomized controlled trials studying individuals with prior history of stroke or TIA suggested that antihypertensive therapy was associated with significant reductions of stroke (odds ratio [OR] 0.76; 95% CI, 0.63-0.92) and myocardial infarction (MI) (OR 0.79; 95% CI, 0.63-0.98) [51] **(Ia/A)** (Table 2). A significant reduction in recurrent strokes was seen in patients treated with diuretics and a combination of diuretics and ACE-Is, but not with β-blockers, or ACE-Is used alone. However, comparisons were limited by the small numbers of trials, patients and events for each drug class, especially for the β-blockers [51]. Overall reduction in stroke and all vascular events were related to the degree of blood pressure lowering achieved.

It is still uncertain whether a particular class of antihypertensive agents provides further benefit to patients after ischemic stroke. The initial results of the Heart Outcomes Prevention Evaluation (HOPE) Study (comparing ramipril versus placebo in a high-risk population) led to the belief that ACE-Is may have a 'vascular protective' effect in addition to their antihypertensive mechanism, maybe by improving endothelial dysfunction, or by not affecting the cerebral auto-regulation, in contrast to other antihypertensive agents [52]. In HOPE, a subset of 1013 patients with a history of stroke or TIA had a 24% risk reduction (95% CI, 5-40) for stroke, MI, or vascular death, despite minimal reduction in blood pressure (average 3/2mm Hg). However, another sub-study of HOPE, using ambulatory blood pressure monitoring found a substantial 10/4mm Hg reduction over 24 hours and a 17/8mm Hg reduction during the night time which implied that the mechanism of ramipril did have a substantial effect on BP control enough to potentially explain stroke risk reduction [53].

Table 2. Meta-analysis of seven large trials analyzing the effects of blood pressure lowering on stroke, myocardial infarction, all vascular events and death [51].

Outcome	Trials	Events	Subjects	Rate in control group %	OR	95% CI	P	Heterogeneity P
Stroke, all	7	1577	15,527	11.5	0.76	0.63-0.92	0.005	0.01
Stroke, fatal	7	329	15,527	2.4	0.76	0.56-1.03	0.08	0.16
Stroke, non-fatal	7	1268	15,527	9.2	0.79	0.65-0.95	0.01	0.042
Myocardial infarction, all	6	555	15,428	4.0	0.79	0.63-0.98	0.03	0.19
Vascular events, all	6	2225	15,428	16.0	0.79	0.66-0.95	0.01	0.002
Death, vascular	7	852	15,527	5.9	0.86	0.70-1.06	0.16	0.066
Death, all	7	1427	15,527	9.6	0.91	0.79-1.05	0.18	0.17

Odds ratio (OR) and 95% confidence intervals (CI) determined using a random effects model

The Perindopril Protection Against Recurrent Stroke Study (PROGRESS) [54] was specifically designed to test the effects of a blood pressure-lowering regimen among 6105 patients with prior stroke or transient ischemic attack. Patients were randomized to receive the ACE-I perindopril alone or the combination of ACE-I plus the diuretic indapamide vs. placebo. After 4 years of follow-up, the active group had a relative stroke risk reduction of 28% (95% CI, 17-38; p<0.0001) and the average blood pressure reduction was 9/4mm Hg. The combination was superior to monotherapy in lowering both blood pressure and stroke risk, but there was no significant benefit when the ACE-I was given alone. The combination reduced blood pressure by an average of 12/5mm Hg and resulted in a 43% (95% CI, 30-54) reduction in the risk of major vascular events.

The ACCESS (Acute Candesartan Cilexetil therapy in stroke Survivors Study) and MOSES (Morbidity and Mortality After Stroke, Eprosartan Compared with Nitrendipine for Secondary Prevention) [55] trials showed a reduction of stroke recurrence risk with angiotensin receptor blockers, but other trials have had less certain results. Telmisartan did not significantly reduce the risk of recurrent stroke or the composite outcome of major cardiovascular events in PRoFESS (Prevention Regimen for Effectively avoiding Secondary Strokes), but on average patients were not followed as long as in other trials [56]. And finally, ONTARGET (Ongoing Telmisartan Alone and in Combination With Ramipril Global Endpoint Trial) showed non-inferiority of telmisartan compared to the ACE-I ramipril, but there was also no advantage of the combination of telmisartan plus ramipril over ramipril alone in preventing cardiovascular events or stroke in patients with vascular disease or diabetes [57]. This latter trial had insufficient power to adequately assess stroke recurrence among the enrolled stroke or TIA patients. The ongoing Secondary Prevention of Small Subcortical Strokes (SPS3) study [58] is evaluating different levels of blood pressure reduction for prevention of recurrent strokes among the lacunar stroke subtype.

Current evidence suggests that effective blood pressure reduction, rather than a particular agent, are required for secondary stroke prevention **(Ib/A)**; ACE-I plus a diuretic is one appropriate first option and an ARB may be similar to an ACE-I **(Ib/A)**. Table 3 shows the recommendations from AHA/ASA regarding hypertension treatment for secondary stroke prevention.

Diabetes mellitus

Diabetes is an independent risk factor for ischemic stroke, with an estimated RR ranging from 1.8-fold to nearly 6-fold, according to case-control and prospective epidemiological studies [59, 60]. Enhanced atherogenesis secondary to glycosylation of end products and generation of free radicals, diversion into the aldolase reductase pathway, vascular smooth muscle cell proliferation, impairment of nitric oxide-mediated vasodilatation and platelet activation have been involved in the increased vascular risk among diabetics [61].

The incidence of microvascular complications of diabetes, such as nephropathy, retinopathy and peripheral neuropathy, is clearly reduced with good glycemic control, as proven by the landmark UK Prospective Diabetes Study (UKPDS) [62] and is recommended for both primary and secondary prevention of stroke and cardiovascular disease. The data on control of macrovascular complications, including stroke, among diabetics is more limited. The UKPDS demonstrated trends in reducing the risk of cardiovascular events with more intensive glycemic control, but failed to reach statistical significance [62]. An even more aggressive glycemic control for patients with type 2 diabetes and vascular disease or multiple vascular risk factors was evaluated in the ACCORD (Action to Control Cardiovascular Risk in Diabetes) trial [63]. The intensive glucose treatment group, targeting a glycosylated hemoglobin A1c (HbA1c) level <6%, was compared to standard programs with a HbA1c goal of 7-7.9%. The study was stopped early for safety reasons, due to

Table 3. Recommendations from the AHA/ASA for hypertension treatment for primary and secondary stroke prevention.

Recommendations from the AHA/ASA for hypertension treatment for primary stroke prevention [6]

♦ Regular screenings for hypertension (at least every 2 years in most adults and more frequently in minority populations and the elderly) and appropriate management (Class I, Level of Evidence A), including dietary changes, lifestyle modification and pharmacological therapy as summarized in JNC7 [40], are recommended.

Recommendations from the AHA/ASA for hypertension treatment for prevention of recurrent strokes [105]

♦ Antihypertensive treatment is recommended for both prevention of recurrent stroke and prevention of other vascular events in persons who have had an ischemic stroke or TIA and are beyond the first 24 hours (Class I, Level of Evidence A).

♦ Since this benefit extends to persons with and without a history of hypertension, this recommendation should be considered for all ischemic stroke and TIA patients (Class IIa, Level of Evidence B).

♦ An absolute target BP level and reduction are uncertain and should be individualized, but benefit has been associated with an average reduction of approximately 10/5mm Hg and normal BP levels have been defined as <120/80mm Hg by JNC7 (Class IIa, Level of Evidence B).

♦ Several lifestyle modifications have been associated with blood pressure reductions and should be included as part of a comprehensive-approach antihypertensive therapy (Class IIb, Level of Evidence C). These modifications include salt restriction, weight loss, consumption of a diet rich in fruits, vegetables and low-fat dairy products, regular aerobic physical activity and limited alcohol consumption.

♦ The optimal drug regimen remains uncertain; however, the available data support the use of diuretics and the combination of diuretics and an ACE-I (Class I, Level of Evidence A).

♦ The choice of specific drugs and targets should be individualized based on the basis of pharmacological properties, mechanism of action and consideration of specific patient characteristics (e.g. extracranial cerebrovascular occlusive disease, renal impairment, cardiac disease, and diabetes) (Class IIa, Level of Evidence B). (New recommendation.)

increased mortality in patients randomized to intensive treatment and no significant differences were observed for the primary outcomes (non-fatal MI, non-fatal stroke or death from a cardiovascular cause) or the secondary outcome (non-fatal stroke). In the similar, independent Action in Diabetes and Vascular Disease (ADVANCE) trial, there was no increase in mortality with very intensive glucose control [64]. Microvascular disease was significantly decreased in the aggressive glycemic control group, but macrovascular complications, including stroke, were not significantly reduced. Finally, no differences between macrovascular and microvascular complications were found in the VA trial among 1791 military veterans with type 2 diabetes who had a prior suboptimal response to treatment [65]. In this trial, the intensive group had a median HbA1c of 6.9% and the standard glucose control group, 8.4%.

In the Prospective Pioglitazone Clinical Trial In Macrovascular Events (PROACTIVE) [66], treatment with pioglitazone in patients with type 2 diabetes and macrovascular disease did not show significant reduction in the primary outcome of all-cause death or cardiovascular events, compared to placebo, but significantly reduced the secondary outcome of fatal and non-fatal stroke (HR 0.53; 95% CI, 0.34-0.85), mainly among patients with prior stroke. A recent meta-analysis of 56 randomized controlled trials of rosiglitazone (at least 24 weeks in duration) with reported cardiovascular adverse events showed a significantly increased risk of MI (OR 1.28; 95% CI, 1.02-1.63; p=0.04), but not cardiovascular mortality (OR 1.03; 95% CI, 0.78-1.36; p=0.86) in relation to rosiglitazone therapy [67]. Another study on 228,000 patients from a national Medicare database has also raised concern regarding an increased risk for stroke, heart failure and all-cause mortality in patients taking rosiglitazone, compared to patients on pioglitazone, who did not have an increase in these cardiovascular events [68].

Overall, these trials have failed to demonstrate significant beneficial effects for stroke risk reduction among higher-risk diabetics with more intensive glycemic control (HbA1C <6.5), but they have not evaluated such treatment regimens earlier in the course of diabetes. Patients with type 2 diabetes have increased prevalence of atherogenic risk factors, as well as increased susceptibility to atherosclerosis. Multiple studies have clearly shown that good control of other vascular risk factors is particularly important in diabetic patients.

The data on the efficacy of risk factor control, particularly blood pressure, is stronger than glucose control for stroke prevention among diabetics (Ib/A). In the UKPDS [69], diabetic patients with controlled BP (mean BP, 144/82mm Hg) had a 44% reduction in risk of stroke compared with diabetic patients with poorer controlled BP (mean BP, 154/87mm Hg, p=0.013).

Thiazide diuretics, β-blockers (BB), ACE-Is and ARBs are all beneficial for reducing cardiovascular events and stroke incidence in patients with diabetes [46, 70-72]. In the Anti-hypertensive and Lipid-Lowering Treatment to prevent Heart Attack Trial (ALLHAT) [73], which included >12,000 diabetic patients, no difference in endpoint for coronary events was found between ACE-Is and diuretics regardless of diabetic status. However, for other vascular events such as stroke, the diuretic, chlorthalidone, was found to be superior to the ACE-I, lisinopril, alone and CCB, amlodipine. The results of the Valsartan Antihypertensive Long-Term Use Evaluation (VALUE) study [72], which included diabetic and non-diabetic patients, found no differences in event rates in the groups treated with a CCB or the ARB, valsartan. Similarly, the HOPE/MicroHOPE trial established the benefits of the ACE-I, ramipril, among those with diabetes and microalbuminuria.

The American Diabetes Association (ADA) recommends that all patients with diabetes and hypertension should be treated with a regimen that includes either an ACE-I or ARB, and the long-term BP goal target should be <130/80mm Hg [74]. The AHA/ASA endorses established guidelines for glycemic control and blood pressure management among diabetic patients who have had a stroke or TIA [40, 75]. Table 4 shows the AHA/ASA recommendations for diabetes and blood sugar control for primary and secondary stroke prevention.

Table 4. Recommendations from the AHA/ASA for diabetes management for primary and secondary stroke prevention [6].

Recommendations from the AHA/ASA for diabetes management and primary stroke prevention [6]

- It is recommended that hypertension be tightly controlled in patients with either type 1 or type 2 diabetes (the JNC7 recommendation of <130/80mm Hg in diabetic patients is endorsed [40]) as part of a comprehensive risk-reduction program (Class I, Level of Evidence A).

- Treatment of adults with diabetes, especially those with additional risk factors, with a statin to lower the risk of a first stroke is recommended (Class I, Level of Evidence A).

- Recommendations to consider treatment of diabetic patients with an ACE-I or ARB, are endorsed.

Recommendations from the AHA/ASA for diabetes management and secondary stroke prevention [105]

- Use of existing guidelines for glycemic control and blood pressure targets in patients with diabetes is recommended for patients who have had a stroke or TIA (Class I, Level of Evidence B). (New recommendation.)

Dyslipidemia

Hypercholesterolemia and other abnormalities of blood lipids are not as strongly correlated with stroke risk as with cardiac disease [76]. However, observational studies have confirmed a positive association of cholesterol level and risk of ischemic stroke and results from trials using statins have shown significant reductions in stroke risk **(Ib/A)**. Three large trials initially designed to evaluate the use of statins in high-risk patients with coronary artery disease, the Scandinavian Simvastatin Survival Study (4S) [77], Long-term Intervention with Pravastatin in Ischemic Disease (LIPID) [78] and Cholesterol And Recurrent Events (CARE) [79] trials, also showed a reduction of stroke outcomes. In 4S, aside from the reduction in primary outcomes of total mortality and cardiac events, stroke risk was also reduced by 30% in patients with a first myocardial infarction and high cholesterol levels. In CARE, patients treated with pravastatin had a 31% stroke risk reduction (95% CI, 3-52; p=0.03) and finally in LIPID, subjects on pravastatin had a 24% reduction in coronary heart disease (CHD) mortality and a 19% reduction in the incidence of stroke (p=0.048). The Heart Protection Study (HPS) [80], a largescale, long-term trial, evaluated the use of simvastatin vs. placebo among over 20,000 patients aged 40-80 years with CHD, other occlusive arterial disease, or diabetes, who were followed up for 5 years. The study showed significant reductions in all-cause mortality, non-fatal myocardial infarction or coronary death and non-fatal or fatal stroke, which was reduced in 25% in among several subgroups of enrolled patients. Benefits with statins were found in different types of high-risk patients, including patients without a previous diagnosis of CHD [81]. In a systematic review and updated meta-analysis of the published randomized trials evaluating the use of statins, Amarenco et al found a relative stroke risk reduction of 21% (OR 0.79 [0.73-0.85]), and for each 10% reduction in LDL-C, the estimated stroke risk reduction was 15% (95% CI, 6.7-23.6) [82].

Most of these studies on hypercholesterolemia had only enrolled very few patients with pre-existent cerebrovascular disease, and the benefits were found mostly among individuals without a prior history of stroke. The Stroke Prevention by Aggressive Reduction in Cholesterol Levels (SPARCL) trial [83] addressed the role of statins in secondary stroke prevention. In this study, 4731 patients without previous CHD who had a stroke or TIA within 6 months prior to enrollment and had LDL-C levels between 100 and 190mg/dL, were randomized to high doses of atorvastatin (80mg/day) or placebo and followed up for 5 years. Mean LDL-C for the treatment group was 73mg/dL and for the placebo group was 129mg/dL and the risk of stroke decreased from 13.1-11.2% (HR 0.84; 95% CI, 0.71-0.99; p=0.03). Acute coronary events were also reduced (HR 0.65; 95% CI, 0.50-0.84; p=0.001). Only 2.2% had a significant increase in liver enzymes and there were no significant differences in the occurrence of myalgias or rhabdomyolysis in the treatment group, compared to placebo. In this study, lower levels of LDL-C resulted in a progressive decrease in stroke and coronary events. Patients with ≥50% reduction in LDL-C had a 35% reduction in combined risk of non-fatal and fatal stroke; and achieving an LDL-C level <70mg/dL was associated with a 28% reduction in stroke (p=0.0018) with no increase in hemorrhagic strokes, compared to LDL-C levels >100mg/dL [84].

Table 5. Recommendations from the AHA/ASA for the management of dyslipidemia and the use of statins for primary and secondary stroke prevention [6].

Recommendations from the AHA/ASA for the management of dyslipidemia and the use of statins for primary stroke prevention [6]

♦ National Cholesterol Education Program III (NCEP III) guidelines [140] for the management of patients who have not had a cerebrovascular event and who have elevated total cholesterol or elevated non-HDL cholesterol in the presence of hypertriglyceridemia are endorsed.

♦ It is recommended that patients with known coronary artery disease (CAD) and high-risk hypertensive patients even with normal LDL cholesterol levels be treated with lifestyle measures and a statin (Class I, Level of Evidence A).

♦ Treatment of adults with diabetes, especially those with additional risk factors, with a statin to lower the risk of a first stroke is recommended (Class I, Level of Evidence A).

♦ Suggested treatments for patients with known CAD and low HDL cholesterol include weight loss, increased physical activity, smoking cessation, and possibly niacin or gemfibrozil (Class IIa, Level of Evidence B).

Recommendations from the AHA/ASA for the management of dyslipidemia and the use of statins in survivors of ischemic stroke or TIA [105]

♦ Statin therapy with intensive lipid-lowering effects is recommended to reduce risk of stroke and cardiovascular events among patients with ischemic stroke or TIA who have evidence of atherosclerosis, an LDL-C level ≥100mg/dL and who are without known CHD (Class I, Level of Evidence B).

♦ For patients with atherosclerotic ischemic stroke or TIA and without known CHD, it is reasonable to target a reduction of at least 50% in LDL-C or a target LDL-C level of <70mg/dL to obtain maximum benefit (Class IIa, Level of Evidence B). (New recommendation.)

♦ Patients with ischemic stroke or TIA with elevated cholesterol or comorbid coronary artery disease should be otherwise managed according to NCEP III guidelines, which include lifestyle modification, dietary guidelines and medication recommendations (Class I; Level of Evidence A).

♦ Patients with ischemic stroke or TIA with low HDL-C may be considered for treatment with niacin or gemfibrozil (Class IIb, Level of Evidence B).

A post hoc analysis showed a small increase in hemorrhagic strokes, from 1.4% to 2.3% (HR 1.6; 95% CI, 1.1-2.6; p<0.02), with atorvastatin. Hemorrhagic strokes were more common in patients with a baseline hemorrhagic stroke, in men and with increasing age, as well as in individuals with uncontrolled hypertension. There was no association between hemorrhage risk and baseline LDL-C levels, or recent LDL-C levels in treated patients. A large meta-analysis evaluating 48,000 patients from multiple statin trials in CHD cohorts showed no increase in the risk of hemorrhagic stroke [85].

There are other medications that have been used to lower lipids including niacin, fibrates, and cholesterol absorption inhibitors. Although these agents may lower cholesterol among stroke or TIA patients, there are sparse data on their efficacy for the prevention of recurrent stroke. They may be considered for patients who are unable to tolerate statins. In older studies, niacin has been associated with a reduction in stroke, such as in the VA HDL Intervention Trial (VA-HIT), where gemfibrozil reduced the rate of total strokes among men with coronary artery disease and low levels of HDL-C (<40mg/dL) [86]. Table 5 shows recommendations from the AHA/ASA for the management of dyslipidemia and the use of statins for primary and secondary stroke prevention.

Lifestyle factors

Smoking

Cigarette smoking increases the risk of stroke by many different mechanisms such as acute effects on thrombus generation, increased burden of atherosclerosis, changes in heart rate, increased mean arterial pressure and cardiac index, and decreased arterial distensibility [87-90]. Multiple epidemiological studies (Framingham, Cardiovascular Health Study, Honolulu Heart Study) have identified cigarette smoking as a potent stroke risk factor, with an associated risk of approximately double for ischemic stroke and a 2- to 4-fold increase for hemorrhagic stroke [91-93] (after adjustment of other risk factors)(IIa/B). In a meta-analysis of 32 studies, the calculated RR in smokers, compared to non-smokers, was 1.9 (95% CI, 1.7-2.2) for ischemic stroke and 2.9 (95% CI, 2.5-3.5) for subarachnoid hemorrhage [94] (IIa/B). Even exposure to environmental tobacco smoke (passive smoking), nearly doubles the risk found for active smoking [95, 96].

Cigarette smoking may also potentiate other stroke risk factors, in a synergistic way. This was clearly seen in the assessment of stroke risk among women using oral contraceptives (OC). When compared to non-smoking, non-OC-using women, the risk of ischemic stroke was 1.3 times greater (95% CI, 0.7-2.1) among women who smoked but did not use OC, 2.1 times greater (95% CI, 1.0-4.5) for non-smoking, OC users and 7.2 times greater (95% CI, 3.2-16.1) for women who smoked and used OC. A synergistic effect was also seen on the risk of hemorrhagic stroke, which was 3.7 times greater (95% CI, 2.4-5.7) for women who smoked and used OC [97, 98].

In terms of primary stroke prevention, a rapid reduction in the risk of stroke and other cardiovascular events is seen after smoking cessation, to a level that approaches those who never smoked [87, 99, 100]. Ethical constraints prevent the performance of randomized, controlled, prospective studies on smoking cessation after stroke, but observational studies have convincingly shown decreased risk of stroke after quitting, and the increased risk that may even disappear after 5 years [101-103].

The use of behavioral and pharmacological combination therapy, such as social support and skills training plus nicotine replacement therapy has been found to be effective for quitting smoking [104]. For primary and secondary stroke prevention, the AHA/ASA recommends abstention from cigarette smoking (non-smokers), smoking cessation for current smokers (Class I, Level of Evidence C for primary prevention; Class I, Level of Evidence C for secondary prevention) and avoidance of environmental tobacco smoke (Class IIa, Level of Evidence C). The use of counseling, nicotine replacement and oral smoking-cessation medications should be considered (Class I, Level of Evidence A) [105].

Alcohol consumption

Alcohol consumption is usually described in number of drinks. An average drink contains about 12g, 15mL, or 0.5oz of alcohol, which is found in one bottle (12oz) of beer, one small glass (4oz) of wine, or one alcoholic (1.5oz liquor) cocktail. There is strong evidence showing that chronic alcoholism and heavy drinking are risk factors for all stroke subtypes [106]. This is true also for recurrence of stroke, as observed in the Northern Manhattan cohort, in which stroke recurrence was significantly increased among those patients with prior heavy alcohol use [107]. But light to moderate alcohol consumption may be protective, at least for ischemic stroke. In a meta-analysis of 35 observational studies of the association between alcohol and stroke, individuals who consumed over five drinks per day had a 69% increased stroke risk (RR 1.69), compared with non-drinkers. But consumption of less than one drink per day was associated with reduced risk (RR 0.80) and an even larger benefit was seen in individuals who consumed one to two drinks per day (RR 0.72) [108]. These studies have suggested a J-shaped association, with protective effect in light or moderate drinkers and an elevated stroke risk with heavy alcohol consumption.

The consensus is that the amount of alcohol ingested is more important than the specific alcoholic beverage [109], but some have suggested that red wine may have added benefits [110]. Increase in HDL, decrease in platelet aggregation, reduced plasma fibrinogen concentration, reduced plasma viscosity, decrease in inflammatory markers and enhancement of insulin sensitivity, which may result in decreased postprandial glucose changes are some of the proposed mechanisms for reduced risk of stroke with light to moderate alcohol consumption [111-115]. Additionally, flavonoids and resveratrol contained in red wine may also provide beneficial effects [116]. Heavy alcohol consumption, on the contrary, induces hypertension, hypercoagulable state, reduced cerebral blood flow and atrial fibrillation (AF) [117-119]. Additionally, brain atrophy associated to heavy alcohol consumption may also increase its vulnerability to vascular events [120, 121].

For clinicians, a primary goal for stroke prevention is to eliminate or reduce alcohol consumption in heavy drinkers. Established screening and counseling methods have been outlined in the US Preventive Services Task Force Update [122].

For primary and secondary stroke prevention, the AHA/ASA recommends that patients who are heavy drinkers should eliminate or reduce their consumption of alcohol (Class I, Level of Evidence A). Light-to-moderate levels of no more than two drinks per day for men and 1 drink per day for non-pregnant women may be considered (Class IIb, Level of Evidence C).

Obesity

Obesity is a state of excess adipose tissue mass. The most widely used method to measure obesity is the body mass index (BMI), defined as weight/height^2 (in kg/m^2). A BMI between 25 and 29.9 Kg/m^2 indicates overweight and a BMI of $\geq$30kg/m^2, obesity. As many as 64% of adults $\geq$20 years of age are overweight and the percent of American adult population with obesity has increased from around 14% between 1976 and 1980, to over 30% between 2003 and 2006 [1] (Figure 3). Extreme obesity has also increased and affects 4.7% of the population. Obesity is more common among women and in the poor, and the prevalence of obesity among children is also rising. Obesity is strongly related to several major vascular risk factors, such as hypertension, diabetes and dyslipidemia.

The Physicians' Health Study showed that an increasing BMI is associated with a steady increase in ischemic stroke, independently of the effects of hypertension, diabetes and cholesterol [123]. Among women data are less consistent, with positive and negative associations [124-126]. Abdominal obesity (defined as a waist circumference of >102cm [40"] in men and 88cm [35"] in women) rather than general obesity seems to be more related to stroke risk [127, 128]. In the Northern Manhattan Study, a significant and independent association between abdominal obesity and ischemic stroke was found in all racial/ethnic groups [127]. After adjustment for other risk factors and BMI, a comparison between the first quartile of waist-to-hip ratio with the third and fourth quartiles gave ORs of 2.4 (95% CI, 1.5-3.9) and 3.0 (95% CI, 1.8-4.8), respectively.

Weight loss significantly improves BP, fasting glucose values, serum lipids and physical endurance. Since obesity is a contributing factor to other risk factors associated with recurrent stroke, weight loss promotion and maintenance of a healthy weight is a priority. Diets such as the Mediterranean diet, rich in fruits and vegetables, can help with weight control and have been associated with reduced risk of stroke, MI and death [129]. However, the relationship between obesity and stroke is complex and has been studied mostly in primary stroke prevention; so far no study has demonstrated weight loss reduces the risk of stroke recurrence [105].

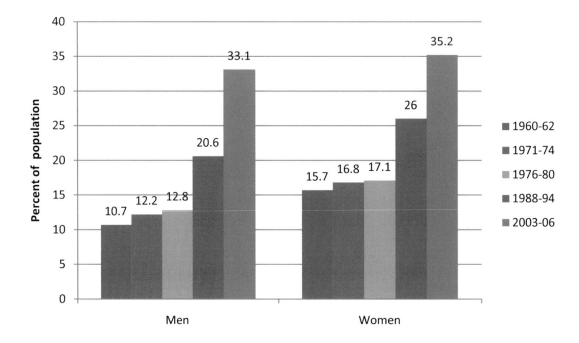

Figure 3. Age-related prevalence of obesity in adults (20-74 years of age), by sex and survey (NHES: 1960-62; NHANES: 1971-74, 1976-80, 1988-94 and 2003-06). Source Health, United States 2002 (NCHS). Heart Disease and Stroke Statistics 2010 Update: A Report from the American Heart Association [1].

For primary stroke prevention, the AHA/ASA recommends that weight reduction may be considered for all overweight patients to maintain the goal of a BMI of between 18.5 and 24.9kg/m^2 and a waist circumference of <35" for women and <40" for men (Class IIb, Level of Evidence C).

Physical activity

There is strong evidence supporting the beneficial effects of physical activity on multiple cardiovascular risk factors, including those for stroke. These beneficial effects have been associated with reduced weight and BP [130, 131], enhanced vasodilatation [132], decreased viscosity and platelet aggregability [133, 134], as well as improved glycemic control and lipidic profiles [135, 136].

A protective effect of physical activity on stroke was clearly seen in a meta-analysis of 18 cohort and five case-control studies. Stroke incidence and mortality was significantly lower in highly active individuals, compared with individuals with low levels of activity (RR 0.73; 95% CI, 0.67-0.79). The effect was also present for individuals who engaged in moderate intensity activity (RR 0.80; 95% CI, 0.74-0.86) [137] and the benefit was found for both ischemic and hemorrhagic strokes. Other studies have also shown benefit in older individuals with vascular risk factors and across different ethnic groups [138, 139]. The implementation of aerobic exercise and strength training to improve cardiovascular fitness after stroke has been supported by several studies and benefits include improved mobility, balance and endurance.

As part of lifestyle modification, physical activity can minimize the need for medical and pharmacological treatments, or enhance treatment targets.

For patients who are capable of engaging in physical activity, the AHA/ASA recommends that at least 30 minutes of moderate-intensity physical exercise, most days of the week, may be considered to reduce risk factors and comorbid conditions that increase the likelihood of first occurrence and recurrence of stroke (Class IIb, Level of Evidence C). For stroke survivors with disability, an oriented supervised therapeutic physical regimen is recommended (Class IIb, Level of Evidence C).

Conclusions

The fact that a 60% decline in death rates from stroke has been observed in the United States and other industrialized nations since 1972, strongly supports that modifiable environmental influences are playing a role [7]. Reduced incidence of stroke as a result of improved detection and treatment of vascular risk factors may explain some of this decline. But despite this progress, stroke still remains a devastating disease, a major burden to individuals, families, communities and to society. Prevention of stroke is much more likely to have an impact on public health and welfare than the most effective, state-of-the art stroke treatment. Appropriate knowledge and management of stroke risk factors are an essential aid to healthcare providers in order to reduce stroke risk.

Key points	Evidence level
◆ Regular screenings for hypertension (at least every 2 years in most adults and more frequently in minority populations and the elderly) and appropriate management of blood pressure are effective for prevention of the first stroke.	Ia/A
◆ Antihypertensive treatment is recommended for prevention of recurrent stroke and other vascular events in persons who have had an ischemic stroke or TIA and are beyond the first 24 hours.	Ia/A
◆ The optimal drug regimen for treatment of hypertension and stroke prevention remains uncertain; however, available data support the use of diuretics and the combination of diuretics and an ACE-I.	Ib/A
◆ The choice of specific drugs and targets of blood pressure should be individualized based on pharmacological properties, mechanism of action and consideration of specific patient characteristics (e.g. extracranial cerebrovascular occlusive disease, renal impairment, cardiac disease and diabetes).	IIa/B
◆ Hypertension should be tightly controlled in patients with either type 1 or type 2 diabetes, as part of a comprehensive risk reduction program for prevention of stroke.	Ib/A
◆ Treatment of adults with diabetes, especially those with additional risk factors, with a statin is effective for prevention of the first stroke.	Ib/A
◆ In patients with known CAD and high-risk hypertensive patients even with normal LDL cholesterol levels, lifestyle measures and the use of a statin are effective for prevention of stroke.	Ib/A
◆ In patients with ischemic stroke or TIA with elevated cholesterol or comorbid coronary artery disease, lifestyle modification, dietary guidelines and medication treatment according to the NCEP III guidelines, are recommended for prevention of stroke.	Ib/A

References

1. Lloyd-Jones D, Adams RJ, Brown TM, *et al*. Heart disease and stroke statistics - 2010 update: a report from the American Heart Association. *Circulation* 2010;121(7): e46-215.
2. Dhamoon MS, Tai W, Boden-Albala B, *et al*. Risk of myocardial infarction or vascular death after first ischemic stroke: the Northern Manhattan Study. *Stroke* 2007; 38(6): 1752-8.
3. Tissue plasminogen activator for acute ischemic stroke. The National Institute of Neurological Disorders and Stroke rt-PA Stroke Study Group. *N Engl J Med* 1995; 333(24): 1581-7.
4. Schwamm L, Fayad P, Acker JE, 3rd, *et al*. Translating evidence into practice: a decade of efforts by the American Heart Association/American Stroke Association to reduce death and disability due to stroke: a presidential advisory from the American Heart Association/American Stroke Association. *Stroke* 2010; 41(5): 1051-65.

5.   Reeves MJ, Arora S, Broderick JP, *et al.* Acute stroke care in the US: results from 4 pilot prototypes of the Paul Coverdell National Acute Stroke Registry. *Stroke* 2005; 36(6): 1232-40.

6.   Goldstein LB, Adams R, Alberts MJ, *et al.* Primary Prevention of Ischemic Stroke: a Guideline from the American Heart Association/American Stroke Association Stroke Council: cosponsored by the Atherosclerotic Peripheral Vascular Disease Interdisciplinary Working Group; Cardiovascular Nursing Council; Clinical Cardiology Council; Nutrition, Physical Activity, and Metabolism Council; and the Quality of Care and Outcomes Research Interdisciplinary Working Group: the American Academy of Neurology affirms the value of this guideline. *Stroke* 2006; 37(6): 1583-633.

7.   Wolf PA. Epidemiology of Stroke. In: *Stroke. Pathopysiology, Diagnosis and Management.* Mohr DW, Grotta JC, Weir B, Wolf PA, Eds. Philadelphia, PA, USA: Churchill Livingstone, 2004: 13-34.

8.   Wolf PA, D'Agostino RB, O'Neal MA, *et al.* Secular trends in stroke incidence and mortality. The Framingham Study. *Stroke* 1992; 23(11): 1551-5.

9.   Brown RD, Whisnant JP, Sicks JD, *et al.* Stroke incidence, prevalence, and survival: secular trends in Rochester, Minnesota, through 1989. *Stroke* 1996; 27(3): 373-80.

10. Towfighi A, Saver JL, Engelhardt R, *et al.* A midlife stroke surge among women in the United States. *Neurology* 2007; 69(20): 1898-904.

11. Bousser MG. Stroke in women: the 1997 Paul Dudley White International Lecture. *Circulation* 1999; 99(4): 463-7.

12. Rossouw JE, Anderson GL, Prentice RL, *et al.* Risks and benefits of estrogen plus progestin in healthy postmenopausal women: principal results From the Women's Health Initiative randomized controlled trial. *JAMA* 2002; 288(3): 321-33.

13. Viscoli CM, Brass LM, Kernan WN, *et al.* A clinical trial of estrogen-replacement therapy after ischemic stroke. *N Engl J Med* 2001; 345(17): 1243-9.

14. Wassertheil-Smoller S, Hendrix SL, Limacher M, *et al.* Effect of estrogen plus progestin on stroke in postmenopausal women: the Women's Health Initiative: a randomized trial. *JAMA* 2003; 289(20): 2673-84.

15. Kurth T, Moore SC, Gaziano JM, *et al.* Healthy lifestyle and the risk of stroke in women. *Arch Intern Med* 2006; 166(13): 1403-9.

16. White H, Boden-Albala B, Wang C, *et al.* Ischemic stroke subtype incidence among whites, blacks, and Hispanics: the Northern Manhattan Study. *Circulation* 2005; 111(10): 1327-31.

17. Qureshi AI, Mendelow AD, Hanley DF. Intracerebral haemorrhage. *Lancet* 2009; 373(9675): 1632-44.

18. Liao D, Myers R, Hunt S, *et al.* Familial history of stroke and stroke risk. The Family Heart Study. *Stroke* 1997; 28(10): 1908-12.

19. Rubattu S, Stanzione R, Gigante B, *et al.* Genetic susceptibility to cerebrovascular accidents. *J Cardiovasc Pharmacol* 2001; 38 Suppl 2: S71-4.

20. Brass LM, Isaacsohn JL, Merikangas KR, *et al.* A study of twins and stroke. *Stroke* 1992; 23(2): 221-3.

21. Scott CH, Sutton MS. Homocysteine: evidence for a causal relationship with cardiovascular disease. *Cardiol Rev* 1999; 7(2): 101-7.

22. Hassan A, Hunt BJ, O'Sullivan M, *et al.* Homocysteine is a risk factor for cerebral small vessel disease, acting via endothelial dysfunction. *Brain* 2004; 127(Pt 1): 212-9.

23. Fodinger M, Horl WH, Sunder-Plassmann G. Molecular biology of 5,10-methylenetetrahydrofolate reductase. *J Nephrol* 2000; 13(1): 20-33.

24. Kalimo H, Viitanen M, Amberla K, *et al.* CADASIL: hereditary disease of arteries causing brain infarcts and dementia. *Neuropathol Appl Neurobiol* 1999; 25(4): 257-65.

25. Hillier CE, Collins PW, Bowen DJ, *et al.* Inherited prothrombotic risk factors and cerebral venous thrombosis. *QJM* 1998; 91(10): 677-80.

26. Deschiens MA, Conard J, Horellou MH, *et al.* Coagulation studies, Factor V Leiden, and anticardiolipin antibodies in 40 cases of cerebral venous thrombosis. *Stroke* 1996; 27(10): 1724-30.

27. De Lucia D, Renis V, Belli A, *et al.* Familial coagulation-inhibiting and fibrinolytic protein deficiencies in juvenile transient ischaemic attacks. *J Neurosurg Sci* 1996; 40(1): 25-35.

28. Bertina RM, Koeleman BP, Koster T, *et al.* Mutation in blood coagulation Factor V associated with resistance to activated protein C. *Nature* 1994; 369(6475): 64-7.

29. Weber M, Hayem G, DeBandt M, *et al.* The family history of patients with primary or secondary antiphospholipid syndrome (APS). *Lupus* 2000; 9(4): 258-63.

30. Goldberg SN, Conti-Kelly AM, Greco TP. A family study of anticardiolipin antibodies and associated clinical conditions. *Am J Med* 1995; 99(5): 473-9.

31. Shetty-Alva N, Alva S. Familial moyamoya disease in Caucasians. *Pediatr Neurol* 2000; 23(5): 445-7.

32. Begelman SM, Olin JW. Fibromuscular dysplasia. *Curr Opin Rheumatol* 2000; 12(1): 41-7.

33. Testai FD, Gorelick PB. Inherited metabolic disorders and stroke part 1: Fabry disease and mitochondrial myopathy, encephalopathy, lactic acidosis, and strokelike episodes. *Arch Neurol* 2010; 67(1): 19-24.

34. Schiffmann R, Kopp JB, Austin HA, 3rd, *et al.* Enzyme replacement therapy in Fabry disease: a randomized controlled trial. *JAMA* 2001; 285(21): 2743-9.

35. Eng CM, Guffon N, Wilcox WR, *et al.* Safety and efficacy of recombinant human alpha-galactosidase A - replacement therapy in Fabry's disease. *N Engl J Med* 2001; 345(1): 9-16.

36. De Schoenmakere G, Chauveau D, Grunfeld JP. Enzyme replacement therapy in Anderson-Fabry's disease: beneficial clinical effect on vital organ function. *Nephrol Dial Transplant* 2003; 18(1): 33-5.

37. Fields LE, Burt VL, Cutler JA, *et al.* The burden of adult hypertension in the United States 1999 to 2000: a rising tide. *Hypertension* 2004; 44(4): 398-404.

38. Burt VL, Whelton P, Roccella EJ, *et al.* Prevalence of hypertension in the US adult population. Results from the Third National Health and Nutrition Examination Survey, 1988-1991. *Hypertension* 1995; 25(3): 305-13.

39. Vasan RS, Beiser A, Seshadri S, *et al.* Residual lifetime risk for developing hypertension in middle-aged women and men: The Framingham Heart Study. *JAMA* 2002; 287(8): 1003-10.

40. Chobanian AV, Bakris GL, Black HR, *et al.* The Seventh Report of the Joint National Committee on Prevention, Detection, Evaluation, and Treatment of High Blood Pressure: the JNC 7 report. *JAMA* 2003; 289(19): 2560-72.

41. Lawes CM, Bennett DA, Feigin VL, *et al.* Blood pressure and stroke: an overview of published reviews. *Stroke* 2004; 35(3): 776-85.

42. Turnbull F. Effects of different blood-pressure-lowering regimens on major cardiovascular events: results of prospectively-designed overviews of randomised trials. *Lancet* 2003; 362(9395): 1527-35.

43. Prevention of stroke by antihypertensive drug treatment in older persons with isolated systolic hypertension. Final results of the Systolic Hypertension in the Elderly Program (SHEP). SHEP Cooperative Research Group. *JAMA* 1991; 265(24): 3255-64.

44. Staessen JA, Fagard R, Thijs L, *et al.* Randomised double-blind comparison of placebo and active treatment for older patients with isolated systolic hypertension. The Systolic Hypertension in Europe (Syst-Eur) Trial Investigators. *Lancet* 1997; 350(9080): 757-64.

45. Douglas JG, Bakris GL, Epstein M, *et al.* Management of high blood pressure in African Americans: consensus statement of the Hypertension in African Americans Working Group of the International Society on Hypertension in Blacks. *Arch Intern Med* 2003; 163(5): 525-41.

46. Major outcomes in high-risk hypertensive patients randomized to angiotensin-converting enzyme inhibitor or calcium channel blocker vs diuretic: The Antihypertensive and Lipid-Lowering Treatment to Prevent Heart Attack Trial (ALLHAT). *JAMA* 2002; 288(23): 2981-97.

47. Black HR, Elliott WJ, Grandits G, *et al.* Principal results of the Controlled Onset Verapamil Investigation of Cardiovascular End Points (CONVINCE) trial. *JAMA* 2003; 289(16): 2073-82.

48. Dahlof B, Devereux RB, Kjeldsen SE, *et al.* Cardiovascular morbidity and mortality in the Losartan Intervention For Endpoint reduction in hypertension study (LIFE): a randomised trial against atenolol. *Lancet* 2002; 359(9311): 995-1003.

49. Neal B, MacMahon S, Chapman N. Effects of ACE inhibitors, calcium antagonists, and other blood-pressure-lowering drugs: results of prospectively designed overviews of randomised trials. Blood Pressure Lowering Treatment Trialists' Collaboration. *Lancet* 2000; 356(9246): 1955-64.

50. Adams HP, Jr., del Zoppo G, Alberts MJ, *et al.* Guidelines for the Early Management of Adults with Ischemic Stroke: a Guideline from the American Heart Association/American Stroke Association Stroke Council, Clinical Cardiology Council, Cardiovascular Radiology and Intervention Council, and the Atherosclerotic Peripheral Vascular Disease and Quality of Care Outcomes in Research Interdisciplinary Working Groups: the American Academy of Neurology affirms the value of this guideline as an educational tool for neurologists. *Stroke* 2007; 38(5): 1655-711.

51. Rashid P, Leonardi-Bee J, Bath P. Blood pressure reduction and secondary prevention of stroke and other vascular events: a systematic review. *Stroke* 2003; 34(11): 2741-8.

52. Yusuf S, Sleight P, Pogue J, *et al.* Effects of an angiotensin-converting-enzyme inhibitor, ramipril, on cardiovascular events in high-risk patients. The Heart Outcomes Prevention Evaluation Study Investigators. *N Engl J Med* 2000; 342(3): 145-53.

53. Svensson P, de Faire U, Sleight P, *et al.* Comparative effects of ramipril on ambulatory and office blood pressures: a HOPE Substudy. *Hypertension* 2001; 38(6): E28-32.

54. PROGRESS, CG. Randomised trial of a perindopril-based blood-pressure-lowering regimen among 6,105 individuals with previous stroke or transient ischaemic attack. *Lancet* 2001; 358(9287): 1033-41.

55. Schrader J, Luders S, Kulschewski A, *et al.* Morbidity and Mortality After Stroke, Eprosartan Compared with Nitrendipine for Secondary Prevention: principal results of a prospective randomized controlled study (MOSES). *Stroke* 2005; 36(6): 1218-26.

56. Yusuf S, Diener HC, Sacco RL, *et al.* Telmisartan to prevent recurrent stroke and cardiovascular events. *N Engl J Med* 2008; 359(12): 1225-37.

57. Yusuf S, Teo KK, Pogue J, *et al.* Telmisartan, ramipril, or both in patients at high risk for vascular events. *N Engl J Med* 2008; 358(15): 1547-59.

58. Secondary Prevention of Small Subcortical Strokes Trial (SPS3). (2010; Available from: http://www.clinicaltrials.gov/ct2/show/study/NCT00059306).

59. Kannel WB, McGee DL. Diabetes and cardiovascular disease. The Framingham study. *JAMA* 1979; 241(19): 2035-8.

60. Burchfiel CM, Curb JD, Rodriguez BL, *et al.* Glucose intolerance and 22-year stroke incidence. The Honolulu Heart Program. *Stroke* 1994; 25(5): 951-7.

61. Beckman JA, Creager MA, Libby P. Diabetes and atherosclerosis: epidemiology, pathophysiology, and management. *JAMA* 2002; 287(19): 2570-81.

62. Intensive blood-glucose control with sulphonylureas or insulin compared with conventional treatment and risk of complications in patients with type 2 diabetes (UKPDS 33). UK Prospective Diabetes Study (UKPDS) Group. *Lancet* 1998; 352(9131): 837-53.

63. Gerstein HC, Miller ME, Byington RP, *et al.* Effects of intensive glucose lowering in type 2 diabetes. *N Engl J Med* 2008; 358(24): 2545-59.

64. Patel A, MacMahon S, Chalmers J, *et al.* Intensive blood glucose control and vascular outcomes in patients with type 2 diabetes. *N Engl J Med* 2008; 358(24): 2560-72.

65. Duckworth W, Abraira C, Moritz T, *et al.* Glucose control and vascular complications in veterans with type 2 diabetes. *N Engl J Med* 2009; 360(2): 129-39.

66. Wilcox R, Bousser MG, Betteridge DJ, *et al.* Effects of pioglitazone in patients with type 2 diabetes with or without previous stroke: results from PROactive (PROspective pioglitAzone Clinical Trial In macroVascular Events 04). *Stroke* 2007; 38(3): 865-73.

67. Nissen SE, Wolski K. Rosiglitazone revisited: an updated meta-analysis of risk for myocardial infarction and cardiovascular mortality. *Arch Intern Med* 2010; 170(14): 1191-201.

68. Graham DJ, Ouellet-Hellstrom R, MaCurdy TE, *et al.* Risk of acute myocardial infarction, stroke, heart failure, and death in elderly Medicare patients treated with rosiglitazone or pioglitazone. *JAMA* 2010; 304(4): 411-8.

69. Tight blood pressure control and risk of macrovascular and microvascular complications in type 2 diabetes: UKPDS 38. UK Prospective Diabetes Study Group. *BMJ* 1998; 317(7160): 703-13.

70. Effects of ramipril on cardiovascular and microvascular outcomes in people with diabetes mellitus: results of the HOPE study and MICRO-HOPE substudy. Heart Outcomes Prevention Evaluation Study Investigators. *Lancet* 2000; 355(9200): 253-9.

71. Shindler DM, Kostis JB, Yusuf S, *et al.* Diabetes mellitus, a predictor of morbidity and mortality in the Studies of Left Ventricular Dysfunction (SOLVD) Trials and Registry. *Am J Cardiol* 1996; 77(11): 1017-20.

72. Weber MA, Julius S, Kjeldsen SE, *et al.* Blood pressure dependent and independent effects of antihypertensive treatment on clinical events in the VALUE Trial. *Lancet* 2004; 363(9426): 2049-51.

73. Hollenberg NK. The Antihypertensive and Lipid-Lowering Treatment to Prevent Heart Attack Trial (ALLHAT). Major outcomes in high-risk hypertensive patients randomized to angiotensin-converting enzyme inhibitor or calcium channel blocker vs diuretic. *Curr Hypertens Rep* 2003; 5(3): 183-5.

74. Summary of revisions for the 2010 Clinical Practice Recommendations. *Diabetes Care* 2010; 33 Suppl 1: S3.

75. Executive summary: standards of medical care in diabetes - 2009. *Diabetes Care* 2009; 32 Suppl 1: S6-12.

76. Gorelick PB. Stroke prevention therapy beyond antithrombotics: unifying mechanisms in ischemic stroke pathogenesis and implications for therapy: an invited review. *Stroke* 2002; 33(3): 862-75.

77. Randomised trial of cholesterol lowering in 4444 patients with coronary heart disease: the Scandinavian Simvastatin Survival Study (4S). *Lancet* 1994; 344(8934): 1383-9.

78. Prevention of cardiovascular events and death with pravastatin in patients with coronary heart disease and a broad range of initial cholesterol levels. The Long-Term Intervention with Pravastatin in Ischaemic Disease (LIPID) Study Group. *N Engl J Med* 1998; 339(19): 1349-57.

79. Sacks FM, Pfeffer MA, Moye LA, *et al.* The effect of pravastatin on coronary events after myocardial infarction in patients with average cholesterol levels. Cholesterol and Recurrent Events Trial investigators. *N Engl J Med* 1996; 335(14): 1001-9.

80. MRC/BHF Heart Protection Study of cholesterol lowering with simvastatin in 20,536 high-risk individuals: a randomised placebo-controlled trial. *Lancet* 2002; 360(9326): 7-22.

81. Collins R, Armitage J, Parish S, *et al.* Effects of cholesterol-lowering with simvastatin on stroke and other major vascular events in 20,536 people with cerebrovascular disease or other high-risk conditions. *Lancet* 2004; 363(9411): 757-67.

82. Amarenco P, Labreuche J, Lavallee P, *et al.* Statins in stroke prevention and carotid atherosclerosis: systematic review and up-to-date meta-analysis. *Stroke* 2004; 35(12): 2902-9.

83. Amarenco P, Bogousslavsky J, Callahan A, 3rd, *et al.* High-dose atorvastatin after stroke or transient ischemic attack. *N Engl J Med* 2006; 355(6): 549-59.

84. Amarenco P, Goldstein LB, Szarek M, *et al.* Effects of intense low-density lipoprotein cholesterol reduction in patients with stroke or transient ischemic attack: the Stroke Prevention by Aggressive Reduction in Cholesterol Levels (SPARCL) trial. *Stroke* 2007; 38(12): 3198-204.

85. Goldstein LB, Amarenco P, Szarek M, *et al.* Hemorrhagic stroke in the Stroke Prevention by Aggressive Reduction in Cholesterol Levels study. *Neurology* 2008; 70(24 Pt 2): 2364-70.

86. Bloomfield Rubins H, Davenport J, Babikian V, *et al.* Reduction in stroke with gemfibrozil in men with coronary heart disease and low HDL cholesterol: The Veterans Affairs HDL Intervention Trial (VA-HIT). *Circulation* 2001; 103(23): 2828-33.

87. Burns DM. Epidemiology of smoking-induced cardiovascular disease. *Prog Cardiovasc Dis* 2003; 46(1): 11-29.

88. Silvestrini M, Troisi E, Matteis M, *et al.* Effect of smoking on cerebrovascular reactivity. *J Cereb Blood Flow Metab* 1996; 16(4): 746-9.

89. Kool MJ, Hoeks AP, Struijker Boudier HA, *et al.* Short- and long-term effects of smoking on arterial wall properties in habitual smokers. *J Am Coll Cardiol* 1993; 22(7): 1881-6.

90. Howard G, Wagenknecht LE, Burke GL, *et al.* Cigarette smoking and progression of atherosclerosis: The Atherosclerosis Risk in Communities (ARIC) Study. *JAMA* 1998; 279(2): 119-24.

91. Wolf PA, D'Agostino RB, Belanger AJ, *et al.* Probability of stroke: a risk profile from the Framingham Study. *Stroke* 1991; 22(3): 312-8.

92. Rodriguez BL, D'Agostino R, Abbott RD, *et al.* Risk of hospitalized stroke in men enrolled in the Honolulu Heart Program and the Framingham Study: a comparison of incidence and risk factor effects. *Stroke* 2002; 33(1): 230-6.

93. Manolio TA, Kronmal RA, Burke GL, *et al.* Short-term predictors of incident stroke in older adults. The Cardiovascular Health Study. *Stroke* 1996; 27(9): 1479-86.

94. Shinton R, Beevers G. Meta-analysis of relation between cigarette smoking and stroke. *BMJ* 1989; 298(6676): 789-94.

95. You RX, Thrift AG, McNeil JJ, *et al.* Ischemic stroke risk and passive exposure to spouses' cigarette smoking. Melbourne Stroke Risk Factor Study (MERFS) Group. *Am J Public Health* 1999; 89(4): 572-5.

96. Bonita R, Duncan J, Truelsen T, *et al.* Passive smoking as well as active smoking increases the risk of acute stroke. *Tob Control* 1999; 8(2): 156-60.

97. Haemorrhagic stroke, overall stroke risk, and combined oral contraceptives: results of an international, multicentre, case-control study. WHO Collaborative Study of Cardiovascular Disease and Steroid Hormone Contraception. *Lancet* 1996; 348(9026): 505-10.

98. Ischaemic stroke and combined oral contraceptives: results of an international, multicentre, case-control study. WHO Collaborative Study of Cardiovascular Disease and Steroid Hormone Contraception. *Lancet* 1996; 348(9026): 498-505.

99. Robbins AS, Manson JE, Lee IM, *et al.* Cigarette smoking and stroke in a cohort of U.S. male physicians. *Ann Intern Med* 1994; 120(6): 458-62.

100. Fagerstrom K. The epidemiology of smoking: health consequences and benefits of cessation. *Drugs* 2002; 62 Suppl 2: 1-9.

101. Kawachi I, Colditz GA, Stampfer MJ, *et al.* Smoking cessation and decreased risk of stroke in women. *JAMA* 1993; 269(2): 232-6.

102. Wolf PA, D'Agostino RB, Kannel WB, *et al.* Cigarette smoking as a risk factor for stroke. The Framingham Study. *JAMA* 1988; 259(7): 1025-9.

103. Wannamethee SG, Shaper AG, Whincup PH, *et al.* Smoking cessation and the risk of stroke in middle-aged men. *JAMA* 1995; 274(2): 155-60.

104. Fiore MC. Treating tobacco use and dependence: an introduction to the US Public Health Service Clinical Practice Guideline. *Respir Care* 2000; 45(10): 1196-9.

105. Furie KL, Kasner SE, Adams RJ, *et al.* Guidelines for the Prevention of Stroke in Patients With Stroke or Transient Ischemic Attack. A Guideline for Healthcare Professionals From the American Heart Association/American Stroke Association. *Stroke* 2011; 42(1): 227-76.

106. Mazzaglia G, Britton AR, Altmann DR, *et al.* Exploring the relationship between alcohol consumption and non-fatal or fatal stroke: a systematic review. *Addiction* 2001; 96(12): 1743-56.

107. Sacco RL, Shi T, Zamanillo MC, *et al.* Predictors of mortality and recurrence after hospitalized cerebral infarction in an urban community: the Northern Manhattan Stroke Study. *Neurology* 1994; 44(4): 626-34.

108. Reynolds K, Lewis B, Nolen JD, *et al.* Alcohol consumption and risk of stroke: a meta-analysis. *JAMA* 2003; 289(5): 579-88.

109. Mukamal KJ, Conigrave KM, Mittleman MA, *et al.* Roles of drinking pattern and type of alcohol consumed in coronary heart disease in men. *N Engl J Med* 2003; 348(2): 109-18.

110. Truelsen T, Gronbaek M, Schnohr P, *et al.* Intake of beer, wine, and spirits and risk of stroke: the Copenhagen City Heart Study. *Stroke* 1998; 29(12): 2467-72.

111. Greenfield JR, Samaras K, Hayward CS, *et al.* Beneficial postprandial effect of a small amount of alcohol on diabetes and cardiovascular risk factors: modification by insulin resistance. *J Clin Endocrinol Metab* 2005; 90(2): 661-72.

112. Imhof A, Woodward M, Doering A, *et al.* Overall alcohol intake, beer, wine, and systemic markers of inflammation in western Europe: results from three MONICA samples (Augsburg, Glasgow, Lille). *Eur Heart J* 2004; 25(23): 2092-100.

113. Jensen T, Retterstol LJ, Sandset PM, *et al.* A daily glass of red wine induces a prolonged reduction in plasma viscosity: a randomized controlled trial. *Blood Coagul Fibrinolysis* 2006; 17(6): 471-6.

114. Mukamal KJ, Mackey RH, Kuller LH, *et al.* Alcohol consumption and lipoprotein subclasses in older adults. *J Clin Endocrinol Metab* 2007; 92(7): 2559-66.

115. Rimm EB, Williams P, Fosher K, *et al.* Moderate alcohol intake and lower risk of coronary heart disease: meta-analysis of effects on lipids and haemostatic factors. *BMJ* 1999; 319(7224): 1523-8.

116. Estruch R, Sacanella E, Badia E, *et al.* Different effects of red wine and gin consumption on inflammatory biomarkers of atherosclerosis: a prospective randomized crossover trial. Effects of wine on inflammatory markers. *Atherosclerosis* 2004; 175(1): 117-23.

117. Hillbom M, Numminen H, Juvela S. Recent heavy drinking of alcohol and embolic stroke. *Stroke* 1999; 30(11): 2307-12.

118. Gorelick PB, Rodin MB, Langenberg P, *et al.* Weekly alcohol consumption, cigarette smoking, and the risk of ischemic stroke: results of a case-control study at three urban medical centers in Chicago, Illinois. *Neurology* 1989; 39(3): 339-43.

119. Djousse L, Levy D, Benjamin EJ, *et al.* Long-term alcohol consumption and the risk of atrial fibrillation in the Framingham Study. *Am J Cardiol* 2004; 93(6): 710-3.

120. Ding J, Eigenbrodt ML, Mosley TH, Jr., *et al.* Alcohol intake and cerebral abnormalities on magnetic resonance imaging in a community-based population of middle-aged adults: the Atherosclerosis Risk in Communities (ARIC) study. *Stroke* 2004; 35(1): 16-21.

121. Mukamal KJ, Longstreth WT, Jr., Mittleman MA, *et al.* Alcohol consumption and subclinical findings on magnetic resonance imaging of the brain in older adults: the cardiovascular health study. *Stroke* 2001; 32(9): 1939-46.

122. U.S. Preventive Services Task Force. Screening and behavioral counseling interventions in primary care to reduce alcohol misuse: recommendation statement. *Ann Intern Med* 2004; 140(7): 554-6.

123. Kurth T, Gaziano JM, Berger K, *et al.* Body mass index and the risk of stroke in men. *Arch Intern Med* 2002; 162(22): 2557-62.
124. Selmer R, Tverdal A. Body mass index and cardiovascular mortality at different levels of blood pressure: a prospective study of Norwegian men and women. *J Epidemiol Community Health* 1995; 49(3): 265-70.
125. Lindenstrom E, Boysen G, Nyboe J. Lifestyle factors and risk of cerebrovascular disease in women. The Copenhagen City Heart Study. *Stroke* 1993; 24(10): 1468-72.
126. DiPietro L, Ostfeld AM, Rosner GL. Adiposity and stroke among older adults of low socioeconomic status: the Chicago Stroke Study. *Am J Public Health* 1994; 84(1): 14-9.
127. Suk SH, Sacco RL, Boden-Albala B, *et al.* Abdominal obesity and risk of ischemic stroke: the Northern Manhattan Stroke Study. *Stroke* 2003; 34(7): 1586-92.
128. Dey DK, Rothenberg E, Sundh V, *et al.* Waist circumference, body mass index, and risk for stroke in older people: a 15-year longitudinal population study of 70-year-olds. *J Am Geriatr Soc* 2002; 50(9): 1510-8.
129. Singh RB, Dubnov G, Niaz MA, *et al.* Effect of an Indo-Mediterranean diet on progression of coronary artery disease in high risk patients (Indo-Mediterranean Diet Heart Study): a randomised single-blind trial. *Lancet* 2002; 360(9344): 1455-61.
130. Thompson PD, Buchner D, Pina IL, *et al.* Exercise and physical activity in the prevention and treatment of atherosclerotic cardiovascular disease: a statement from the Council on Clinical Cardiology (Subcommittee on Exercise, Rehabilitation, and Prevention) and the Council on Nutrition, Physical Activity, and Metabolism (Subcommittee on Physical Activity). *Circulation* 2003; 107(24): 3109-16.
131. Kokkinos PF, Narayan P, Colleran JA, *et al.* Effects of regular exercise on blood pressure and left ventricular hypertrophy in African-American men with severe hypertension. *N Engl J Med* 1995; 333(22): 1462-7.
132. Endres M, Gertz K, Lindauer U, *et al.* Mechanisms of stroke protection by physical activity. *Ann Neurol* 2003; 54(5): 582-90.
133. Koenig W, Sund M, Doring A, *et al.* Leisure-time physical activity but not work-related physical activity is associated with decreased plasma viscosity. Results from a large population sample. *Circulation* 1997; 95(2): 335-41.
134. Rauramaa R, Salonen JT, Seppanen K, *et al.* Inhibition of platelet aggregability by moderate-intensity physical exercise: a randomized clinical trial in overweight men. *Circulation* 1986; 74(5): 939-44.
135. Kohrt WM, Kirwan JP, Staten MA, *et al.* Insulin resistance in aging is related to abdominal obesity. *Diabetes* 1993; 42(2): 273-81.
136. Dylewicz P, Przywarska I, Szczesniak L, *et al.* The influence of short-term endurance training on the insulin blood level, binding, and degradation of 125I-insulin by erythrocyte receptors in patients after myocardial infarction. *J Cardiopulm Rehabil* 1999; 19(2): 98-105.
137. Lee CD, Folsom AR, Blair SN. Physical activity and stroke risk: a meta-analysis. *Stroke* 2003; 34(10): 2475-81.
138. Fossum E, Gleim GW, Kjeldsen SE, *et al.* The effect of baseline physical activity on cardiovascular outcomes and new-onset diabetes in patients treated for hypertension and left ventricular hypertrophy: the LIFE study. *J Intern Med* 2007; 262(4): 439-48.
139. Sacco RL, Gan R, Boden-Albala B, *et al.* Leisure-time physical activity and ischemic stroke risk: the Northern Manhattan Stroke Study. *Stroke* 1998; 29(2): 380-7.
140. Grundy SM, Cleeman JI, Merz CN, *et al.* Implications of recent clinical trials for the National Cholesterol Education Program Adult Treatment Panel III guidelines. *Circulation* 2004; 110(2): 227-39.

Chapter 3

Antithrombotic therapies in stroke prevention

James F. Meschia MD, Professor of Neurology
and Chair of the Cerebrovascular Division
Mayo Clinic, Jacksonville, Florida, USA

Introduction

Ischemic stroke constitutes about 85% of all strokes. In addition to controlling risk factors such as hypertension and hyperlipidemia, the use of antithrombotic agents is the standard of care in preventing recurrent stroke in patients with ischemic stroke. Aspirin has been used for this purpose for decades. Other antithrombotic agents like clopidogrel have been tested for stroke prevention alone or in combination with aspirin. This chapter summarizes the evidence for various approaches to antithrombotic therapy in general and for specific clinical situations like preventing stroke at the time of placement of a carotid stent.

Aspirin

No antithrombotic agent has been systematically studied more than aspirin. That aspirin prevents death, myocardial infarction, and stroke is incontrovertible. Overall, aspirin reduces the risk of cardiovascular events by about 25% [1] **(Ia/A)**. Aspirin is ubiquitous and inexpensive. Also adding to the appeal of the drug is that aspirin has a broad therapeutic index. Direct comparison trials have failed to establish the superiority of one dose of aspirin over another. The Dutch TIA trial showed no difference in efficacy in stroke prevention between 30 and 283mg/d [2]. The UK-TIA trial showed no significant difference in efficacy in stroke prevention between 300 and 1200mg/day [3]. Overall, aspirin appears to be effective in preventing vascular events at any dose above 30mg/day [4] **(Ia/A)**. As demonstrated by the UK-TIA trial, though the efficacy of low- and high-dose aspirin appears to be comparable, gastrointestinal side effects are more frequent with high-dose aspirin.

Preventing early recurrent stroke is an important goal following an acute ischemic stroke. Patients are at relatively high risk of recurrence shortly after an acute ischemic stroke. Patients can ill-afford recurrent stroke as recurrent stroke has devastating consequences regarding cognitive impairment [5] and mortality [6]. Mega-trials like the International Stroke Trial (IST) [7] and the Chinese Acute Stroke Trial (CAST) [8] have shown that aspirin is both safe and effective when administered in the acute post-stroke period. A meta-analysis of antiplatelet trials for acute ischemic stroke showed that for every 1000 patients treated with aspirin given at a dose of 160mg daily and initiated within 48 hours of stroke, 13 patients would avoid death or dependency [9] **(Ia/A)**.

While it is generally recommended that aspirin be given within 48 hours after stroke to begin the process of early secondary stroke prevention, there is one notable exception: patients who have received thrombolytic therapy. Acute ischemic stroke treatment trials like the Multicenter Acute Stroke Trial – Italy (MAST-I) have shown an interaction between thrombolysis and aspirin use with regard to symptomatic intracranial hemorrhage [10]. The NINDS rt-PA trial protocol forbade the use of concomitant antiplatelet or anticoagulant therapy for the first 24 hours after randomization [11]. Largely because of the design of the NINDS rt-PA trial, current evidence-based guidelines pertaining to acute stroke treatment with intravenous thrombolytic agents recommend against the co-administration of aspirin or other antiplatelet agent for the first 24 hours **(IV/C)**.

Aspirin non-responsiveness

First-time and recurrent vascular events can occur at standard clinical doses of aspirin. It is unrealistic to expect any antithrombotic agent to completely prevent thrombotic or thromboembolic clinical events. However, because clinical events can occur despite consistent use of therapeutic doses of aspirin, this has led to the concept of aspirin resistance or, perhaps more appropriately, aspirin non-responsiveness. Potential explanations for clinical non-responsiveness include a too low dose of aspirin for the given patient, non-compliance with prescribed therapy, poor absorption of aspirin, or an underlying genetic predisposition to aspirin ineffectiveness. The diverse array of platelet function assays in clinical use includes whole blood platelet function tests, bleeding time, and light transmission aggregometry. Recent meta-analyses suggest that diverse assays of platelet function that are commercially available can differentiate aspirin responders from non-responders in a clinically meaningful way. A meta-analysis of 20 studies totaling 2930 patients with cardiovascular disease assessed the clinical implications of aspirin non-responsiveness across diverse platelet functional assays [12]. Studies included patients with acute coronary syndrome, cerebrovascular disease, post-coronary artery bypass grafting, and percutaneous coronary intervention. Doses of aspirin ranged from 81-1500mg daily. An average of 28% of participants was considered aspirin-resistant. A total of 39% of aspirin-resistant patients compared with 16% of aspirin-sensitive patients had a cardiovascular event (odds ratio [OR] 3.85; 95% CI, 3.08-4.80; p<0.001). The odds ratio for death was 5.99 (95% CI, 2.28-15.72; p<0.003). No dose-response relationship was found between aspirin resistance and cardiovascular outcome. Concomitant therapy with clopidogrel or an inhibitor of platelet glycoprotein IIb-IIIa provided no benefit to patients identified as aspirin-resistant. The study raises several important points. First, it appears that diverse platelet function assays are detecting a biologically and clinically meaningful phenomenon, though the relative merits of the individual platelet function assays are not well known. Secondly, varying the dose of aspirin over typical clinical ranges does not appear to negate the adverse consequences of aspirin non-responsiveness. Finally, simply adding clopidogrel to aspirin may not solve the problem of aspirin non-responsiveness. A smaller meta-analysis of aspirin resistance reached the same conclusion regarding the elevated risk and cardiovascular events associated with resistance [13].

Triflusal

Triflusal is chemically related to acetylsalicylic acid (aspirin). It inhibits cyclo-oxygenase 1 (prostaglandin G/H synthase 1; PTGS1). It appears to have no significant effect on arachidonic acid metabolism in endothelial cells [14]. A meta-analysis that included four trials of patients with stroke or TIA found triflusal to be equivalent to aspirin in terms of preventing serious vascular events (OR 1.02; 95% CI, 0.83-1.26), but triflusal was significantly safer in terms of causing any major hemorrhage (OR 2.42; 95% CI, 1.56-3.77) [15]. The 2008 European Stroke Organization Stroke guidelines consider triflusal an acceptable first-line antiplatelet therapy for stroke prevention **(I/A)**.

Cilostazol

Cilostazol is an antiplatelet therapy that inhibits phosphodiesterase III. A meta-analysis of 12 double-blind, placebo-controlled trials included two trials in patients with cerebrovascular events (n=1187) [16]. The quality of all the trials was judged to be high (Jadad scale = 5). The analysis was done on group rather than individual data. Serious bleeding and cardiac events were not significantly different between cilostazol and placebo. However, there was a 42% risk reduction in cerebrovascular events (p<0.001). The results of CSPS II have been presented in abstract form [17]. CSPS was a randomized, double-blind trial comparing cilostazol to aspirin. The primary endpoint was the composite of cerebral infarction, cerebral hemorrhage, and subarachnoid hemorrhage. Every patient had a history of prior cerebral infarction. The hazard ratio in favor of cilostazol was 0.743 (95% CI, 0.564-0.981). This suggests that cilostazol is superior to aspirin when weighing both risks and benefits.

Thienopyridines

Ticlopidine and clopidogrel are both thienopyridines that have been tested as to their ability to prevent recurrent stroke and other vascular events in patients who have had previous stroke or TIA. In a meta-analysis that involved ten trials and 26,865 high vascular risk patients, a thienopyridine produced a modest but significant reduction in the odds of serious vascular events (11.6% vs. 12.5%), corresponding to avoidance of ten serious vascular events per thousand patients treated for approximately 2 years [18] (Ia/A). Thienopyridines significantly reduced gastrointestinal adverse effects relative to aspirin. However, this advantage was offset by an increased risk in skin rash and diarrhea and, in the case of ticlopidine, neutropenia. The risk of neutropenia from ticlopidine and the mandated monitoring of complete blood counts when initiating ticlopidine have made the drug an unpopular choice of therapy from the perspective of both the patient and prescribing clinician. Ticlopidine has largely been supplanted by clopidogrel.

Recent pharmacogenomic studies have shown that functional variants in the cytochrome P450 (CYP) genes can alter the effectiveness of clopidogrel. In a study of healthy subjects who were treated with clopidogrel, carriers of at least one CYP2C19 reduced-function allele had a relative reduction of about one third in plasma exposure to the active metabolite of clopidogrel as compared with non-carriers [19]. The reduced-function allele was present in approximately 30% of the study population. Among clopidogrel-treated subjects in the TRITON-TIMI 38 study, carriers had a relative increase of 53% in the composite primary efficacy outcome of risk of death from cardiovascular causes, myocardial infarction, or stroke, as compared with non-carriers (12.1% vs. 8.0%; p=0.01). The risk of in-stent thrombosis was increased by a factor of 3 (p=0.02). Simply increasing the maintenance dose of clopidogrel above the standard 75mg/d dose may not be effective in every patient [20]. The new thienopyridine, prasugrel, has less dependence on CYP2C19 oxidation than clopidogrel. While prasugrel potentially may be a therapeutic alternative for patients who are resistant to clopidogrel, it is presently indicated only for the reduction of thrombotic cardiovascular events, including stent thrombosis, in patients with acute coronary syndrome. There is no reliable information regarding its safety or efficacy in secondary prevention of stroke.

Vitamin K antagonists

Warfarin

In patients with recent ischemic stroke or TIA, warfarin reduces the risk of recurrent stroke or systemic embolism by about 61% compared to placebo in patients with atrial fibrillation [21] (Ia/A). The risk of stroke needs to outweigh the risk of warfarin-related serious hemorrhage. If there are no contraindications to anticoagulation, patients should be offered therapy if they have congestive heart failure, hypertension, age >75 years, diabetes, prior stroke, or TIA (i.e. a CHADS2 score >0) [22].

Direct thrombin inhibitors

Examples of direct thrombin inhibitors include ximelagatran and dabigatran. Hepatotoxicity of ximelagatran makes it unsuitable as a replacement for warfarin for preventing stroke in patients with atrial fibrillation [23]. The RE-LY trial randomly compared warfarin (INR target of 2.0 to 3.0) to dabigatran at doses of either 110mg or 150mg [24]. The dabigatran treatment regimen at a dose of 150mg proved superior to warfarin. Results are not generalizable to patients with liver disease or renal failure (<30ml/min).

Combination antiplatelet therapy

Aspirin and dipyridamole

Combination antiplatelet therapy has also been assessed in various randomized clinical trials in the stroke/TIA population. A meta-analysis involving research completed through 2006 compared aspirin to the combination of aspirin and dipyridamole in either the immediate- or extended-release form [25]. The meta-analysis was limited to a patient population with previous non-cardioembolic stroke or TIA. Six randomized controlled trials met inclusion criteria with a total of 7648 patients. The study found a significant reduction in relative risk of non-fatal ischemic and hemorrhagic stroke for dipyridamole with aspirin compared to aspirin alone (RR 0.77; 95% CI, 0.67-0.8). There was also significant reduction in the overall risk of stroke, myocardial infarction and all vascular death (RR 0.85; 95% CI, 0.76-0.94) **(Ia/A)**. Although a significant difference between aspirin alone and aspirin plus immediate-release dipyridamole was not observed, this may well have been related to the reduction in statistical power for summarized trial data with immediate-release as compared to extended-release preparations.

Independent meta-analysis of dipyridamole plus aspirin versus aspirin alone for secondary prevention after a transient ischemic attack or stroke also concluded that the combination of the two antiplatelet agents was slightly superior to aspirin alone for the prevention of stroke and other vascular events [26]. Subgroup analyses showed consistent results with the overall analysis for subgroups defined by age, sex, qualifying event (TIA or stroke), hypertension, diabetes, immediate-release vs. extended-release dipyridamole, or large- vs. small-vessel stroke. Investigators also explored the effects of baseline risk. They used two risk models, one of which had been developed in the Dutch TIA Trial [27]. The meta-analysis did not find relative efficacy for prevention of vascular events to be related to estimated baseline risk. However, the risk models did not have strong discriminatory abilities, with values for the areas under the receiver operating curves of 0.59 and 0.62.

Aspirin and clopidogrel

The Management of Atherothrombosis with Clopidogrel and High-risk patients (MATCH) trial was a randomized, double-blind, placebo-controlled trial comparing aspirin at 75mg per day with placebo in 7599 high-risk patients with recent stroke or TIA and at least one additional vascular risk factor, who were already receiving clopidogrel at 75mg daily [28]. Only 13 patients were enrolled within 24 hours of onset of symptoms. Patients were followed for

18 months. The primary endpoint was the composite of ischemic stroke, myocardial infarction, vascular death, or re-hospitalization for acute ischemia. A total of 15% of patients on combination therapy reached an endpoint compared to 16.7% for the clopidogrel-only group. This resulted in a non-significant relative risk reduction of 6.4%, and an absolute risk reduction of 1%. The risk of life-threatening bleeding nearly doubled from 1.3% in the group receiving clopidogrel alone compared to 2.6% in the group receiving the combination of aspirin and clopidogrel (Ib/A).

The Clopidogrel for High Atherothrombotic Risk and Ischemic Stabilization, Management and Avoidance (CHARISMA) trial was a randomized, double-blind, placebo-controlled trial of clopidogrel at 75mg per day plus low-dose aspirin at 75-162mg per day versus placebo plus low-dose aspirin performed in 15,603 individuals followed for a median of 28 months [29]. The primary endpoint in the study was the composite of myocardial infarction, stroke, or death from cardiovascular causes. The rate of the primary efficacy endpoint was 6.8% with combination therapy and 7.3% with aspirin alone. This resulted in a non-significant relative risk of 0.93. The rate of the primary endpoint among patients with multiple risk factors was 6.6% with combination therapy and 5.5% with aspirin alone, resulting in a non-significant relative risk reduction of 1.2 (Ib/A). The rate of death from cardiovascular causes was higher with combination therapy (3.9% vs. 2.2%; p=0.01). In the subgroup of patients with clinically evident atherothrombosis, the rate was 6.9% with combination therapy and 7.9% with aspirin alone, corresponding to a relative risk of 0.88 (p=0.046).

The Prevention Regimen for Effectively Avoiding Secondary Strokes (PRoFESS) was a 2 x 2 factorial, double-blind trial of low-dose aspirin at 25mg combined with extended-release dipyridamole (ERDP) at 200mg given twice daily versus clopidogrel at 75mg daily, and of telmisartan at 80mg once daily versus placebo in patients with recent ischemic stroke [30]. Patients were included if they had a recent ischemic stroke within 120 days before randomization and were over the age of 50 years. The primary outcome was recurrent stroke of any cause. The secondary outcome was a composite of stroke, myocardial infarction, or death for vascular causes. Primary and secondary outcomes and episodes of major bleeding were adjudicated by central committee. A total of 20,333 patients were enrolled from 695 centers and 35 countries. The mean age of participants was 66.1 years. Approximately one third of patients were women. The mean time from qualifying stroke to randomization was 15 days. There was a greater level of compliance in the clopidogrel group. When defining compliance as taking medication more than 75% of the time, 76.8% of the clopidogrel group was compliant versus 69.6% of the aspirin-ERDP group. Permanent discontinuation of study medication due to headache was more frequent among patients in the aspirin-ERDP group than the clopidogrel group (5.9% vs. 0.9%). This higher rate of discontinuation because of headache observed in the aspirin-ERDP group occurred despite counseling of patients and providing them with the option of adjusting the dose of medication over several days. Acetaminophen is not an effective way of preventing the headache associated with initiation of aspirin-ERDP [31].

The primary outcome of recurrent stroke occurred in 9% (916/10,181) of the aspirin-ERDP group and 8.8% (898/10,151) of the clopidogrel group, resulting in a hazard ratio for aspirin-ERDP of 1.01 (0.92-1.11) **(Ib/A)**. The composite secondary outcome occurred in 13.1% of each group. With regard to safety, intracranial hemorrhage occurred in 1.4% (147/10,181) of the aspirin-ERDP group versus 1% (103/10,151) of the clopidogrel group, resulting in a hazard ratio for aspirin-ERDP of 1.42 (1.11-1.83). Trial investigators concluded that there was no evidence that either of the two treatments were superior to the other for the prevention of recurrent stroke.

A subgroup analysis of PRoFESS was performed to assess the effect of combined aspirin and extended-release dipyridamole versus clopidogrel on functional outcomes and recurrence in acute mild ischemic stroke [32]. Of the 10,181 individuals randomized to aspirin and ERDP, 672 were randomized within 72 hours of onset of stroke. Of the 10,151 individuals who were randomized to clopidogrel, 688 were randomized within 72 hours of onset of stroke. The mean NIH Stroke Scale score was 2.9 points for the aspirin-ERDP group and 3.1 points for the clopidogrel group in this subgroup analysis. The mildness of the strokes included in this analysis likely resulted from the inclusion criterion that patients needed to have a baseline modified Rankin Scale of 3 or less. Combined death or dependency based on a modified Rankin Scale at 30 days did not differ between treatment groups. The rates of death, major bleeding, and serious adverse events did not differ between treatment groups.

In a separate substudy of PRoFESS, investigators looked for differences between treatment groups in post-stroke disability at 3 months in patients with recurrent stroke [33]. Modified Rankin scores did not differ significantly between patients with recurrent stroke who were treated with aspirin and ERDP versus clopidogrel. Also, there was no significant difference in the median Mini-Mental State Exam (MMSE) scores, the percentage of patients with an MMSE score of 24 points or less, or the percentage of patients with a drop in MMSE of 3 points or more between the 1-month visit and the penultimate visit. The fact that recurrent stroke did not yield different functional outcomes for the different treatment groups may reflect that the strokes (hemorrhagic and ischemic) may have been comparable in size, severity and location for the two groups.

Neither MATCH nor CHARISMA focused on acute secondary prevention. However, both of the trials showed in subgroup analyses that treatment effects tended to be greatest for those individuals treated most acutely after onset of stroke symptoms [34]. The Fast Assessment of Stroke and Transient ischemic attack to prevent Early Recurrence (FASTER) trial was a pilot randomized, double-blind trial that compared clopidogrel (300mg loading dose followed by 75mg/d) and aspirin (81mg/d) versus placebo and aspirin (81mg/d) [35]. Patients were required to have an NIHSS score of 3 or less at the time of randomization. Randomization occurred within 24 hours of onset of symptoms. A total of 392 patients were enrolled. The trial was stopped early because of failure to recruit patients at the pre-specified minimum. A total of 7.1% of patients in the clopidogrel group had a stroke within 90 days compared with 10.8% in the placebo group (p=0.19).

There have been two multicenter randomized surrogate-endpoint trials of combination aspirin and clopidogrel versus aspirin alone for the prevention of ultrasound-detected microembolic signals (MES). The Clopidogrel and Aspirin for Reduction of Emboli in Symptomatic carotid Stenosis (CARESS) trial screened 230 patients with symptomatic carotid arterial stenosis greater than 50% using transcranial Doppler [36]. A total of 110 patients (47.8%) had detectable MES during the initial screening. Of these, 107 were randomized to receive either a combination of clopidogrel and aspirin or aspirin alone. On day 7 post-randomization, 43.8% of dual-therapy patients were MES-positive compared with 72.7% of monotherapy patients (relative risk reduction 39.8%; p=0.0046). MES frequency was greater in the 17 patients with recurrent ipsilateral cerebrovascular events compared with the 90 patients who did not have events (p=0.0003).

The CLAIR trial was an open-label, blinded-endpoint trial of aspirin at 75-160mg daily with or without clopidogrel at a 300mg load followed by 75mg/day in patients with symptomatic cerebral or carotid stenosis [37]. A total of 100 patients were randomized. Unlike CARESS, which focused on cervical carotid stenosis, nearly all of the participants in CLAIR had symptomatic intracranial stenosis. There was a 42% relative risk reduction in the detection of at least one microembolic signal at day 2 for the combined therapy (p=0.025). The study was not powered to detect differences in clinically relevant endpoints like stroke or cerebral hemorrhage.

Peri-operative antiplatelet therapy for carotid endarterectomy

Aspirin versus endarterectomy

Antiplatelet therapy plays a crucial role in the peri-operative medical management of patients undergoing carotid endarterectomy. A small randomized trial of aspirin versus endarterectomy was performed across the Mayo Clinic hospital system [38]. It soon became apparent that it was not safe to withhold aspirin from this patient population. Patients in the surgical group were discouraged from taking aspirin unless there were other indications for its use. In accordance with the recommendations of the Data and Safety Monitoring Committee, the study was stopped early because of safety concerns in the surgical arm. Myocardial infarction, a secondary endpoint, was significantly more frequent in the surgical arm. Only 35 patients were randomized to the aspirin group, and only 36 patients were randomized to the surgical treatment group. Timing of the myocardial infarctions did not support the concept of rebound hypercoagulability. Subsequent phase III randomized clinical trials of endarterectomy for asymptomatic stenosis included systematic use of aspirin or other antiplatelet agents in both the medical and surgical groups.

Peri-operative aspirin versus placebo

A study conducted in Lund, Sweden, randomized 232 patients undergoing carotid endarterectomy to either low-dose aspirin at 75mg/d or placebo [39]. Treatment started on the evening of surgery and then daily thereafter for the next 6 months. Patients were followed for 1 year. Peri-operative and postoperative stroke with symptoms lasting more than 1 week were significantly lower in the aspirin group **(Ib/A)**. Importantly, intra-operative bleeding did not differ between groups. It is of interest to note that among the patients treated with aspirin, the surgeons could do no better than chance in terms of guessing whether or not the patients were receiving aspirin. This study helped show that choosing between aspirin and endarterectomy is really a false choice as patients who undergo surgery can safely receive aspirin as well.

Peri-operative low- versus high-dose aspirin

A retrospective analysis of the NASCET trial suggested that patients did better with higher doses of aspirin peri-operatively. This led to the ASA and Carotid Endarterectomy (ACE) trial. ACE was an international randomized, double-blind, controlled trial assessing four different doses of aspirin: 81, 325, 650 and 1300mg [40]. It was considered unethical to have a placebo group. Patients were to initiate the medication before surgery and then daily for 3 months. The combined rate of stroke, myocardial infarction and death was lower in the low-dose groups (81 and 325mg/d) versus the high-dose groups (650 and 1300mg/d) at 30 days (5.4% vs. 7.0%; p=0.07). The combined rate of stroke, myocardial infarction and death was lower in the low-dose groups versus the high-dose groups at 3 months (6.2% vs. 8.4%; p=0.03). There was a trend toward more hemorrhagic strokes in the high-dose group.

Peri-operative aspirin versus aspirin and clopidogrel

Attempts at further inhibition of platelet aggregation as a means of preventing postoperative stroke have included trials of combination therapy. No phase III trials of combination therapy have been completed as yet. A pilot randomized, double-blind trial of the combination of aspirin and clopidogrel versus aspirin alone was completed in 100 individuals undergoing carotid endarterectomy using surrogate endpoints [41]. Every patient received 150mg/d of aspirin for 4 weeks before surgery. Patients were randomized to either placebo or clopidogrel 75mg 12 hours before surgery. Continuous transcranial Doppler (TCD) monitoring of blood flow velocity in the middle cerebral artery was performed for the duration of the surgery and for 3 hours afterward. The trial found a significant ten-fold reduction in risk of having >20 transcranial Doppler-detected MES postoperatively. Peri-operative morbidity and mortality were unaffected by the addition of clopidogrel. However, the addition of clopidogrel significantly prolonged surgical closure times. For closure times of 40 minutes or longer, the percentage of patients requiring additional closure time was 30% in the combination group versus only 8% in the placebo group (p=0.004).

Peri-operative antiplatelet therapy for carotid artery stenting

Clopidogrel was tested against heparin in the peri-stenting period in a randomized clinical trial of 120 patients. Prior to the procedure, all patients were taking aspirin at 75mg/day. Patients in the clopidogrel group were given a loading dose of 300mg 6-12 hours before the procedure followed by 75mg 2 hours prior to the procedure. Patients were then given 75mg/day for the next 28 days following stent placement. The neurological complication rate was 25% for the heparin group and 0% for the clopidogrel group (p=0.02) [42] **(Ib/A)**. Aspirin/clopidogrel combination therapy was also standard medical therapy for stented patients in the CREST trial [43].

The glycoprotein IIb/IIIa antagonist, abciximab, has been tested in small pilot studies of carotid stenting. A randomized trial of 74 patients who underwent elective carotid stenting tested an abciximab bolus dose of 0.25mg/kg and found a periprocedural ischemic event rate of 19% in the active treatment group versus 8% in the control group [44]. All patients received standard therapy that consisted of aspirin, clopidogrel and heparin. The study was too small to draw firm conclusions on the use of abciximab in this setting.

Antiplatelet therapy for atrial fibrillation

Antiplatelet therapy has not proven superior to warfarin for preventing cardioembolism in patients with atrial fibrillation who have at least a moderate risk of embolization. Compared to aspirin, warfarin reduces the risk of stroke by about 45% [45]. Recently, combination therapy with aspirin and clopidogrel has been tested in the atrial fibrillation population. The ACTIVE-W trial randomized patients with atrial fibrillation and at least one additional risk factor for stroke to aspirin and clopidogrel or warfarin to a target International Normalized Ratio (INR) of 2-3 [46]. A total of 6706 patients were randomized. The composite of stroke, non-CNS embolus, myocardial infarction, and vascular death occurred at a rate of 5.6% per year for the combination antiplatelet group and 3.93% per year for the warfarin group (p=0.0003), demonstrating the clear superior efficacy of adjusted-dose warfarin in this population. However, not every patient with atrial fibrillation is a good candidate for warfarin therapy due to reasons such as risk of falling, bleeding or non-compliance. For this patient population deemed warfarin ineligible, there was a trial that assessed the effects of adding clopidogrel to aspirin. In the ACTIVE trial, 7554 patients were randomized to clopidogrel (75mg/d) or placebo in addition to aspirin [47]. Patients were followed for a median of 3.6 years. Major vascular events occurred at a rate of 6.8% per year for the combination antiplatelet therapy group as opposed to 7.6% per year for the group on aspirin alone (p=0.01). However, the benefits in favor of combination therapy were offset by the risk of major bleeding, which occurred at a rate of 2% per year with combination therapy and 1.3% per year for aspirin monotherapy (p <0.001).

Antiplatelet therapy for symptomatic intracranial stenosis

There has been only one major randomized, multicenter clinical trial to assess the relative efficacy of warfarin versus aspirin for prevention of stroke in patients with symptomatic intracranial disease [48]. The Warfarin-Aspirin Symptomatic Intracranial Disease (WASID) trial enrolled patients at 59 sites across North America. Inclusion criteria included transient ischemic attack or non-disabling stroke within 90 days before randomization. Patients were required to have angiographically confirmed stenosis of 50-99% in a major intracranial large artery, and they needed to be at least 40 years of age. A double-dummy design was used to maintain the treatment blind. Warfarin was adjusted to a target INR of 2-3. High-dose aspirin was used (650mg twice daily). The primary endpoint was the composite of ischemic stroke, brain hemorrhage, or death from vascular causes other than stroke. Patients were followed for an average of 1.8 years. There was no efficacy separation. The primary endpoint occurred in 22.1% of patients in the aspirin group compared to 21.8% of patients of the warfarin group (p=ns). However, complications were more frequent in the warfarin group. Major hemorrhage occurred in 8.3% of patients in the warfarin group compared to 3.2% of patients in the aspirin group (p=0.01) **(Ib/A)**. Myocardial infarction or sudden death occurred in 7.3% of patients in the warfarin group compared to 2.9% of patients in the aspirin group (p=0.02). Death occurred in 9.7% of patients in the warfarin group compared to 4.3% of patients in the aspirin group. INRs <2 were associated with higher risk of ischemic stroke (p <0.001). INRs >3 were associated with higher risk of major hemorrhage (p <0.001). Based on WASID, there is little rationale for opting for warfarin over high-dose aspirin for this patient population in patients with no contraindication to aspirin.

Conclusions

All of the following have been shown to reduce the risk of stroke:

- aspirin at doses from 30mg/d to 650mg BID;
- clopidogrel at 75mg/day;
- aspirin 25mg and extended-release dipyridamole 200mg one tab BID;
- triflusal at 600mg/day.

Regarding combination aspirin and clopidogrel:

- the risk of hemorrhage outweighs the benefits of thromboprophylaxis for most patients;
- a short course of combination therapy is indicated for patients undergoing carotid stenting.

Key points	Evidence level
◆ Aspirin, combination aspirin and extended-release dipyridamole, triflusal and clopidogrel are all acceptable for preventing stroke in patients with non-cardioembolic stroke or TIA.	Ia/A
◆ Aspirin from doses of 30mg/d to 650mg twice daily are comparably effective in preventing stroke.	Ia/A
◆ The combination of aspirin and extended-release dipyridamole is slightly more effective than aspirin alone in preventing recurrent stroke in patients with non-cardioembolic stroke.	Ia/A
◆ Clopidogrel and combination aspirin and extended-release dipyridamole are comparable in preventing stroke, but the latter has a higher risk of hemorrhage.	Ib/A
◆ The combination of aspirin and clopidogrel is not recommended for routine use in stroke prophylaxis due to increased hemorrhage risk.	Ib/A
◆ High-dose aspirin therapy (650mg BID) is recommended over warfarin for preventing stroke in patients with intracranial arterial stenosis.	Ib/A
◆ Limited-duration combination antiplatelet therapy with aspirin and clopidogrel may be effective in preventing stroke in patients who are about to undergo carotid arterial stenting.	Ib/A
◆ Aspirin and other antiplatelet agents should be avoided in the first 24 hours after administering IV rt-PA for acute ischemic stroke.	IV/C
◆ For patients with acute ischemic stroke who are not candidates for IV rt-PA, aspirin should be given within 48 hours of onset of symptoms.	Ia/A
◆ Gene testing for variants in the CYP2C19 gene should be considered for patients who have a stroke or TIA while taking clopidogrel and an alternative antiplatelet agent should be used by individuals found to be genetically resistant.	IV/C

References

1. Antiplatelet Trialists' Collaboration. Collaborative overview of randomised trials of antiplatelet therapy - I: prevention of death, myocardial infarction, and stroke by prolonged antiplatelet therapy in various categories of patients. *BMJ* 1994; 308: 81-106.

2. A comparison of two doses of aspirin (30mg vs. 283mg a day) in patients after a transient ischemic attack or minor ischemic stroke. The Dutch TIA Trial Study Group. *N Engl J Med* 1991; 325: 1261-6.

3. Farrell B, Godwin J, Richards S, Warlow C. The United Kingdom Transient Ischaemic Attack (UK-TIA) aspirin trial: final results. *J Neurol Neurosurg Psychiatry* 1991; 54: 1044-54.

4. Algra A, van Gijn J. Aspirin at any dose above 30mg offers only modest protection after cerebral ischaemia. *J Neurol Neurosurg Psychiatry* 1996; 60: 197-9.

5. Pendlebury ST, Rothwell PM. Prevalence, incidence, and factors associated with pre-stroke and post-stroke dementia: a systematic review and meta-analysis. *Lancet Neurol* 2009; 8: 1006-18.

6.   Jorgensen HS, Nakayama H, Reith J, *et al*. Stroke recurrence: predictors, severity, and prognosis. The Copenhagen Stroke Study. *Neurology* 1997; 48: 891-5.

7.   The International Stroke Trial (IST): a randomised trial of aspirin, subcutaneous heparin, both, or neither among 19,435 patients with acute ischaemic stroke. International Stroke Trial Collaborative Group. *Lancet* 1997; 349: 1569-81.

8.   CAST: randomised placebo-controlled trial of early aspirin use in 20,000 patients with acute ischaemic stroke. CAST (Chinese Acute Stroke Trial) Collaborative Group. *Lancet* 1997; 349: 1641-9.

9.   Sandercock PA, Counsell C, Gubitz GJ, Tseng MC. Antiplatelet therapy for acute ischaemic stroke. *Cochrane Database Syst Rev* 2008: CD000029.

10.   Randomised controlled trial of streptokinase, aspirin, and combination of both in treatment of acute ischaemic stroke. Multicentre Acute Stroke Trial - Italy (MAST-I) Group. *Lancet* 1995; 346: 1509-14.

11.   The National Institute of Neurological Disorders and Stroke rt-PA Stroke Study Group. Tissue plasminogen activator for acute ischemic stroke. *N Engl J Med* 1995; 333: 1581-7.

12.   Krasopoulos G, Brister SJ, Beattie WS, Buchanan MR. Aspirin 'resistance' and risk of cardiovascular morbidity: systematic review and meta-analysis. *BMJ* 2008; 336: 195-8.

13.   Snoep JD, Hovens MM, Eikenboom JC, *et al*. Association of laboratory-defined aspirin resistance with a higher risk of recurrent cardiovascular events: a systematic review and meta-analysis. *Arch Intern Med* 2007; 167: 1593-9.

14.   Anninos H, Andrikopoulos G, Pastromas S, *et al*. Triflusal: an old drug in modern antiplatelet therapy. Review of its action, use, safety and effectiveness. *Hellenic Journal of Cardiology* 2009; 50: 199-207.

15.   Hankey G, Costa J, Ferro J, *et al*. Triflusal for preventing serious vascular events in people at high risk. *Stroke* 2006; 37: 2193-5.

16.   Uchiyama S, Demaerschalk BM, Goto S, *et al*. Stroke prevention by cilostazol in patients with atherothrombosis: meta-analysis of placebo-controlled randomized trials. *J Stroke Cerebrovasc Dis* 2009; 18: 482-90.

17.   Shinohara Y, CSPS Group. Cilostazol shows superiority to aspirin for secondary stroke prevention: the results of CSPS II. International Stroke Conference, San Antonio, TX, 2010.

18.   Sudlow CL, Mason G, Maurice JB, *et al*. Thienopyridine derivatives versus aspirin for preventing stroke and other serious vascular events in high vascular risk patients. *Cochrane Database Syst Rev* 2009: CD001246.

19.   Mega JL, Close SL, Wiviott SD, *et al*. Cytochrome p-450 polymorphisms and response to clopidogrel. *N Engl J Med* 2009; 360: 354-62.

20.   Pena A, Collet JP, Hulot JS, *et al*. Can we override clopidogrel resistance? *Circulation* 2009; 119: 2854-7.

21.   Hart RG, Pearce LA, Aguilar MI. Meta-analysis: antithrombotic therapy to prevent stroke in patients who have nonvalvular atrial fibrillation. *Ann Intern Med* 2007; 146: 857-67.

22.   Gage BF, Waterman AD, Shannon W, *et al*. Validation of clinical classification schemes for predicting stroke: results from the National Registry of Atrial Fibrillation. *JAMA* 2001; 285: 2864-70.

23.   Diener HC. Stroke prevention using the oral direct thrombin inhibitor ximelagatran in patients with non-valvular atrial fibrillation. Pooled analysis from the SPORTIF III and V studies. *Cerebrovasc Dis* 2006; 21: 279-93.

24.   Connolly SJ, Ezekowitz MD, Yusuf S, *et al*. Dabigatran versus warfarin in patients with atrial fibrillation. *N Engl J Med* 2009; 361: 1139-51.

25.   Verro P, Gorelick PB, Nguyen D. Aspirin plus dipyridamole versus aspirin for prevention of vascular events after stroke or TIA: a meta-analysis. *Stroke* 2008; 39: 1358-63.

26.   Halkes PH, Gray LJ, Bath PM, *et al*. Dipyridamole plus aspirin versus aspirin alone in secondary prevention after TIA or stroke: a meta-analysis by risk. *J Neurol Neurosurg Psychiatry* 2008; 79: 1218-23.

27.   Predictors of major vascular events in patients with a transient ischemic attack or nondisabling stroke. The Dutch TIA Trial Study Group. *Stroke* 1993; 24: 527-31.

28.   Diener HC, Bogousslavsky J, Brass LM, *et al*. Aspirin and clopidogrel compared with clopidogrel alone after recent ischaemic stroke or transient ischaemic attack in high-risk patients (MATCH): randomised, double-blind, placebo-controlled trial. *Lancet* 2004; 364: 331-7.

29.   Bhatt DL, Fox KA, Hacke W, *et al*. Clopidogrel and aspirin versus aspirin alone for the prevention of atherothrombotic events. *N Engl J Med* 2006; 354: 1706-17.

30.   Sacco RL, Diener HC, Yusuf S, *et al*. Aspirin and extended-release dipyridamole versus clopidogrel for recurrent stroke. *N Engl J Med* 2008; 359: 1238-51.

31. Lipton RB, Bigal ME, Kolodner KB, *et al.* Acetaminophen in the treatment of headaches associated with dipyridamole-aspirin combination. *Neurology* 2004; 63: 1099-101.

32. Bath PM, Cotton D, Martin RH, *et al.* Effect of combined aspirin and extended-release dipyridamole versus clopidogrel on functional outcome and recurrence in acute, mild ischemic stroke: PRoFESS subgroup analysis. *Stroke* 2010; 41: 732-8.

33. Diener HC, Sacco RL, Yusuf S, *et al.* Effects of aspirin plus extended-release dipyridamole versus clopidogrel and telmisartan on disability and cognitive function after recurrent stroke in patients with ischaemic stroke in the Prevention Regimen for Effectively Avoiding Second Strokes (PRoFESS) trial: a double-blind, active and placebo-controlled study. *Lancet Neurol* 2008; 7: 875-84.

34. Johnston S, Lavallée P, Meseguer E, *et al.* Fast Assessment of Stroke and Transient ischaemic attack to prevent Early Recurrence (FASTER): a randomised controlled pilot trial. *Lancet Neurol* 2007; 6: 941-3.

35. Kennedy J, Hill M, Ryckborst K, *et al.* Fast Assessment of Stroke and Transient ischaemic attack to prevent Early Recurrence (FASTER): a randomised controlled pilot trial. *Lancet Neurol* 2007; 6: 961-9.

36. Markus HS, Droste DW, Kaps M, *et al.* Dual antiplatelet therapy with clopidogrel and aspirin in symptomatic carotid stenosis evaluated using Doppler embolic signal detection: the Clopidogrel and Aspirin for Reduction of Emboli in Symptomatic Carotid Stenosis (CARESS) trial. *Circulation* 2005; 111: 2233-40.

37. Wong KS, Chen C, Fu J, *et al.* Clopidogrel plus aspirin versus aspirin alone for reducing embolisation in patients with acute symptomatic cerebral or carotid artery stenosis (CLAIR study): a randomised, open-label, blinded-endpoint trial. *Lancet Neurol* 2010; 9: 489-97.

38. Results of a randomized controlled trial of carotid endarterectomy for asymptomatic carotid stenosis. Mayo Asymptomatic Carotid Endarterectomy Study Group. *Mayo Clin Proc* 1992; 67: 513-8.

39. Lindblad B, Persson NH, Takolander R, Bergqvist D. Does low-dose acetylsalicylic acid prevent stroke after carotid surgery? A double-blind, placebo-controlled randomized trial. *Stroke* 1993; 24: 1125-8.

40. Taylor DW, Barnett HJ, Haynes RB, *et al.* Low-dose and high-dose acetylsalicylic acid for patients undergoing carotid endarterectomy: a randomised controlled trial. ASA and Carotid Endarterectomy (ACE) Trial Collaborators. *Lancet* 1999; 353: 2179-84.

41. Payne DA, Jones CI, Hayes PD, *et al.* Beneficial effects of clopidogrel combined with aspirin in reducing cerebral emboli in patients undergoing carotid endarterectomy. *Circulation* 2004; 109: 1476-81.

42. McKevitt F, Randall M, Cleveland T, *et al.* The benefits of combined anti-platelet treatment in carotid artery stenting. *Eur J Vasc Endovasc Surg* 2005; 29: 522-7.

43. Brott TG, Hobson RW, 2nd, Howard G, *et al.* Stenting versus endarterectomy for treatment of carotid-artery stenosis. *N Engl J Med* 2010; 363: 11-23.

44. Hofmann R, Kerschner K, Steinwender C, *et al.* Abciximab bolus injection does not reduce cerebral ischemic complications of elective carotid artery stenting: a randomized study. *Stroke* 2002; 33: 725.

45. van Walraven C, Hart R, Singer D, *et al.* Oral anticoagulants vs aspirin in nonvalvular atrial fibrillation: an individual patient meta-analysis. *JAMA* 2002; 288: 2441.

46. Site H. Clopidogrel plus aspirin versus oral anticoagulation for atrial fibrillation in the Atrial fibrillation Clopidogrel Trial with Irbesartan for prevention of Vascular Events (ACTIVE W): a randomised controlled trial. *Lancet* 2006; 367: 1903-12.

47. Connolly SJ, Pogue J, Hart RG, *et al.* Effect of clopidogrel added to aspirin in patients with atrial fibrillation. *N Engl J Med* 2009; 360: 2066-78.

48. Chimowitz MI, Lynn MJ, Howlett-Smith H, *et al.* Comparison of warfarin and aspirin for symptomatic intracranial arterial stenosis. *N Engl J Med* 2005; 352: 1305-16.

Chapter 4

Anticoagulant therapy in prevention of ischemic stroke

Harold P. Adams, Jr., MD, Professor of Neurology
Division of Cerebrovascular Diseases
Department of Neurology, Carver College of Medicine
University of Iowa Health Care Stroke Center
University of Iowa, Iowa City, Iowa, USA

Introduction

For more than half a century, anticoagulants have been prescribed with the goal of lowering the risk of ischemic stroke among high-risk patients. Several different medications including heparin, low-molecular-weight (LMW) heparins or heparinoid, or vitamin K antagonists, have been given as an acute intervention or as a long-term therapy to prevent ischemic stroke or recurrent ischemic stroke. Warfarin is the most commonly tested and administered vitamin K antagonist oral anticoagulant. New medications, such as direct thrombin inhibitors, are being developed.

The oral anticoagulants (vitamin K antagonists) lead to depletion of several vitamin K-dependent coagulation factors including proteins C and S and Factors II, VII, IX, and X [1]. While a parenteral formulation of warfarin is available, most patients take the medication orally. There is a lag of several days from the initiation of therapy before the anticoagulant effects are noted. Because levels of proteins C and S are reduced before those of the prothrombotic coagulation factors, a transient hypercoagulable state leading to skin necrosis and the purple toe syndrome are potential complications [2]. The doses of warfarin are adjusted on a regular basis in response to the level of anticoagulation as measured by the International Normalized Ratio (INR). Doses are individualized to patients' responses. Some patients may have genetic mutations including polymorphisms of the P450 gene or vitamin K1 epoxide reductase which may lead to hypersensitivity or resistance to warfarin [3-5]. Concomitant diseases or the use of medications may affect responses to the oral anticoagulants, with either augmentation or lessening of effects being found. The widespread use of the INR, which is based on a mathematical formula adjusting the patient's and control prothrombin times for the reagents used by the laboratory, has greatly eased management of the medication. For most indications, the desired level of INR is 2-3 (1 being no effect). Bleeding is the most frequent and serious complication of the use of oral anticoagulants. Patients with a history of stroke, particularly those with a prior brain hemorrhage, are at highest risk. Other risk factors for bleeding complications include serious comorbid diseases, such as cancer or gastrointestinal disease, advancing age, poor balance or incoordination, a high risk for falls, dementia, alcohol or drug abuse, poor compliance with the treatment regimen, and the non-availability of laboratory monitoring. The antidotes for warfarin include supplemental vitamin K and administration of clotting factors. Because vitamin K is essential for formation of bone matrix, osteopenia and pathological fractures are potential complications. In addition, the risk of birth defects is considerable and as a result, pregnant women are not given oral anticoagulants [6].

Unfractionated heparin and the low-molecular-weight (LMW) heparins are mixtures of glycosaminoglycans that are of biological origin [7]. The LMW heparins are fractionated subunits of traditional heparin and they have more restricted antithrombotic actions. These agents are given intravenously or subcutaneously. When given with a bolus dose, they have immediate antithrombotic effects [8]. Heparin works primarily via antithrombin and heparin co-factor II to inhibit thrombin and activated Factors X and XI. The LMW heparins have more selective actions on Factor X. The medications may be administered in an intravenous infusion using a weight-based nomogram with subsequent adjustments [9, 10]. The level of anticoagulant effects of heparin is measured by the activated partial thromboplastin time (aPTT). The desired level presumably is approximately two times control. Because the aPTT is not affected by the LMW heparins, their activity may be measured by the level of inhibition of Factor Xa activity [11]. Subcutaneous administration of lower doses of heparin (5000 units twice a day) may not require monitoring. The effects of the heparin diminish rapidly after stopping the medication and the duration of action of the LMW heparins is approximately 12 hours. Although they are more expensive, the LMW heparins are easier to use on a long-term basis. Bleeding is the most frequent and serious complication. The anticoagulant effects of heparin may be reversed with protamine sulfate but there is no antidote for the LMW heparins. In addition, heparin is antigenic and heparin-associated thrombocytopenia leading to arterial thrombosis is a potential complication. Though less common than with unfractionated heparin, this complication may occur with the LMW heparin.

Anticoagulants may be prescribed in an acute care situation, such as a recent ischemic stroke or transient ischemic attack (TIA). In this setting, the goals of treatment are:

- halt neurological worsening of the acute stroke by inhibiting the growth of an intravascular thrombus or by helping maintenance of collateral flow; and
- prevent early recurrent stroke by lessening the risk of repeated embolism arising from a thrombus within the heart or a proximal artery.

The ultimate goal of anticoagulant therapy would be to improve neurological outcomes. In addition, anticoagulants are prescribed to seriously ill, bedridden patients with the aim of preventing deep vein thrombosis and secondary pulmonary embolism; important complications that may cause morbidity or mortality after stroke. Parenteral anticoagulants following by long-term administration of oral agents are used to treat most patients with cerebral venous thrombosis.

Anticoagulants also are prescribed on a long-term basis with the goal of preventing thromboembolism. These medications may be used for primary prevention among high-risk persons who have not had any neurological symptoms. They also may be administered to prevent recurrent ischemic stroke. In many cases, anticoagulants are prescribed as an alternative to antiplatelet agents. There are a number of factors that influence decisions about the use of anticoagulants. For example, the presumed vascular territory (carotid circulation vs. vertebrobasilar circulation) may impact on decisions about administering either anticoagulants or antiplatelet agents. The presumed etiology of the neurological symptoms also affects choices about the use of antithrombotic medications; anticoagulants may be given to patients with stroke symptoms secondary to cardioembolism, large artery atherosclerosis, some non-atherosclerotic vasculopathies such as dissection, or prothrombotic disorders. In addition, the selection of antithrombotic therapy may be altered by the patient's responses to previous therapies or decisions about surgical or endovascular interventions. For example, anticoagulants may be prescribed as an alternative to or in combination with antiplatelet medications to those patients who have had recurrent symptoms despite antithrombotic treatment. In some instances, an antiplatelet agent may be prescribed for one indication, such as treatment of coronary artery disease, and the anticoagulant is prescribed for another reason, such as prevention of a cardioembolic event.

Despite their widespread use, the role of anticoagulant medications in the prevention of stroke is the subject of considerable controversy. There are concerns about the safety of these medications among persons at high risk for stroke that are elderly. Anticoagulants are associated with the real risk of serious hemorrhage including intracranial bleeding that cannot be divorced from their potential therapeutic effects. There is uncertainty about the efficacy of these agents in preventing ischemic events in the several situations in which they are prescribed. Because these agents have biological responses that require monitoring, there have been issues about the timing and types of laboratory assessments to maintain an adequate benefit-risk ratio. Because of the problems associated with the use of anticoagulants, alternative medical therapies have been sought. Antiplatelet agents, such as aspirin, are now used in a wide variety of situations that, in the past, were considered as indications for anticoagulation. New medications, such as the direct thrombin inhibitors, are being developed in part because of the perceived deficiencies of the traditional anticoagulants. While this chapter evaluates the utility of anticoagulants in preventing stroke both in an acute situation and on a longer-term basis, it emphasizes the latter because this is the area that has the most robust data supporting the use of these medications.

Early administration of anticoagulants to patients with acute cerebrovascular disease

For many years, parenteral anticoagulants (unfractionated heparin or LMW heparin) were prescribed to patients with a recent TIA or ischemic stroke [12]. Patients with a recent (in the previous 24-48 hours) or crescendo (several events within a few days) TIA may have an indication for emergency administration of anticoagulants, most commonly heparin, based on the assumption that they are at an extremely high risk for ischemic stroke. In a survey of neurologists in North America, Al-Sadat et al [13] reported that 47% of American neurologists believed that a patient with multiple TIAs should be treated with heparin. A French study reported that high doses of heparin were given to 28% of 203 patients with TIA that were admitted to a stroke unit [14]. Despite the widespread use of heparin, there are uncertainties about the level of anticoagulation, the desired dosing, the use of a weight-based regimen, or the use of a bolus dose to initiate treatment [8, 10, 15]. In addition, there are doubts about the safety of emergency administration of heparin for patients with recent TIA. Petty et al [16] reported a complication rate of 0.3/100 patient-days with the use of heparin. Overall, the rate of complications of the interim course of heparin was higher than the rates of complications for the long-term administration of either warfarin or aspirin. Surprisingly, prospective studies testing the efficacy of heparin or LMW heparin in this situation are limited. One small prospective randomized clinical trial tested the utility of an interim course (average of 5.8 days) of heparin or aspirin in preventing stroke among patients with recent (within 7 days) TIA [17]. Recurrent TIA happened in 8 of 27 patients treated with heparin and 7 of 28 patients given aspirin. On the other hand, strokes were diagnosed in 1 patient in the heparin group and 4 patients in the aspirin group **(Ib/A)**.

Given that a TIA is, in fact, an ischemic stroke that has spontaneous clinical resolution, the data looking at the utility of anticoagulants in treating patients with acute ischemic stroke are relevant. Besides preventing early recurrent thromboembolic events, early administration of heparin or another parenteral anticoagulant has been prescribed in an attempt to halt neurological worsening and to improve outcomes after stroke. The utility of heparin was evaluated by clinical studies performed in the 1960s; because these studies were performed before the development of modern brain imaging and may have included patients with primary brain hemorrhage in the studies, they are no longer relevant. In a series of reports published in the mid-1980s, the Cerebral Embolism Study Group described the potential utility of heparin in preventing early recurrent stroke [18-20]. The relatively small studies suggested that heparin might be useful. Subsequently, several clinical trials tested intravenous or subcutaneous administration of heparin or the LMW heparins [21-34] (Tables 1-2). Some included a bolus dose and monitoring of the level of anticoagulation with adjustments in response to the levels. While the trials included randomization in treatment assignment, several did not include blinded assessment of responses. A few trials tested anticoagulants in comparison to placebo and others compared the anticoagulant to aspirin, usually in a dose of 300-325mg/day.

Overall, the trials show that emergency administration of heparin is associated with a modest increase in the risk of serious intracranial or extracranial bleeding (Table 1). The likelihood of bleeding is higher than administration of antiplatelet agents but it is less than with the use of thrombolytic agents. The intracranial bleeding largely involves symptomatic hemorrhagic transformation of the original infarction. The increased risk of bleeding complications is sufficiently small that treatment could be justified if these agents demonstrate evidence of efficacy. Overall, the trials do not demonstrate a benefit in lowering the risk of neurological worsening or improving outcomes. The data on the ability of the anticoagulants

Table 1. Hemorrhagic complications among patients treated with anticoagulants in acute ischemic stroke.

Study	Agent	Intracranial		Extracranial	
Chamorro	Heparin	7/83	8.4%	-	
Camerlingo	Heparin	2/45	4.4%	0/45	0
IST	LD heparin	16/2429	0.7%	10/2429	0.4%
	LD heparin	43/2426	1.8%	33/2426	1.4%
Camerlingo	Heparin	13/208	6.2%	6/208	2.9%
RAPID	Heparin	2/32	6.3%	-	
TOAST	Danaparoid	19/638	2.9%	25/638	3.9%
FISS	LD nadroparin	0/100	0	4/100	4.0%
	HD nadroparin	0/101	0	6/101	5.2%
FISS-bis	LD nadroparin	10/271	3.7%	-	
	HD nadroparin	15/245	6.1%	-	
HAEST		6/224	2.7%	13/224	5.8%
TOPAS	LD	2/99	2.0%	1/99	1.0%
	MD	1/102	0.9%	0	0
	HD	2/103	1.9%	0	0
	SD	4/100	4.0%	5/100	6.0%
TAIST	LD	3/507	0.6%	2/507	0.4%
	HD	7/486	1.4%	4/486	0.8%
FISS-3		1/180	0.5%	25/180	14%

LD = low dose; MD = medium dose; HD = high dose; SD = highest dose; Chamorro [157]; Camerlingo [24]; Camerlingo [29]; IST = International Stroke Trial [23]; RAPID = Rapid Anticoagulation to Prevent Ischemic Damage [158]; FISS = Fraxiparine Ischemic Stroke Study [22]; FISS-bis = Second Fraxiparine Ischemic Stroke Study [27]; FISS-3 = Fraxiparine Ischemic Stroke Study-3 [159]; TOAST = Trial of Org 10172 in Acute Stroke Treatment [30]; HAEST = Heparin in Acute Embolic Stroke Trial [25]; TOPAS = Therapy of Patients with Acute Stroke [160]; TAIST = Tinzaparin in Acute Ischemic Stroke Trial [161]

Table 2. Effect of anticoagulants on prevention of early recurrent stroke.

Trial	Agent	Anticoagulant		Control	
All subjects					
IST	LD heparin	78/2429	1.6%	214/4859	2.2%
	HD heparin	86/2426	1.8%	-	
FISS	Nadroparin	3/203	1.5%	5/105	4.7%
TOAST	Danaparoid	7/638	1.1%	7/628	1.1%
TOPAS	Certoparin	13/414	3.1%	-	
TAIST	Tinzaparin	60/993	4.0%	15/491	3.1%
FISS-3	Nadroparin	8/180	4.0%	8/173	5.0%
Subjects with presumed cardioembolism					
IST	Heparin	44/1557	2.8%	79/1612	4.9%
TOAST	Danaparoid	0/143	0	2/123	1.6%
HAEST	Dalteparin	19/224	8.6%	17/225	7.5%
TAIST	Tinzaparin	4/256	1.6%	2/112	1.8%

IST = International Stroke Trial [23]; LD = low dose; HD = high dose; FISS-3 = Fraxiparine Ischemic Stroke Study-3 [22, 159]; TOAST = Trial of Org 10172 in Acute Stroke Treatment [30]; TOPAS = Therapy of Patients with Acute Stroke [160]; TAIST = Tinzaparin in Acute Ischemic Stroke Trial [161]; HAEST = Heparin in Acute Embolic Stroke Trial [25]

in lowering the risk of early recurrent thromboembolic events are included in Table 2. Because there has been a particular concern about the risk of early recurrent cardioembolic stroke, these data have been reported separately. Unfortunately, the data do not show efficacy of early anticoagulation in lowering the risk of early recurrent thromboembolic events (Ia/A). There is no real difference in responses to unfractionated heparin or the LMW heparins [35, 36]. As a result, current guidelines do not recommend the administration of heparin or LMW heparins with the aim of preventing early recurrent events among patients with acute ischemic stroke [37-40].

Parenteral anticoagulant treatment has been used as a transition to long-term treatment with oral medications. In some circumstances, the therapy is prescribed to persons perceived to be at an extremely high risk for embolic events, such as those with an intracardiac thrombus detected by echocardiography. Data supporting this course of action are not available **(IV/C)**. An interim course of heparin or a LMW heparin often is used to forestall any thromboembolic events that may be induced by the effects of warfarin. Most patients tolerate the initiation of anticoagulant therapy with oral medication, particularly when lower doses of warfarin are used [41, 42]. Hallevi *et al* [43] did a retrospective review of 204 patients with recent cardioembolic stroke who received no specific antithrombotic treatment, aspirin only, aspirin followed by warfarin, or bridging with either heparin or a LMW heparin before treatment with warfarin. Only two recurrent strokes occurred but symptomatic hemorrhages or other serious bleeding occurred with the parenteral anticoagulants. They concluded that warfarin could be safely started without bridging therapy. These are the only data to provide guidance as to the utility of this management option in patients with cerebrovascular disease **(III/B)**. Thus, the need for a short course of a parenteral anticoagulant as a supplement when starting oral anticoagulants is not established.

A bridging course of heparin or a LMW heparin also may be used as a peri-procedural therapy to maintain anticoagulation for patients with high-risk vascular lesions and who need a surgical procedure [44-46]. The warfarin would be halted a few days before the operation and the parenteral medication would be started. The heparin or LMW heparin would be halted a few hours before surgery and restarted postoperatively when the surgeon believes it is safe to resume treatment. Thereafter, the oral anticoagulant therapy would be reinstituted. Daniels *et al* [45] evaluated the outcomes among 556 patients with mechanical heart valves who had an interim course of heparin or LMW heparin. Three cases of ischemic stroke occurred. A multicenter registry of patients with mechanical valves evaluated the frequency of events among 73 patients who received interim heparin and 172 who had a bridging course of LMW heparin [47]. Most of the patients treated with LMW heparin were outpatients. They found that the bridging therapy could be performed with reasonable safety and it was not associated with a high risk of thromboembolic events **(Ib/A)**. Current guidelines recommend bridging parenteral anticoagulant therapy for patients having surgical procedures and who need to have their warfarin temporarily halted [48].

Because of the high teratogenic risk of the vitamin K antagonists, parenteral anticoagulants are prescribed to pregnant women with high-risk cardiac lesions, such as mechanical mitral valves [49, 50].

In contrast to the lack of data supporting the usefulness of parenteral anticoagulants in reducing the risk of recurrent stroke or improving neurological outcomes after ischemic stroke, the results of clinical trials testing the utility of heparin or LMW heparin in preventing deep vein thrombosis among patients with a paralyzed leg following a stroke are robust [51-53] **(Ia/A)**. The doses of subcutaneously administered heparin or LMW heparin are relatively low and the risk of bleeding complications also is not high. Current guidelines recommend that these agents be used to lower the risk of venous thromboembolism in patients with either a recent stroke, particularly if the patient has a paralyzed leg or if the patient is immobile [37, 38].

Treatment of patients with cerebral venous thrombosis

Cerebral venous thrombosis is an uncommon cause of neurological dysfunction. Because these events usually are subacute, diagnosis is often delayed [54]. The usual presentation is a subacute course of headache, seizures, focal neurological signs, and evidence of increased intracranial pressure [55, 56]. Besides causing brain ischemia, stagnation of the venous flow also may induce intracerebral hemorrhage. Because the pathology involves the venous system and often is due to a coagulation disorder that may promote thrombosis, anticoagulants often are prescribed, even in the presence of intracranial bleeding. The prognosis of patients with cerebral venous thrombosis is influenced by the location of the thrombosis (deep is worse than superficial venous occlusion), the extent of the brain injury (decreased consciousness is a poor prognostic sign), and the presence of hemorrhage [57-59].

Patients usually are treated with early administration of a parenteral anticoagulant and a longer-term course of oral anticoagulants [57, 60, 61]. Unless the patient has a hypercoagulable disorder, the oral anticoagulants usually are prescribed for approximately 6 months. Thereafter, these persons often are given an antiplatelet agent such as aspirin. Persons with an inherited or acquired prothrombotic disorder may be treated with oral anticoagulants on a lifetime basis. While current guidelines include recommendations for anticoagulation in this situation, supporting data are limited (Ib/A-III/B). Given the relatively low frequency of the disorder, it is difficult to recruit a sufficiently large number of patients to provide solid information. In a randomized blinded trial, Einhaupl et al [62] compared outcomes among ten patients treated with heparin to those found in ten control patients. Complete recovery was found in eight of the patients given heparin and one control patient. Three patients in the control group died while no deaths were reported among the heparin-treated patients. A Dutch trial tested treatment with nadroparin (180 anti Xa units daily) to control in 59 patients [63]. No bleeding complications were noted but outcomes were similar in the two treatment groups. In an observational study, Brucker et al [64] treated 42 patients with heparin for 3 weeks followed by oral anticoagulants. On follow-up, partial or complete recanalization of the venous system was found in 36 patients. Forty patients improved and only one patient died. In a retrospective review of their experience using an adjusted-dose regimen of heparin in 79 patients, Mehraein et al [65] reported that a decreased level of consciousness at the time of initiation of treatment was associated with poor outcomes. Eight of 15 comatose patients died while all of the 64 patients with relatively normal consciousness survived. Other predictors of a poor outcome included advanced age or the presence of intracranial bleeding on brain imaging.

More recently, physicians have used thrombolytic agents administered directly into the intravenous thrombus or a mechanical intervention to emergently restore flow in critically ill patients [66, 67]. These therapies have been prescribed to those patients who have not responded to anticoagulants. Following the intravascular treatment, patients may be treated with antiplatelet agents or anticoagulants. At present, information regarding these treatments is largely based on case reports or small clinical series. There is a real need for additional clinical research to define the role of anticoagulants in the early and long-term management of cerebral venous thrombosis.

Long-term prevention of ischemic stroke among persons with arterial diseases

For many years, oral anticoagulants were prescribed to patients with intracranial or extracranial large artery diseases, including atherosclerosis or dissection. The rationales include:

- prevention of artery-to-artery thromboembolism; and
- forestalling arterial occlusion with secondary flow-related ischemia.

A popular hypothesis is that severe arterial stenoses with resultant low flow would induce formation of clotting-factor-rich thrombi that are similar to those found with venous disease. The latter might be forestalled with the use of warfarin. In particular, warfarin has been used to treat patients with intracranial stenoses or lesions in the vertebrobasilar circulation. Unfortunately, data supporting the differential development of clots as affected by the severity of arterial stenosis are not available. In addition, warfarin has been used as an adjunct to antiplatelet agents for patients who have had recurrent symptoms despite therapy. Warfarin also has been used as a monotherapy when the patient is judged to have 'failed' treatment with antiplatelet agents.

Trials have tested oral anticoagulants versus aspirin in preventing recurrent ischemic events among patients with atherosclerotic arterial disease or cryptogenic stroke (Table 3). Subjects with both extracranial and intracranial lesions were enrolled. The results are complementary; there are no data that warfarin is superior to aspirin [68-72]. An analysis of subgroups in the Warfarin-Aspirin Recurrent Stroke Study found that warfarin was not superior to aspirin in any subset of patients with arterial disease and recent stroke [73]. In addition, another trial found that combination of warfarin and aspirin was not more effective in preventing stroke than antiplatelet therapy among patients with peripheral arterial disease [74]. These data provide no evidence to support the administration of warfarin to prevent stroke and other ischemic events among patients with arterial disease (I/A).

Intracranial or extracranial dissections are the second most common large artery disease that causes ischemic stroke or TIA. Dissections may occur in either the carotid or vertebrobasilar circulation and may happen spontaneously or be secondary to trauma of variable severity. Despite the lack of availability of supporting data, experts and guidelines often recommend a course of oral anticoagulants to prevent recurrent ischemic events [39]. However, the overall prognosis of patients with arterial dissections generally is favorable [75]. Recently, Swiss investigators reported the results of a non-randomized study from a single center [76]. They found that the prognoses of their patients generally were good and that responses were similar whether they were treated with warfarin or aspirin (IIa/B). Based on a systemic review and meta-analysis of 34 non-randomized studies, Menon et al [77] concluded that there were no significant differences in responses to anticoagulants or antiplatelet agents (IIa/B). A clinical trial comparing the safety and efficacy of aspirin or warfarin in prevention of recurrent ischemic events among patients with extracranial arterial dissections is underway [78]. Until these data become available there appears to be little reason to favor oral anticoagulants over the use of aspirin.

Table 3. Trials of oral anticoagulant therapy for the prevention of stroke in patients with arterial disease.

Trial	INR level	Warfarin		Aspirin		p-value
SPIRIT	3-4	81/651	12.4%	36/665	5.4%	-
WARSS	1.4-2.8	196/1103	17.8%	176/1103	16%	0.25
WASID	2-3	63/289	22.1%	62/280	21.8%	0.83
ESPRIT	2-3	99/536	19%	98/532	18%	-

SPIRIT = Stroke Prevention in Reversible Ischemia Trial (primary outcomes were vascular death, serious bleeding, recurrent stroke, or myocardial infarction; major difference was more hemorrhage with warfarin) [162]; WARSS = Warfarin-Aspirin Recurrent Stroke Study, (primary outcomes were recurrent ischemic stroke or death) [68]; WASID = Warfarin-Aspirin Symptomatic Intracranial Disease trial (primary outcomes were stroke, brain hemorrhage, or vascular death) [163]; ESPRIT = European/Australasian Stroke Prevention in Reversible Ischemia Trial (primary outcomes were vascular death, ischemic stroke, major bleeding, or myocardial infarction) [71]

With the development of transesophageal echocardiography, physicians' ability to detect advanced atherosclerotic lesions in the aorta improved considerably. Besides being a potential source for emboli, the presence of aortic lesions also is a marker of generalized atherosclerosis [79]. These lesions are found most commonly among older patients and those with risk factors for accelerated atherosclerosis [80]. Atheromatous changes in the aorta, particularly plaques that are greater than 4mm in thickness or those associated with intra-luminal mobility, are recognized as an important cause of thromboembolism [80, 81]. Because of the perceived high risk for embolization, which may be as high as with atrial fibrillation or severe stenosis of the internal carotid artery, anticoagulants and antiplatelet agents have been prescribed [80]. Still, data demonstrating superiority of either treatment approach are lacking [81]. A retrospective study of 519 patients with severe plaque formation in the thoracic aorta found no difference in the risk of embolic events with treatment using either aspirin or oral anticoagulants [82]. At present, data do not provide clear guidance about the use of antiplatelet agents or anticoagulants in preventing embolic events among persons with advanced aortic atherosclerosis **(IIa/B-IV/C)**.

Data about the utility of warfarin in the prevention of ischemic events among children with arterial causes of brain ischemia are limited [83]. A collaborative German-American registry evaluated the usefulness of anticoagulants in children with acute arteriopathies other than moyamoya [84]. They reported that recurrent events occurred within 1 year in 14% of the children. Their conclusion was that warfarin could be given with reasonable safety to children with arterial diseases causing stroke. Additional research demonstrating potential efficacy is needed to determine if this is an indication for warfarin.

Long-term prevention of ischemic stroke among persons with cardiac sources of embolism

The cardiac diseases that may lead to ischemic stroke are divided into higher- and lower-risk lesions based on the associated relative risk for thromboembolism. The high-risk cardiac lesions include structural diseases such as a recent myocardial infarction (especially anterior wall), mechanical prosthetic valves particularly at the mitral position, and rheumatic mitral stenosis (Table 4). The detection of an intra-atrial or intraventricular thrombus on cardiac

Table 4. Cardiac causes of cerebral embolism – higher and uncertain risk lesions.	
Higher-risk cardiac lesions	**Uncertain or lower-risk cardiac lesions**
Acute myocardial infarction (anterior wall in particular)	Lone atrial fibrillation
	Akinetic or hypokinetic left ventricular segment
Rheumatic mitral stenosis	
	Left ventricular aneurysm
Mechanical prosthetic valve (mitral position in particular)	
	Mitral annulus calcification
Atrial fibrillation complicating structural cardiac disease	Mitral valve prolapse
Left atrial, left atrial appendage, or ventricular thrombus	Bioprosthetic mitral or aortic valve
	Bicuspid aortic valve
Infective endocarditis	Calcific aortic stenosis
Non-bacterial thrombotic (marantic) endocarditis	Lambl excrescence
	Mitral valve strands
Libman-Sacks endocarditis	Aneurysm of the sinus of Valsalva
Atrial myxoma	Patent foramen ovale
Dilated cardiomyopathy	Atrial septal aneurysm
	Atrial septal defect
	Sick sinus syndrome
	Idiopathic hypertrophic subaortic stenosis

imaging also is associated with a high risk of embolic events. Treatment of persons with infective endocarditis or atrial myxoma differs from that prescribed to other high-risk cardiac lesions. Surgical resection is recommended for the treatment of myxoma. Because of the concern for infective aneurysms of the brain that may lead to intracranial hemorrhage, antithrombotic agents are not recommended for the management of patients with embolic events secondary to infective endocarditis [85]. An exception to this rule would be the presence of another high-risk cardiac lesion, such as a mechanical prosthetic valve, that would mandate long-term anticoagulant therapy. The risk for cerebral thromboembolism has not been clearly established or appears to be relatively low with several other cardiac abnormalities (Table 4).

While lone atrial fibrillation is accompanied by a relatively low risk of thromboembolic events, the presence of atrial fibrillation complicating structural cardiac disease usually is associated with a further increase in the risk of ischemic stroke. Atrial fibrillation is the cardiac lesion most commonly found among persons with stroke. It is a particularly important cause of thromboembolism among persons older than 75; in this group, atrial fibrillation is the highest predictor of ischemic stroke. The development of the CHADS2 score is useful in forecasting the risk of thromboembolic events and in helping decisions about the administration of antithrombotic agents to prevent stroke [86]. The components of the CHADS2 score are:

- history of congestive heart failure – 1 point;
- hypertension – 1 point;
- age older than 75 – 1 point;
- diabetes mellitus – 1 point; and
- neurological symptoms (stroke) – 2 points.

A total score of 2 or more points is considered an indication for administration of oral anticoagulants. Based on this scale, virtually all patients with atrial fibrillation and a history of a TIA or stroke would be optimally treated with oral anticoagulants.

While systemic bleeding, particularly gastrointestinal bleeding, is the most common type of hemorrhage, the most feared bleeding complications involve intracranial hemorrhage (either intracerebral or subdural hematomas) [87]. Petty et al [88] calculated that cumulative risks of serious bleeding complications of warfarin were 1% at 6 months, 5% at 1 year, and 7% at 3 years. However, the study probably reflects data from patients treated before the widespread implementation of the INR. In one recent study of 13,559 patients with atrial fibrillation taking warfarin for prevention of thromboembolic events, 72 serious bleeding episodes (35 fatal) involved intracranial hemorrhages and 98 extracranial hemorrhages (5 fatal) [87]. In a spin-off report, investigators in one study reported that the annual incidence of bleeding complications with warfarin was approximately 2% [89]. Patients and those with heart failure, renal disease, hepatic disease, and diabetes had an increased risk of serious bleeding events. In a single-center study, Jacobs et al [90] evaluated the safety and efficacy of warfarin in a population of elderly patients with atrial fibrillation including those with dementia or a risk for falls. Those patients with an increased fall risk or dementia had the highest rates of bleeding. However, advanced age is not a contraindication for treatment. Mant *et al* [91] performed a randomized trial that enrolled subjects aged older than 75. The desired level of anticoagulation was an INR of 2-3; only two intracranial hemorrhages were diagnosed among the 488 subjects. Rash *et al* [92] enrolled 75 patients with atrial fibrillation and who were aged 80-90. They found that adjusted-dose aspirin (INR: 2-3) actually was better tolerated than the aspirin 300mg/day. Singer *et al* [86] evaluated the impact of the level of anticoagulation (as measured by the INR) on the frequency of serious bleeding complications. They noted that the risk of serious hemorrhage was relatively stable at all levels below an INR value of 3.6. With higher levels of INR, the risk of intracranial hemorrhage increased by an odds ratio of 3.56.

Data about the utility of anticoagulants in preventing cerebral embolism among higher-risk cardiac lesions are robust. Numerous clinical trials have tested the efficacy and safety of oral anticoagulants in patients with atrial fibrillation not associated with mitral stenosis. Evidence about the usefulness of anticoagulants for prevention of embolization among persons with the uncertain or lower-risk cardiac abnormalities is less clear.

Several trials tested adjusted-dose warfarin in the prevention of embolism in patients with atrial fibrillation who did not have neurological symptoms [91, 93-103] (Table 4). One trial enrolled patients who had a prior TIA or ischemic stroke [104]. An adjusted-dose regimen of warfarin was compared to placebo, aspirin, aspirin and low (fixed)-dose warfarin, aspirin and clopidogrel, or indobufen (Table 5). The desired levels of anticoagulation as measured by the INR in the trials have ranged from 1.4-2.8 to 2.0-4.5. Some of the more recent clinical trials enrolled subjects who previously had been taking warfarin without complication [101]. More recently, adjusted-dose oral anticoagulant therapy has been compared to the direct oral thrombin inhibitors, ximelagatran or dabigatran [105-110].

In general, the adjusted-dose regimen of warfarin is superior to other interventions in lowering the risk of thromboembolic events among a broad range of patients with atrial fibrillation, including those with previous neurological symptoms. The absolute reduction in risk with adjusted-dose warfarin with the desired INR of 2-3 is a decline from 4.5% to 1.4% annually [111] (Ia/A)(Table 5). Based on meta-analyses of the data from the many trials, the relative risk reduction in stroke with warfarin is approximately 68% (95% CI, 50%-79%) [111, 112]. While the number of systemic embolic events is relatively low, evidence also supports the use of anticoagulants for preventing these events [113]. While the risk of bleeding is increased with the use of adjusted doses of warfarin, overall the risk-benefit ratio strongly supports the use of oral anticoagulants [113]. Current guidelines include recommendations for the use of oral anticoagulants to prevent ischemic stroke and other thromboembolic events [38, 111, 114]. Patients with atrial fibrillation and a CHADS score of 0 or 1 may be treated with antiplatelet agents [115].

There are other potential indications for the use of oral anticoagulants among patients with atrial fibrillation, including a short-term course of treatment (approximately 4 weeks before and 2 weeks after treatment) to lower the risk of embolic events among patients with atrial fibrillation who are treated with pharmacological or electrical cardioversion [114, 116]. Warfarin

Table 5. Trials of adjusted-dose warfarin patients with atrial fibrillation – annual rates of embolic events.

	INR	OAC	Control	RRR	p-value
Comparison to placebo					
AFASAK-1	2.8-4.2	2.7%	6.2%	56%	<0.05
SPAF-1	2.0-4.5	2.3%	7.4%	67%	0.01
BAATAF	1.5-2.7	0.4%	3.0%	86%	0.002
CAFA	2.0-3.0	3.4%	4.6%	26%	0.25
SPINAF	1.4-2.8	0.9%	4.3%	79%	0.001
EAFT	2.5-4.0	8.5%	16.5%	47%	0.001
Comparison to aspirin or aspirin/clopidogrel					
AFASAK-1	2.8-4.2	2.7%	5.2%	48%	<0.05
SPAF-2	2.0-4.5				
≤75 years		1.3%	1.9%	33%	0.24
>75 years		3.6%	4.8%	27%	0.39
AFASAK-2	2.0-3.0	3.4%	2.7%	-21%	NS
Hellemons	2.5-3.5	2.5%	3.1%	19%	NS
BAFTA	2.0-3.0	1.8%	3.8%	52%	0.003
ACTIVE - W	2.0-3.0	3.9%	5.6%	44%	0.003
Comparison to low fixed-dose anticoagulant with/without antiplatelet agent					
AFASAK-2	2.0-3.0	3.4 %	3.9%	13%	NS
		-	3.2%	-6%	NS
SPAF-3	2.0-3.0	1.9%	7.9%	74%	<0.0001
Hellemons	2.5-3.5	2.5%	2.2%	-14%	NS
Pengo	3.0	3.6%	6.2%	42%	0.29

AFASAK (1 or 2) = Copenhagen Atrial Fibrillation Aspirin and Anticoagulant Therapy studies 1 and 2 [93]; SPAF (I, II, III) = Stroke Prevention Atrial Fibrillation studies I, II, III [95-97, 164]; BAATAF = Boston Area Anticoagulation Trial for Atrial Fibrillation [94]; CAFA = Canadian Atrial Fibrillation Anticoagulation study [98]; SPINAF = Veterans Affairs Stroke Prevention in Non-rheumatic Atrial Fibrillation study [165]; EAFT = European Atrial Fibrillation Trial [104]; BAFTA: Birmingham Atrial Fibrillation Treatment of the Aged study [91]; ACTIVE - W = Atrial Fibrillation Clopidogrel Trial with Irbesartan for prevention of Vascular Events - Warfarin [115]; Hellemons [166]; Pengo [167] also is prescribed as a periprocedural therapy for patients with atrial fibrillation who are treated with catheter ablation.

Oral anticoagulants also are recommended for the treatment of patients with other cardiac disorders that are considered as having a high likelihood of being a source of cerebral embolization [39, 117-121]. In comparison to research evaluating the utility of oral anticoagulants in preventing thromboembolic events among patients with atrial fibrillation, data describing safety and efficacy for these situations are less extensive. While anticoagulants are given to persons with dilated cardiomyopathies, evidence about their usefulness is not available [121, 122]. Massie *et al* [123] performed a randomized trial that compared aspirin (162mg/day), clopidogrel (75mg/day) or warfarin (INR 2.5-3 target) among 1587 patients with reduced cardiac ejection fractions with the goal of preventing death, non-fatal myocardial infarction or stroke. Warfarin was associated with fewer strokes but the frequency of the composite primary endpoint was similar in the three groups **(Ia/A)**. Another clinical trial is testing aspirin or warfarin among patients with dilated cardiomyopathy [124]. While it is reasonable to prescribe warfarin to a patient with a dilated cardiomyopathy, additional information is needed to determine whether this approach is correct.

Vaitkus and Barnathan [125] did a meta-analysis of studies looking at the impact of anticoagulation on the formation of mural thrombosis and embolization after acute anterior myocardial infarction. The medications reduced the risk of mural thrombosis by approximately 32% and the frequency of embolization by approximately 20% **(Ia/A)**. Currently, long-term administration of oral anticoagulants is recommended for the treatment of patients with anterior wall myocardial infarction, particularly if an intraventricular thrombus is detected [121].

The relative risk of thromboembolic events among persons with rheumatic mitral stenosis and atrial fibrillation is approximately 17 times of similar aged healthy persons [39, 120]. Concomitant left atrial enlargement, left atrial turbulence, or left ventricular dysfunction also increases the risk of embolism [126]. Although data from clinical trials are limited, long-term anticoagulation is recommended [38, 39, 120, 126]. A small Thai study compared oral anticoagulation (INR 1.5-3) or aspirin (75mg/day) among persons with mitral stenosis and atrial fibrillation; the anticoagulants were found to be superior in preventing cardioembolic stroke [127]. An Italian study compared low intensity (INR goal 2) or moderate intensity (INR goal 3) anticoagulation among patients with mitral stenosis and atrial fibrillation [102]. The numbers of ischemic and hemorrhagic events were similar in the two groups and the authors concluded that the lower level of anticoagulation could be used. Perez-Gomez *et al* [128] compared the combination of warfarin and antiplatelet agents to warfarin monotherapy and reported that the combination of agents was superior when patients had a history of thromboembolism **(Ia/A)**. Another study demonstrated that low-dose anticoagulation was effective in lowering the risk of thromboembolic events among patients with mitral regurgitation [129].

The risk of embolic stroke is high among persons with mechanical prosthetic valves. While embolic events occur among those patients taking warfarin, anecdotal evidence suggests that the risk was reduced considerably. As a result, anticoagulants are prescribed to patients among persons with mechanical valves, especially mitral valve prostheses [130]. Azar *et al* [131] reported that anticoagulation (INR goal 3) reduced the risk of embolic events from 1.2 to 0.7/100 patient years. The results of early studies of anticoagulants in patients with mechanical prosthetic cardiac valves may not be completely relevant because the evolution of the prostheses means that modern valves may have a low potential for thromboembolism [132]. Still, current guidelines recommend the use of oral anticoagulants for patients with mechanical valves [39, 85] **(Ia/A)**.

Patients perceived as having an especially high risk for cardiac thromboembolism may be treated with the combination of warfarin and aspirin or dipyridamole [85]. Patients who have embolic events despite treatment with therapeutic levels of anticoagulation also may receive adjunctive treatment with aspirin or dipyridamole. While data from clinical trials and meta-analyses are limited, current evidence suggests that adding aspirin (75-81mg/day) is effective and safe [133, 134]. However, current guidelines recommend that patients be treated with a combination of medications if they are perceived as not having a high risk for bleeding complications [85] **(Ia/A)**.

The risk of thromboembolic events appears to be less among patients with bioprosthetic valves, especially in the aortic position; thus, current guidelines recommend long-term treatment with antiplatelet agents instead of anticoagulants [85]. In some instances, patients are prescribed warfarin for a few months prior to conversion to aspirin therapy. In a small study that compared aspirin (100mg/day) or warfarin (INR goal 2-3) for 3 months followed by aspirin 100mg daily, Colli *et al* [135] found that the rates of ischemic and bleeding events were similar. They concluded that the interim course of warfarin therapy was not needed **(IIa/B)**.

Thromboembolic events, including ischemic stroke, are ascribed to a number of congenital or acquired cardiac disorders that appear not to have the same associated risk as the previously described lesions (Table 4). Management of persons with these cardiac abnormalities is controversial in part because there are limited or no data about the benefit-risk ratio for treatment options including anticoagulants. A patent foramen ovale (PFO) is commonly detected by contrast-enhanced echocardiography among persons with stroke, especially among younger patients with otherwise cryptogenic events. The scenario would be a paradoxical embolism of a piece of thrombus that has arisen in a vein and traverses the heart through the right-to-left shunt. However, the prevalence of PFO among healthy persons may be as high as 20% and thus, the discovery of the PFO in a patient with a stroke is not surprising. The cause-and-effect relationship between PFO and stroke has not been established [136]. The risk of cerebrovascular complications has not been correlated with the size of the PFO [137]. Conflicting data are present about the impact of a concomitant atrial septal aneurysm [137, 138]. While the presence of a PFO may be an important finding in persons younger than 55, it also may be relevant among older persons [139]. Because the thrombi presumably would be of venous origin, the use of anticoagulants makes sense. Other treatment options include antiplatelet agents, endovascular placement of a closure device, or direct surgical repair. A clinical trial that compared aspirin or warfarin therapy among patients with PFO and cryptogenic stroke did not demonstrate a benefit from anticoagulant therapy [137]. Based on a systemic review of the available data, a panel of the American Academy of Neurology concluded that there was insufficient evidence to state whether aspirin or warfarin was superior in preventing ischemic stroke among patients with a PFO [140]. Guidelines currently recommend that aspirin be prescribed to most patients with cryptogenic stroke and PFO [85] **(Ia/A)**.

Okajima *et al* [141] evaluated the impact of the thickness of mitral and aortic valves as detected by echocardiography on the risk of recurrent events; they found that these abnormalities were not associated with an increased risk of new cerebrovascular events regardless of treatment with either warfarin or aspirin. Echocardiographic detection of valvular strands also appears not to be associated with an increased risk of recurrent ischemic events [124]. Because of the low risk for thromboembolism, current guidelines recommend that no antithrombotic therapy or aspirin be given to patients with mitral valve prolapse and who have not had any embolic events [85, 126]. Patients with calcific aortic stenosis also are not treated with antithrombotic agents [85] **(IIa/B)**.

Other antithrombotic agents are being tested for the prevention of thromboembolism in patients with heart disease [142]. Ximelagatran was compared to adjusted-dose warfarin for the prevention of embolic events among persons with atrial fibrillation [107-109]. The risk of ischemic events was lower among the warfarin-treated subjects and no major difference in major bleeding complications was found between the two treatment groups. However, when an aggregation of minor and major bleeding was analyzed, significantly fewer events were reported among the group that received ximelagatran. While the trial found that ximelagatran was not inferior to warfarin, it was associated with an increased risk of hepatic problems that limits its use. A pooled analysis of trials of ximelagatran found that the agent was at least as effective as warfarin for the prevention of stroke among patients with atrial fibrillation [106]. The addition of ximelagatran to aspirin was tested in comparison to aspirin monotherapy for the prevention of ischemic events in patients with recent myocardial infarction and atrial fibrillation [143]. They reported that the combination was effective in reducing the risk of death, myocardial infarction or stroke. More recently, another direct thrombin antagonist, dabigatran, was tested in clinical trials. In a three-arm study, two different doses of dabigatran were compared to adjusted warfarin in a trial that enrolled 18,113 patients with atrial fibrillation [144]. The lower dose of dabigatran (110mg/day) was associated with embolic rates that were similar to that achieved with warfarin but the rate of major bleeding was less. The higher dose of the medication (150mg/day) produced a rate of thromboembolic events that was less than warfarin but the bleeding risk was similar to the anticoagulant. In another trial, Ezekowitz *et al* [145] compared the combination of dabigatran and aspirin to warfarin among patients with atrial fibrillation. They found bleeding complications were increased with the highest doses of dabigatran and ischemic events occurred with the lower doses of the medication. Dabigatran has not been associated with an increased risk of hepatotoxicity. It is possible that this medication will be approved as an alternative to adjusted-dose warfarin **(Ia/A)**.

Idraparinux, a synthetic analogue of heparin that must be given parenterally, binds to antithrombin and inactivates Factor Xa. The medication may be injected once a week because of its long duration of action [146]. It was compared to an adjusted-dose warfarin regimen (INR 2-3) for the prevention of embolic events among patients with atrial fibrillation. There was no difference in the rates of ischemic events between the two treatment groups, but there was a significantly higher rate of serious bleeding with idraparinux. As a result, it is likely that idraparinux will not be an alternative to warfarin. Orally or subcutaneously administered inhibitors of Factor Xa are being evaluated as an alternative to warfarin. These agents include rivaroxaban, apixaban, edoxaban, and idrabiotaparinux [146]. Tecarfarin is an antagonist to vitamin K epoxide reductase, which may have fewer interactions with food and other medications than warfarin [146]. A trial of tecarfarin is underway [147].

Long-term prevention of ischemic stroke among persons with hypercoagulable disorders

Acquired or inherited disorders of coagulation that promote thrombotic venous or arterial occlusions may account for a small number of ischemic strokes. Some of these diseases are treated with specific interventions, such as children with sickle cell disease being treated with blood transfusions [148]. Those patients with thrombocytosis may be given antiplatelet agents. However, patients with the more common hypercoagulable disorders such as the presence of Factor V Leiden, the prothrombin gene mutation, or antiphospholipid antibodies often are prescribed warfarin for the prevention of recurrent venous and arterial thromboembolic events. In particular, anticoagulants have been recommended to prevent deep vein thrombosis, cerebral venous thrombosis, and pulmonary embolism among affected patients. The utility of warfarin for the prevention of arterial thromboembolic events is less clear.

The presence of elevated levels of antiphospholipid antibodies and the definition of the antiphospholipid antibody syndrome is the subject of considerable controversy [149]. Recently, a large multinational European trial reported the frequency of ischemic events among 1000 patients with antiphospholipid antibody syndrome; recurrent thromboembolic events occurred in 166 patients during a 5-year period of follow-up; 24 were strokes [150]. Because of the perceived high risk of thromboembolism, anticoagulants often are recommended. However, there are concerns that monitoring of the level of anticoagulation among patients taking warfarin may not be accurate; the presence of the antibodies may affect the prothrombin times. Alternative methods for measuring therapeutic effects of warfarin, such as direct levels of thrombin, may be needed. Despite these limitations, many physicians prescribe warfarin to achieve relatively high INR levels (up to 4.5). The utility of warfarin or antiplatelet agents among patients who have elevations of antiphospholipid antibodies has been evaluated. In a randomized trial, Finazzi et al [151] tested moderate (INR 2-3) or high (INR 3-4.5) degrees of anticoagulation in 109 cases with antiphospholipid antibody syndrome. They found that the higher level of anticoagulation was not superior. The Antiphospholipid Antibodies and Stroke Study was a spin-off project of another larger trial that was comparing aspirin or adjusted-dose warfarin for the prevention of recurrent ischemic cerebrovascular events [152]. The trial enrolled 1770 subjects; 720 had the presence of antiphospholipid antibodies and/or a lupus anticoagulant. The presence of the antiphospholipid antibodies was not associated with an increased risk of ischemic stroke. The rates of new ischemic events were similar among the subjects who received aspirin or warfarin. Another study evaluated the interactions between the presence of a PFO, thickening of cardiac valves and the presence of antiphospholipid antibodies; the study showed no effect of the combination of factors on the response to treatment [153]. Systemic reviews and meta-analyses of secondary prophylaxis among patients with antiphospholipid antibodies provide conflicting conclusions [154, 155]. One review concluded that warfarin was the desired intervention to prevent thromboembolism among patients with antiphospholipid antibody syndrome [155]. They recommended that the desired INR level for patients with venous events should be 2-3 and the optimal INR for patients with arterial events would be greater than 3. Conversely, Lim *et al* [154] concluded that warfarin is not superior to aspirin in preventing recurrent ischemic events among patients with cerebrovascular disease and the presence of antiphospholipid antibody syndrome **(I/A)**. Current guidelines state that either aspirin or warfarin may be given to patients with antiphospholipid antibody syndrome and stroke. Given the uncertainty about the data and the conflicting recommendations, additional research is needed to define the role of warfarin for preventing stroke in this situation.

Administration of LMW heparin has been used to prevent venous thromboembolism among persons with cancer, another situation that can be associated with an acquired hypercoagulable state [156]. Among the disorders associated with cancer are disseminated intravascular coagulation and non-bacterial thrombotic endocarditis. While patients with these complications of cancer and other serious diseases are often treated with parenteral or oral anticoagulants, there are no results from clinical trials that help guide treatment decisions. In some circumstances, patients with cancer also receive oral anticoagulants.

Conclusions

For several years, the role of anticoagulants in the management of patients with ischemic cerebrovascular disease has been controversial. Fortunately, clinical trials have demonstrated the utility of these medications in some circumstances, in particular for long-term prevention of thromboembolism among patients with heart disease and for prevention of deep vein thrombosis among patients who are bedridden after stroke. Conversely, these agents have not been established as safe or effective in preventing stroke among persons with arterial diseases nor have they been found to be effective in halting neurological worsening, forestalling early recurrent stroke, or improving outcomes following stroke.

Key points	Evidence level
◆ Little evidence of efficacy of anticoagulants to prevent stroke in patients with recent TIA.	Ib/A
◆ No evidence of efficacy of anticoagulants to prevent early recurrent stroke in patients with recent stroke including those with cardioembolic events.	Ia/A
◆ No evidence of efficacy of anticoagulants to improve neurological outcomes after ischemic stroke.	Ia/A
◆ No evidence of efficacy of anticoagulants to halt neurological worsening after acute ischemic stroke.	Ia/A
◆ No evidence of utility of an interim course of parenterally administered anticoagulants during a transition to oral anticoagulants among persons with recent stroke.	IV/C
◆ Some evidence of utility of bridging or interim therapy for patients with mechanical heart valves and other high-risk lesions when having surgery.	Ib/A
◆ Some evidence that warfarin without bridging treatment with parenteral anticoagulants can be given after stroke.	III/B
◆ Anticoagulants are useful in preventing deep vein thrombosis in patients immobilized after stroke.	Ia/A
◆ The usefulness of anticoagulants in preventing recurrent stroke among persons with hypercoagulable disorders is not established.	Ib/A-III/B
◆ Anticoagulants are not as effective as antiplatelet agents in preventing stroke secondary to arterial disease.	Ia/A
◆ The role of anticoagulants in preventing stroke among persons with arterial dissections is uncertain.	IIa/B
◆ Long-term adjusted-dose (INR 2-3) oral anticoagulation is indicated for preventing stroke among most patients with atrial fibrillation.	Ia/A
◆ Long-term anticoagulants are not indicated in the treatment of low-risk patients with atrial fibrillation (CHADS score 0-1).	Ia/A
◆ The combination of low-dose fixed-dose oral anticoagulation alone or in combination is not indicated for preventing stroke among patients with atrial fibrillation.	Ia/A
◆ Long-term adjusted-dose (INR 2-3) oral anticoagulation is indicated for preventing stroke among patients with a recent high-risk myocardial infarction, particularly if an intraventricular thrombus is present.	Ia/A
◆ Long-term adjusted-dose (INR 2-3) oral anticoagulation is indicated for preventing stroke among persons with rheumatic mitral stenosis and atrial fibrillation.	Ia/A
◆ Long-term adjusted oral (INR 2.5-3.5) oral anticoagulation alone or in combination with antiplatelet agents is indicated for preventing stroke among persons with prosthetic heart valves.	Ia/A

Continued

Key points *continued*	Evidence level
◆ Long-term adjusted-dose oral anticoagulation is not needed for patients with bioprosthetic valves, particularly those in the aortic position.	Ia/A
◆ Long-term adjusted-dose oral anticoagulation is not superior to antiplatelet therapy for preventing stroke among persons with patent foramen ovale.	Ia/A
◆ Dabigatran is an alternative to adjusted-dose oral anticoagulation (INR 2-3) in preventing stroke among persons with atrial fibrillation.	Ia/A
◆ While anticoagulants are indicated to prevent venous thromboembolism among persons with genetic or acquired hypercoagulable disorders, their utility in preventing arterial events is not established.	Ib/A

References

1. Hirsh J, Dalen JE, Anderson DR, Poller L, Bussey H, Ansell J, Deykin D. Oral anticoagulants: mechanism of action, clinical effectiveness, and optimal therapeutic range. *Chest* 2001; 119: 8S-21S.

2. Essex DW, Wynn SS, Jin DK. Late-onset warfarin-induced skin necrosis: case report and review of the literature. *Am J Hematol* 1998; 57: 233-7.

3. Linder MW, Looney S, Adams JE, III, Johnson N, Antonino-Green D, Lacefield N, Bukaveckas BL, Valdes R, Jr. Warfarin dose adjustments based on CYP2C9 genetic polymorphisms. *J Thromb Thrombolysis* 2002; 14: 227-32.

4. Fregin A, Rost S, Wolz W, Krebsova A, Muller CR, Oldenburg J. Homozygosity mapping of a second gene locus for hereditary combined deficiency of vitamin K-dependent clotting factors to the centromeric region of chromosome 16. *Blood* 2002; 100: 3229-32.

5. Hulse ML. Warfarin resistance: diagnosis and therapeutic alternatives. *Pharmacotherapy* 1996; 16: 1009-17.

6. Ginsberg JS, Greer I, Hirsh J. Use of antithrombotic agents during pregnancy. *Chest* 2001; 119: 122S-31.

7. Hirsh J, Anand SS, Halperin JL, Fuster V. Guide to anticoagulant therapy: heparin. *Circulation* 2001; 103: 2994-3018.

8. Toth C. The use of bolus of intravenous heparin while initiating heparin therapy in anticoagulation following transient ischemic attack or stroke does not lead to increased morbidity or mortality. *Blood Coagulation & Fibrinolysis* 2003; 14: 463-8.

9. Raschke RA, Reilly BM, Guidry JR, Fontana JR, Srinivas S. The weight-based heparin dosing nomogram compared with a 'standard care' nomogram. A randomized controlled trial. *Ann Intern Med* 1993; 119: 874-81.

10. Toth C, Voll C. Validation of a weight-based nomogram for the use of intravenous heparin in transient ischemic attack or stroke. *Stroke* 2002; 33: 670-4.

11. Laposata M, Green D, Van Cott EM, Barrowcliffe TW, Goodnight SH, Sosolik RC. College of American Pathologists Conference XXXI on laboratory monitoring of anticoagulant therapy: the clinical use and laboratory monitoring of low-molecular-weight heparin, danaparoid, hirudin and related compounds, and argatroban. *Arch Pathol Lab Med* 1998; 122: 799-807.

12. Marsh EE, Adams HP, Jr., Biller J, Wasek P, Banwart K, Mitchell V, Woolson R. Use of antithrombotic drugs in the treatment of acute ischemic stroke: a survey of neurologists in practice in the United States. *Neurology* 1989; 39: 1631-4.

13. Al-Sadat A, Sunbulli M, Chaturvedi S. Use of the intravenous heparin by North American neurologists: do the data matter? *Stroke* 2002; 33: 1574-7.

14. Calvet D, Lamy C, Touze E, Oppenheim C, Meder JF, Mas J-L. Management and outcome of patients with transient ischemic attack admitted to a stroke unit. *Cerebrovasc Dis* 2007; 24: 80-5.

15. Kang K, Kim DW, Park HK, Yoon BW. Optimal dosing of intravenous unfractionated heparin bolus in transient ischemic attack or stroke. *Clin Appl Thromb Hemost* 2010; 16: 126-31.

16. Petty GW, Brown RD, Jr., Whisnant JP, Sicks JD, O'Fallon WM, Wiebers DO. Frequency of major complications of aspirin, warfarin, and intravenous heparin for secondary stroke prevention. *Ann Intern Med* 1999; 130: 14-22.

17. Biller J, Bruno A, Adams HP, Jr., Godersky JC, Loftus CM, Mitchell VL, Banwart KJ, Jones MP. A randomized trial of aspirin or heparin in hospitalized patients with recent transient ischemic attacks. A pilot study. *Stroke* 1989; 20: 441-7.

18. Cerebral Embolism Study Group. Immediate anticoagulation of embolic stroke: brain hemorrhage and management options. *Stroke* 1984; 15: 779-89.

19. Cerebral Embolism Study Group. Cardioembolic stroke, early anticoagulation, and brain hemorrhage. *Arch Intern Med* 1987; 147: 636-40.

20. Cerebral Embolism Study Group. Immediate anticoagulation and embolic stroke. A randomized trial. *Stroke* 1983; 14: 668-76.

21. Kay R, Wong KS, Woo J. Pilot study of low-molecular-weight heparin in the treatment of acute ischemic stroke. *Stroke* 1994; 25: 684-5.

22. Kay R, Wong KS, Yu YL, Chan YW, Tsoi TH, Ahuja AT, Chan FL, Fong KY, Law CB, Wong A. Low-molecular-weight heparin for the treatment of acute ischemic stroke. *N Engl J Med* 1995; 333: 1588-93.

23. International Stroke Trial Collaborative Group The International Stroke Trial (IST): a randomised trial of aspirin, subcutaneous heparin, both, or neither among 19,435 patients with acute ischaemic stroke. *Lancet* 1997; 349: 1569-81.

24. Camerlingo M, Casto L, Censori B, Ferraro B, Gazzaniga GC, Cesana B, Mamoli A. Immediate anticoagulation with heparin for first-ever ischemic strokes in the carotid artery territories observed within 5 hours of onset. *Arch Neurol* 1994; 51: 462-7.

25. Berge E, Abdelnoor M, Nakstad PH, Sandset PM, and on behalf of the HAEST Study Group. Low-molecular-weight heparin versus aspirin in patients with acute ischaemic stroke and atrial fibrillation: a double-blind randomised study. *Lancet* 2000; 355: 1205-10.

26. Diener HC, Ringelstein EB, von Kummer R, Langohr HD, Bewermeyer H, Landgraf H, Hennerici M, Welzel D, Grave M, Brom J, Weidinger G, and for the Therapy of Patients with Acute Ischemic Stroke (TOPAS) Investigators. Treatment of acute ischemic stroke with the low-molecular-weight heparin certoparin. *Stroke* 2001; 32: 22-9.

27. Chamorro A. Heparin in acute ischemic stroke: the case for a new clinical trial. *Cerebrovasc Dis* 1999; 9 Suppl 3: 16-23.

28. Bath P, Leonard-Bee J, Bath F. Low-molecular-weight heparin versus aspirin for acute ischemic stroke: a systematic review. *J Stroke Cerebrovasc Dis* 2002; 11: 55-62.

29. Camerlingo M, Salvi P, Belloni G, Gamba T, Cesana BM, Mamoli A. Intravenous heparin started within the first 3 hours after onset of symptoms as a treatment for acute nonlacunar hemispheric cerebral infarctions. *Stroke* 2005; 36: 2415-20.

30. The Publications Committee for the Trial of ORG 10172 in Acute Stroke Treatment (TOAST) Investigators. Low-molecular-weight heparinoid, ORG 10172 (danaparoid), and outcome after acute ischemic stroke: a randomized controlled trial. *JAMA* 1998; 279: 1265-72.

31. Wong KS, Chen C, Ng, PW, Tsoi TH, Li HL, Fong WC, Yeung J, Wong CK, Yip KK, Gao H, Wong HB. Low-molecular-weight heparin compared with aspirin for the treatment of acute ischaemic stroke in Asian patients with large artery occlusive disease: a randomised study. *Lancet Neurology* 2007; 6: 407-13.

32. Chamorro A. Heparin in acute ischemic stroke revisited. *Rev Neurol* (Paris) 2008; 164: 815-8.

33. Adams HP, Jr. Emergent use of anticoagulation for treatment of patients with ischemic stroke. *Stroke* 2002; 33: 856-61.

34. Coull BM, Williams LS, Goldstein LB, Meschia JF, Heitzman D, Chaturvedi S, Johnston KC, Starkman S, Morgenstern LB, Wilterdink JL, Levine SR, Saver JL. Anticoagulants and antiplatelet agents in acute ischemic stroke. Report of the Joint Stroke Guideline Development Committee of the American Academy of Neurology and the American Stroke Association (a division of the American Heart Association). *Neurology* 2002; 59: 13-22.

35. Counsell C, Sandercock P. Low-molecular-weight heparins or heparinoids versus standard unfractionated heparin for acute ischemic stroke (Cochrane review). *Stroke* 2002; 33: 1925-6.

36. Sandercock P, Counsell C, Stobbs SL. Low-molecular-weight heparins or heparinoids versus standard unfractionated heparin for acute ischaemic stroke. *Cochrane Database of Systematic Reviews* 2005; 2: CD 000119.

37. Adams HP, Jr., del Zoppo G, Alberts MJ, Bhatt DL, Brass L, Furlan A, Grubb RL, Higashida RT, Jauch EC, Kidwell C, Lyden PD, Morgenstern LB, Qureshi AI, Rosenwasser RH, Scott PA, Wijdicks EFM. Guidelines for the early management of adults with ischemic stroke: a guideline from the American Heart Association/American Stroke Association Stroke Council, Clinical Cardiology Council, Cardiovascular Radiology and Intervention Council, and the Atherosclerotic Peripheral Vascular Disease and Quality of Care Outcomes in Research Interdisciplinary Working Groups: the American Academy of Neurology affirms the value of this guideline as an educational tool for neurologists. *Stroke* 2007; 38: 1655-711.

38. The European Stroke Organisation (ESO) Executive Committee and the ESO Writing Committee. Guidelines for management of ischaemic stroke and transient ischaemic attack 2008. *Cerebravascular Diseases* 2008; 25: 457-507.

39. Sacco RL, Adams R, Albers G, Alberts MJ, Benavente O, Furie K, Goldstein LB, Gorelick P, Halperin J, Harbaugh R, Johnston SC, Katzan I, Kelly-Hayes M, Kenton EJ, Marks M, Schwamm LH, Tomsick T. Guidelines for Prevention of Stroke in Patients With Ischemic Stroke or Transient Ischemic Attack: A Statement for Healthcare Professionals From the American Heart Association/American Stroke Association Council on Stroke: Co-Sponsored by the Council on Cardiovascular Radiology and Intervention: The American Academy of Neurology affirms the value of this guideline. *Stroke* 2006; 37: 577-617.

40. Adams RJ, Albers G, Alberts MJ, Benavente O, Furie K, Goldstein LB, Gorelick P, Halperin J, Harbaugh R, Johnston SC, Katzan I, Kelly-Hayes M, Kenton EJ, Marks M, Sacco RL, Schwamm LH. Update to the AHA/ASA Recommendations for the Prevention of Stroke in Patients With Stroke and Transient Ischemic Attack. *Stroke* 2008; 39: 1647-52.

41. Crowther MA, Ginsberg JB, Kearon C, Harrison L, Johnson J, Massicotte MP, Hirsh J. A randomized trial comparing 5mg and 10mg warfarin loading doses. *Arch Intern Med* 1999; 159: 46-8.

42. Harrison L, Johnston M, Massicotte MP, Crowther M, Moffat K, Hirsh J. Comparison of 5mg and 10mg loading doses in initiation of warfarin therapy. *Ann Intern Med* 1997; 126: 133-6.

43. Hallevi H, *et al.* Anticoagulation after cardioembolic stroke: to bridge or not to bridge? *Arch Neurol* 2008; 65: 1169-73.

44. Grant PJ, Brotman DJ, Jaffer AK. Perioperative anticoagulant management. *Med Clin North Am* 2009; 93: 1105-21.

45. Daniels PR, McBane RD, Litin SC, Ward SA, Hodge DO, Dowling NF, Heit JA. Peri-procedural anticoagulation management of mechanical prosthetic heart valve patients. *Thromb Res* 2009; 124: 300-5.

46. Hanania G. Role of heparin in the antithrombotic treatment of valvulopathies. *J Heart Valve Dis* 2004; 13: 339-43.

47. Spyropoulos AC, Turpie AG, Dunn AS, Kaatz S, Douketis J, Jacobson A, Petersen H, REGIMENT Investigators. Perioperative bridging therapy with unfractionated heparin or low-molecular-weight heparin in patients with mechanical prosthetic heart valves on long-term oral anticoagulants (from the REGIMENT Registry). *Am J Cardiol* 2008; 102: 883-9.

48. Douketis JD, Johnson JA, Turpie AG. Low-molecular-weight heparin as bridging anticoagulation during interruption of warfarin: assessment of a standardized periprocedular anticoagulation regimen. *Arch Intern Med* 2004; 164: 1319-26.

49. Yinon Y, Siu SC, Warshafsky C, Maxwell C, McLeod A, Colman JM, Sermer M, Silversides CK. Use of molecular-weight heparin in pregnant women with mechanical heart valves. *Am J Cardiol* 2009; 104: 1259-63.

50. Helms AK, Drogan O, Kittner SJ. First trimester stroke prophylaxis in pregnant women with a history of stroke. *Stroke* 2009; 40: 1158-61.

51. Sandercock PA, van den Belt AG, Lindley RI, Slattery, J. Antithrombotic therapy in acute ischaemic stroke: an overview of the completed randomised trials. *J Neurol Neurosurg Psychiatry* 1993; 56: 17-25.

52. Sherman DG, Albers GW, Bladin C, Fieschi C, Gabbai AA, O'Riordan W, Pineo GF, Kase CS, and on behalf of the PREVAIL Investigators. The efficacy and safety of enoxaparin versus unfractionated heparin for the prevention of venous thromboembolism after acute ischaemic stroke (PREVAIL Study): an open-label randomised comparison. *Lancet* 2007; 369: 1347-55.

53. Sherman DG. Prevention of venous thromboembolism, recurrent stroke, and other vascular events after acute ischemic stroke: the role of low-molecular-weight heparin and antiplatelet therapy. *J Stroke Cerebrovasc Dis* 2006; 15: 250-9.

54. Ferro JM, Canhão P, Stam J, Bousser MG, Barinagarrementeria F, Massaro A, Ducrocq X, Kasner SE, ISCVT Investigators. Delay in the diagnosis of cerebral vein and dural sinus thrombosis: influence on outcome. *Stroke* 2009; 40: 3133-8.

55. Ferro JM, Correia M, Rosas MJ, Pinto AN, Neves G, and for the Cerebral Venous Thrombosis Portuguese Collaborative Study Group. Seizures in cerebral vein and dural sinus thrombosis. *Cerebrovasc Dis* 2003; 15: 78-83.

56. Ferro JM, Canhão P, Bousser MG, Stam J, Barinagarrementeria F, and ISCVT Investigators. Early seizures in cerebral vein and dural sinus thrombosis: risk factors and role of antiepileptics. *Stroke* 2008; 39: 1152-8.

57. Ferro JM, Canhão P, Stam J, Bousser M-G, Barinagarrementeria F, and for the ISCVT Investigators. Prognosis of cerebral vein and dural sinus thrombosis. Results of the International Study on Cerebral Vein and Dural Sinus Thrombosis (ISCVT). *Stroke* 2004; 35: 664-70.

58. Canhão P, Ferro JM, Lindgren AG, Bousser MG, Stam J, Barinagarrementeria F, and ISCVT Investigators. Causes and predictors of death in cerebral venous thrombosis. *Stroke* 2005; 36: 1720-5.

59. Girot M, Ferro JM, Canhão P, Stam J, Bousser MG, Barinagarrementeria F, Leys D and ISCVT Investigators. Predictors of outcome in patients with cerebral venous thrombosis and intracerebral hemorrhage. *Stroke* 2007; 38: 337-42.

60. Stam J. Thrombosis of the cerebral veins and sinuses. *N Engl J Med* 2005; 352: 1791-8.

61. Stam J, de Bruijn SFTM, deVeber G. Anticoagulation for cerebral sinus thrombosis. *Cochrane Database of Systematic Reviews* 2002: CD002005.

62. Einhaupl KM, Villringer A, Meister W, Mehraein S, Gamer C, Pellkofer M, Habert RL, Pfister HW, Schmiedek P. Heparin treatment in sinus venous thrombosis. *Lancet* 1991; 338: 597-600.

63. de Bruijn SF, de Haan RJ, Stam J. Clinical features and prognostic factors of cerebral venous sinus thrombosis in a prospective series of 59 patients. For The Cerebral Venous Sinus Thrombosis Study Group. *J Neurol Neurosurg Psychiatry* 2001; 70: 105-8.

64. Brucker AB, Vollert-Rogenhofer H, Wagner M, Stieglbauer K, Felber S, Trenkler J, Deisenhammer E, Aichner F. Heparin treatment in acute cerebral sinus venous thrombosis: a retrospective clinical and MR analysis of 42 cases. *Cerebrovasc Dis* 1998; 8: 331-7.

65. Mehraein S, Schmidtke K, Villringer A, Valdueza JM, Masuhr F. Heparin treatment in cerebral sinus and venous thrombosis: patients at risk of fatal outcome. *Cerebrovasc Dis* 2003; 15: 17-21.

66. Canhão P, Falcao F, Ferro JH. Thrombolytics for cerebral sinus thrombosis. *Cerebrovasc Dis* 2003; 15: 159-66.

67. Stam J, Majoie CBLM, van Delden OM, van Lienden KP, Reekers JA. Endovascular thrombectomy and thrombolysis for severe cerebral sinus thrombosis: a prospective study. *Stroke* 2008; 39: 1487-90.

68. Mohr JP, Thompson JL, Lazar RM, Levin B, Sacco RL, Furie KL, Kistler JP, Albers GW, Pettigrew LC, Adams HP, Jr., Jackson CM, Pullicino P. A comparison of warfarin and aspirin for the prevention of recurrent ischemic stroke. *N Engl J Med* 2001; 345: 1444-51.

69. Algra A, De Schryver EL, van Gijn J, Kappelle LJ, Koudstaal PJ. Oral anticoagulants versus antiplatelet therapy for preventing further vascular events after transient ischemic attack or minor stroke of presumed arterial origin. *Stroke* 2003; 34: 234-5.

70. Algra, A. Medium intensity oral anticoagulants versus aspirin after cerebral ischaemia of arterial origin (ESPRIT): a randomised controlled trial. *Lancet Neurology* 2007; 6: 115-24.

71. ESPIRIT Study Group, Halkes P, van Gijn J, Kappelle LJ, Koudstaal PJ, Algra A. Aspirin plus dipyridamole versus aspirin alone after cerebral ischaemia of arterial origin (ESPRIT): randomised controlled trial. *Lancet* 2006; 367: 1665-73.

72. Chimowitz MI, Lynn MJ, Howlett-Smith H, Stern BJ, Hertzber VS, Frankel MR, Levine SR, Chaturvedi S, Kasner SE, Benesch CG, Sila CA, Jovin TG, Romano JG. Comparison of warfarin and aspirin for symptomatic intracranial arterial stenosis. *N Engl J Med* 2006; 353: 1305-16.

73. Sacco RL, Prabhakaran S, Thompson JLP, Murphy A, Sciacca RR, Levin B, Mohr JP, WARSS Investigators. Comparison of warfarin versus aspirin for the prevention of recurrent stroke or death: subgroup analyses from the Warfarin-Aspirin Recurrent Stroke Study. *Cerebrovasc Dis* 2006; 22: 4-12.

74. Anand SS, Yusuf S. Oral anticoagulants in patients with coronary heart disease. *J Am Coll Cardiol* 2003; 41: 62S-9.

75. Debette S, Leys D. Cervical-artery dissections: predisposing factors, diagnosis, and outcome. *Lancet Neurology* 2009; 8: 668-78.

76. Georgiadis D, Arnold M, von Buedingen HC, Valko P, Sarikaya H, Rousson V, Mattle HP, Bousser MG, Baumgartner RW. Aspirin vs anticoagulation in carotid artery dissection: a study of 298 patients. *Neurology* 2009; 72: 1810-15.

77. Menon R, Kerry S, Norris JW, Markus HS, *et al*. Treatment of cervical artery dissection: a systematic review and meta-analysis. *J Neurol Neurosurg Psychiatry* 2008; 79: 1122-7.

78. The CADISS Trial Investigators antiplatelet therapy vs. anticoagulation in cervical artery dissection: rationale and design of the Cervical Artery Dissection in Stroke Study (CADISS). *Int J Stroke* 2007; 2: 292-6.

79. Thenappan T, Ali Raza J, Movahed A. Aortic atheromas: current concepts and controversies - a review of the literature. *Echocardiography* 2008; 25: 198-207.

80. Zavala JA, Amarenco P, Davis SM, Jones EF, Young D, Macleod MR, Horky LL, Donnan GA. Aortic arch atheroma. *Int J Stroke* 2006; 1: 74-80.

81. Di Tullio MR, Russo C, Jin Z, Sacco RL, Mohr JP, Homma S, Patent Foramen Ovale in Cryptogenic Stroke Study Investigators. Aortic arch plaques and risk of recurrent stroke and death. *Circulation* 2009; 119: 2376-82.

82. Tunick PA, Nayar AC, Goodkin GM, Mirchandani S, Francescone S, Rosenzweig BP, Freedberg RS, Katz ES, Applebaum RM, Kronzon I, and NYU Atheroma Group. Effect of treatment on the incidence of stroke and other emboli in 519 patients with severe thoracic aortic plaque. *Am J Cardiol* 2002; 90: 1320-5.

83. Roach ES, Golomb MR, Adams R, Biller J, Daniels S, deVeber G, Ferriero D, Jones BV, Kirkham FJ, Scott RM, Smith ER. Management of stroke in infants and children: a scientific statement from a special writing group of the American Heart Association Stroke Council and the Council on Cardiovascular Disease in the Young. *Stroke* 2008; 39: 2644-91.

84. Bernard TJ, Goldenberg NA, Tripputi M, Manco-Johnson MJ, Niederstadt T, Nowak-Gottl U. Anticoagulation in childhood-onset arterial ischemic stroke with nonmoyamoya arteriopathy: findings from the Colorado and German (COAG) Collaboration. *Stroke* 2009; 40(8): 2869-71.

85. Salem DN, O'Gara PT, Madias C, Pauker SG, and American College of Chest Physicians. Valvular and structural heart disease: American College of Chest Physicians, Evidence-Based Clinical Practice Guidelines (8th Edition). *Chest* 2008; 133: 593S-629.

86. Singer DE, Chang Y, Fang MC, Borowsky LH, Pomernacki NK, Udaltsova N, Go AS. Should patient characteristics influence target anticoagulation intensity for stroke prevention in nonvalvular atrial fibrillation?: the ATRIA Study. *Circ Cardiovasc Qual Outcomes* 2009; 2: 297-304.

87. Fang MC, Go AS, Chang Y, Hylek EM, Henault LE, Jensvold NG, Singer DE. Death and disability from warfarin-associated intracranial and extracranial hemorrhages. *Am J Med* 2007; 120: 700-5.

88. Petty GW, Lennihan L, Mohr JP, Hauser WA, Weitz J, Owen J, Towey C. Complications of long-term anticoagulation. *Ann Neurol* 1988; 23: 570-4.

89. Dimarco JP, Flaker G, Waldo AL, Corley SD, Greene HL, Safford RE, Rosenfeld LE, Mitrani G, Nemeth M, and AFFIRM Investigators. Factors affecting bleeding risk during anticoagulant therapy in patients with atrial fibrillation: observations from the atrial fibrillation follow-up investigation of rhythm management (AFFIRM) study. *Am Heart J* 2005; 149: 650-6.

90. Jacobs LG, Billett HH, Freeman K, Dinglas C, Jumaquio L. Anticoagulation for stroke prevention in elderly patients with atrial fibrillation, including those with falls and/or early-stage dementia: a single-center, retrospective, observational study. *Am J Geriatr Pharmacother* 2009; 7: 159-66.

91. Mant J, Hobbs FD, Fletcher K, Roalfe A, Fitzmaurice D, Lip GY, Murray E, BAFTA investigators, and Midland Research Practices Network (MidReC). Warfarin versus aspirin for stroke prevention in an elderly community population with atrial fibrillation (the Birmingham Atrial Fibrillation Treatment of the Aged Study, BAFTA): a randomised controlled trial. *Lancet* 2007; 370: 493-503.

92. Rash A, Downes T, Portner R, Yeo WW, Morgan N, Channer KS. A randomised controlled trial of warfarin versus aspirin for stroke prevention in octogenarians with atrial fibrillation (WASPO). *Age Ageing* 2007; 36: 117-9.

93. Petersen P, Boysen G, Godtfredsen J, Andersen ED, Andersen B. Placebo-controlled, randomised trial of warfarin and aspirin for prevention of thromboembolic complications in chronic atrial fibrillation. The Copenhagen AFASAK study. *Lancet* 1989; 1: 175-9.

94. The Boston Area Anticoagulation Trial for Atrial Fibrillation Investigators. The effect of low-dose warfarin on the risk of stroke in patients with nonrheumatic atrial fibrillation. *N Engl J Med* 1990; 323: 1505-11.

95. Stroke Prevention in Atrial Fibrillation Investigators. Stroke Prevention in Atrial Fibrillation study. Final results. *Circulation* 1991; 84: 527-39.

96. Stroke Prevention in Atrial Fibrillation Investigators. Warfarin versus aspirin for prevention of thromboembolism in atrial fibrillation: Stroke Prevention in Atrial Fibrillation II Study. *Lancet* 1994; 343: 687-91.

97. Stroke Prevention in Atrial Fibrillation Investigators. Adjusted-dose warfarin versus low-intensity, fixed-dose warfarin plus aspirin for high-risk patients with atrial fibrillation: Stroke Prevention in Atrial Fibrillation III randomised clinical trial. *Lancet* 1996; 348: 633-8.

98. Connolly SJ, Laupacis A, Gent M, Roberts RS, Cairns JA, Joyner C. Canadian Atrial Fibrillation Anticoagulation (CAFA) Study. *J Am Coll Cardiol* 1991; 18: 349-55.

99. Gullov AL, Koefoed BG, Petersen P, Pedersen TS, Andersen ED, Godtfredsen J, Boysen G. Fixed minidose warfarin and aspirin alone and in combination vs. adjusted-dose warfarin for stroke prevention in atrial fibrillation: Second Copenhagen Atrial Fibrillation, Aspirin, and Anticoagulation Study. *Arch Intern Med* 1998; 158: 1513-21.

100. Morocutti C, Amabile G, Fattapposta F, Nicolosi A, Matteoli S, Trappolini M, Cataldo G, Milanesi G, Lavezzari M, Pamparana F, Coccheri S. Indobufen versus warfarin in the secondary prevention of major vascular events in nonrheumatic atrial fibrillation. SIFA (Studio Italiano Fibrillazione Atriale) Investigators. *Stroke* 1997; 28: 1015-21.

101. ACTIVE Investigators, Connolly SJ, Pogue J, Hart RG, Hohnloser SH, Pfeffer M, Chrolavicius S, Yusuf S. Effect of clopidogrel added to aspirin in patients with atrial fibrillation. *N Engl J Med* 2009; 360: 2066-78.

102. Pengo V, Barbero F, Biasiolo A, Pegoraro C, Noventa F, Ilceto S. Prevention of thromboembolism in patients with mitral stenosis and associated atrial fibrillation: effectiveness of low intensity (INR target 2) oral anticoagulant treatment. *Thromb Haemost* 2003; 89: 760-4.

103. Poli D, Antonucci E, Grifoni E, Abbate R, Gensini GF, Prisco D. Stroke risk in atrial fibrillation patients on warfarin. Predictive ability of risk stratification schemes for primary and secondary prevention. *Thromb Haemost* 2009; 101: 367-72.

104. EAFT (European Atrial Fibrillation Trial) Study Group. Secondary prevention in non-rheumatic atrial fibrillation after transient ischaemic attack or minor stroke. *Lancet* 1993; 342: 1255-62.

105. Petersen P, Grind M, Adler J, and SPORTIF II Investigators. Ximelagatran versus warfarin for stroke prevention in patients with nonvalvular atrial fibrillation. SPORTIF II: a dose-guiding tolerability, and safety study. *J Am Coll Cardiol* 2003; 41: 1445-51.

106. Akins PT, Feldman HA, Zoble RG, Newman D, Spitzer SG, Diener HC, Albers GW. Secondary stroke prevention with ximelagatran versus warfarin in patients with atrial fibrillation: pooled analysis of SPORTIF III and V clinical trials. *Stroke* 2007; 38: 874-80.

107. Albers GW, Diener HC, Frison L, Grind M, Nevinson M, Partridge S, Halperin JL, Horrow J, Olsson SB, Petersen P, Vahanian A, and SPORTIF Executive Steering Committee for the SPORTIF V Investigators. Ximelagatran vs. warfarin for stroke prevention in patients with nonvalvular atrial fibrillation: a randomized trial. *JAMA* 2005; 293: 690-8.

108. Diener H-C and Executive Steering Committee on behalf of the SPORTIF III and V Investigators. Stroke prevention using the oral direct thrombin inhibitor ximelagatran in patients with non-valular atrial fibrillation. *Cerebrovasc Dis* 2006; 21: 279-93.

109. Ford GA, Choy AM, Deedwania P, Karalis DG, Lindholm CJ, Pluta W, Frison L, Olsson SB, and on behalf of the SPORTIF III. Direct thrombin inhibition and stroke prevention in elderly patients with atrial fibrillation: experience from the SPORTIF III and V trials. *Stroke* 2007; 38: 2965-71.

110. Connolly SJ, Ezekowitz MD, Yusuf S, Eikelboom J, Oldgren J, Parekh A, Pogue J, Reilly PA, Themeles E, Varrone J, Wang S, Xavier D, Diaz R, Lewis BS, Darius H, Diener HC, Joyner CD, Wallentin L, RE-LY Steering Committee and Investigators. Dabigatran versus warfarin in patients with atrial fibrillation. *N Engl J Med* 2009; 361: 1139-51.

111. Sacco RL, Adams R, Albers G, Alberts MJ, Benavente O, Furie K, Goldstein LB, Gorelick P, Halperin J, Harbaugh R, Johnston SC, Katzan I, Kelly-Hayes M, Kenton EJ, Marks M, Schwamm LH, Tomsick T. Guidelines for Prevention of Stroke in Patients With Ischemic Stroke or Transient Ischemic Attack: A Statement for Healthcare Professionals from the American Heart Association/American Stroke Association Council on Stroke: Co-Sponsored by the Council on Cardiovascular Radiology and Intervention: The American Academy of Neurology affirms the value of this guideline. *Stroke* 2006; 37: 577-617.

112. Aguilar MI, Hart R. Oral anticoagulants versus antiplatelet therapy for preventing stroke in patients with nonvalvular atrial fibrillation and no history of stroke or transient ischemic attacks. *Stroke* 2008; 39: 1399-400.

113. Andersen LV, Vestergaard P, Deichgraeber P, Lindholt JS, Mortensen LS, Frost L. Warfarin for the prevention of systemic embolism in patients with nonvalvular atrial fibrillation: a meta-analysis. *Heart* 2008; 94; 1607-13.

114. Singer DE, Albers GW, Dalen JE, Fang MC, Go AS, Halperin JL, Lip GY, Manning WJ. Antithrombotic therapy in atrial fibrillation: American College of Chest Physicians Evidence-Based Clinical Practice Guidelines (8th Edition). *Chest* 2008; 133: 546S-92.

115. Healey JS, Hart RG, Pogue J, Pfeffer MA, Hohnloser SH, De Caterina R, Flaker G, Yusuf S, Connolly SJ. Risks and benefits of oral anticoagulation compared with clopidogrel plus aspirin in patients with atrial fibrillation according to stroke risk: the Atrial Fibrillation Clopidogrel Trial With Irbesartan for Prevention of Vascular Events (ACTIVE-W). *Stroke* 2008; 39: 1482-6.

116. Gallagher MM, Hennessy BJ, Edvardsson N, Hart CM, Shannon MS, Obel OA, Al-Saady NM, Camm AJ. Embolic complications of direct current cardioversion of atrial arrhythmias: association with low intensity of anticoagulation at the time of cardioversion. *J Am Coll Cardiol* 2002; 40: 926-33.

117. Albers GW, Amarenco P, Easton JD, Sacco RL, Teal P. Antithrombotic and thrombolytic therapy for ischemic stroke: American College of Chest Physicians evidence-based clinical practice guidelines (8th edition). *Chest* 2008; 133: 630S-69.

118. Hart RG. Atrial fibrillation and stroke prevention. *N Engl J Med* 2003; 349: 1015-6.

119. Feinberg WM, Albers GW, Barnett HJ. Guidelines for the management of transient ischemic attacks. *Stroke* 1994; 25: 1320-35.

120. Salem DN, Levine HJ, Pauker SG, Eckman MH, Daudelin DH. Antithrombotic therapy in valvular heart disease. *Chest* 1998; 114: 590S-601.

121. McCabe DJ, Rakhit RD. Antithrombotic and interventional treatment options in cardioembolic transient ischaemic attack and ischaemic stroke. *J Neurol Neurosurg Psychiatry* 2007; 78: 14-24.

122. Pullicino P, Thompson JLP, Mohr JP, Sacco RL, Freudenberger R, Levin B, Homma S. Oral anticoagulation in patients with cardiomyopathy or heart failure in sinus rhythm. *Cerebrovasc Dis* 2008; 26: 322-7.

123. Massie BM, Collins JF, Ammon SE, Armstrong PW, Cleland JGF, Ezekowitz M, Jafri SM, Krol WF, O'Connor CM, Teo K, Warren SR, and for the WATCH Trial Investigators. Randomized trial of warfarin, aspirin, and clopidogrel in patients with chronic heart failure. *Circulation* 2009; 119: 1616-24.

124. Homma S, Di Tullio MR, Sciacca RR, Sacco RL, Mohr JP, and PICSS Investigators. Effect of aspirin and warfarin therapy in stroke patients with valvular strands. *Stroke* 2004; 35: 1436-42.

125. Vaitkus PT, Barnathan ES. Embolic potential, prevention and management of mural thrombus complicating anterior myocardial infarction: a meta-analysis. *J Am Coll Cardiol* 1993; 22: 1004-9.

126. Voller H. Antithrombotic therapy in native heart valve disease. *J Heart Valve Dis* 2004; 13: 325-8.

127. Poungvarin N, Opartkiattikul N, Chaithiaraphan S, Viriyavejakul A. A comparative study of coumadin and aspirin for primary cardioembolic stroke and thromboembolic preventions of chronic rheumatic mitral stenosis with atrial fibrillation. *J Med Assoc Thai* 1994; 77: 1-6.

128. Perez-Gomez F, Salvador A, Zumalde J, Iriarte JA, Berjon J, Alegria E, Almeria C, Bover R, Herrera D, Fernandez C. Effect of antithrombotic therapy in patients with mitral stenosis and atrial fibrillation: a sub-analysis of NASPEAF randomized trial. *Eur Heart J* 2006; 27: 960-7.

129. Wada Y, Mizushige K, Ohmori K, Iwado Y, Kohno M, Matsuo H. Prevention of cerebral thromboembolism by low-dose anticoagulant therapy in atrial fibrillation with mitral regurgitation. *J Cardiovasc Pharmacol* 2001; 37: 422-6.

130. Tiede DJ, Nishimura RA, Gastineau DA, Mullany CJ, Orszulak TA, Schaff HV. Modern management of prosthetic valve anticoagulation. *Mayo Clin Proc* 1998; 73: 665-80.

131. Azar AJ, Koudstaal PJ, Wintzen AR, van Bergen PF, Jonker JJ, Deckers JW. Risk of stroke during long-term anticoagulant therapy in patients after myocardial infarction. *Ann Neurol* 1996; 39: 301-7.

132. Stewart RA. Clinical trials in heart valve disease. *Curr Opin Cardiol* 2009; 24: 279-87.

133. O'Connor CM, Gattis WA, Hellkamp AS, Langer A, Larsen RL, Harrington RA, Berkowitz SD, O'Gara PT, Kopecky SL, Gheorghiade M, Daly R, Califf RM, Fuster V. Comparison of two aspirin doses on ischemic stroke in post-myocardial infarction patients in the warfarin (Coumadin) Aspirin Reinfarction Study (CARS). *Am J Cardio* 2001; 88: 541-6.

134. Massel D, Little SH. Risks and benefits of adding anti-platelet therapy to warfarin among patients with prosthetic heart valves: a meta-analysis. *J Am Coll Cardiol* 2001; 37: 569-78.

135. Colli A, Fragnito C, Nicolini F, Borrello B, Saccani S, D'Amico R, Beghi C. Comparing warfarin with aspirin after biological aortic valve replacement: a prospective study. *Circulation* 2004; 110: 496-500.

136. Meissner I. The management of patients with patent foramen ovale and stroke. *Curr Treat Options Neurol* 2005; 7: 483-90.

137. Homma S, Sacco R, Di Tuillo M, Sciacca R, Mohr JP, and for the PFO in Cryptogenic Stroke Study (PICSS) Investigators. Effect of medical treatment in stroke patients with patent foramen ovale. Patent Foramen Ovale In Cryptogenic Stroke Study. *Circulation* 2002; 105: 2625-31.

138. Mas JL, Arquizan C, Lamy C, Zuber M, Cabanes L, Derumeaux G, Coste J, and Patent Foramen Ovale and Atrial Septal Aneurysm Study Group. Recurrent cerebrovascular events associated with patent foramen ovale, atrial septal aneurysm, or both. *N Engl J Med* 2001; 345: 1740-6.

139. Handke M, Harloff A, Olschewski H, Hetzel A, Geibel A. Patent foramen ovale and cryptogenic stroke in older patients. *N Engl J Med* 2007; 357: 2262-8.

140. Messe SR, Silverman IE, Kizer JR, Homma S, Zahn C, Gronseth G, Kasner SE, and Quality Standards Subcommittee of the American Academy of Neurology Practice parameter: recurrent stroke with patent foramen ovale and atrial septal aneurysm: report of the Quality Standards Subcommittee of the American Academy of Neurology. *Neurology* 2004; 62: 1042-50.

141. Okajima K, Abe Y, Suzuki K, Salameh MJ, Di Tullio MR, Jin Z, Sacco RL, Mohr JP, Homma S. Impact of valvular thickness on stroke recurrence in medically treated patients with stroke. *Cerebrovasc Dis* 2007; 24: 375-80.

142. Sobieraj-Teague M, O'Donnell M, Eikelboom J. New anticoagulants for atrial fibrillation. *Semin Thromb Hemost* 2009; 35: 515-24.

143. Tangelder MJ, Frison L, Weaver D, Wilcox RG, Bylock A, Emanuelsson H, Held P, Oldgren J. Effect of ximelagatran on ischemic events and death in patients with atrial fibrillation after acute myocardial infarction in the efficacy and safety of the oral direct thrombin inhibitor ximelagatran in patients with recent myocardial damage (ESTEEM) trial. *Am Heart J* 2008; 155: 382-7.

144. Connolly SJ, Ezekowitz MD, Yusuf S, Eikelboom J, Oldgren J, Parekh A, Pogue J, Reilly PA, Themeles E, Varrone J, Wang S, Alings M, Xavier D, Zhu J, Diaz R, Lewis BS, Darius H, Diener H-C, Joyner CD, Wallentin L, and the RE-LY Steering Committee and Investigators. Dabigatran versus warfarin in patients with atrial fibrillation. *N Engl J Med* 2009; 361: 1139-51.

145. Ezekowitz MD, Koti MJ, Fulton B. Reducing stroke rates in patients with atrial fibrillation. How long can we go? *Circulation* 2009; 120: 1169-70.

146. Hankey GJ, Eikelboom JW. Antithrombotic drugs for patients with ischaemic stroke and transient ischaemic attack to prevent recurrent major vascular events. *Lancet Neurol* 2010; 9: 273-84.

147. Ellis DJ, Usman MH, Milner PG, Canafax DM, Ezekowitz MD. The first evaluation of a novel vitamin K antagonist, tecarfarin (ATI-5923), in patients with atrial fibrillation. *Circulation* 2009; 120: 1029-35.

148. Adams RJ, Pavlakis S, Roach ES. Sickle cell disease and stroke: primary prevention and transcranial Doppler. *Ann Neurol* 2003; 54: 559-63.

149. Baker WF Jr., Bick RL, Fareed J. Controversies and unresolved issues in antiphospholipid syndrome pathogenesis and management. *Hematol Oncol Clin North Am* 2008; 22: 155-74.

150. Cervera R, Khamashta MA, Shoenfeld Y, Camps MT, Jacobsen S, Kiss E, Zeher MM, Tincani A, Kontopoulou-Griva I, Galeazzi M, Bellisai F, Meroni PL, Derksen RH, de Groot PG, Gromnica-Ihle E, Baleva M, Mosca M, Bombardieri S, Houssiau F, Gris JC, Quere I, Hachulla E, Vasconcelos C, Roch B, Fernandez-Nebro A, Piette J-C, Espinosa G, Bucciarelli S, Pisoni CN, Bertolaccini ML, Boffa MC, Hughes GR, and Euro-Phospholipid Project Group. Morbidity and mortality in the antiphospholipid syndrome during a 5-year period: a multicentre prospective study of 1000 patients. *Ann Rheum Dis* 2009; 68: 1428-32.

151. Finazzi G, Marchioli R, Brancaccio V, Wisloff F, Musial J, Baudo F, Berrettini M, Testai FD, D'Angelo A, Tognoni G, Barbui T. A randomized clinical trial of high-intensity warfarin vs. conventional antithrombotic therapy for the prevention of recurrent thrombosis in patients with the antiphospholipid syndrome (WAPS). *J Thromb Haemost* 2005; 3: 848-53.

152. Levine SR, Brey RL, Tilley BC, Thompson JL, Sacco RL, Sciacca RR, Murphy A, Lu Y, Costigan TM, Rhine C, Levin B, Triplett DA, Mohr JP, and APASS Investigators. Antiphospholipid antibodies and subsequent thrombo-occlusive events in patients with ischemic stroke. *JAMA* 2004; 291: 576-84.

153. Rajamani K, Chaturvedi S, Jin Z, Homma S, Brey RL, Tilley BC, Sacco RL, Thompson JL, Mohr JP, Levine SR, and PICSS-APASS Investigators. Patent foramen ovale, cardiac valve thickening, and antiphospholipid

antibodies as risk factors for subsequent vascular events: the PICSS-APASS Study. *Stroke* 2009; 40: 2337-42.

154. Lim W, Crowther MA, Eikelboom JW. Management of antiphospholipid antibody syndrome: a systematic review. *JAMA* 2006; 295: 1050-7.

155. Ruiz-Irastorza G, Khamashta MA, Hunt BJ, Escudero A, Cuadrado MJ, Hughes GR. Bleeding and recurrent thrombosis in definite antiphospholipid syndrome: analysis of a series of 66 patients treated with oral anticoagulation to a target International Normalized Ratio of 3.5. *Arch Intern Med* 2002; 162: 1164-9.

156. Debourdeau P, Elalamy I, de Raignac A, Meria P, Gornet JM, Amah Y, Korte W, Marty M, Farge D. Long-term use of daily subcutaneous low-molecular-weight heparin in cancer patients with venous thromboembolism: Why hesitate any longer? *Support Care Cancer* 2008; 16: 1333-41.

157. Chamorro A, Vila N, Saiz A, Alday M, Tolosa E. Early anticoagulation after large cerebral embolic infarction: a safety study. *Neurology* 1995; 45: 861-5.

158. Chamorro A, Busse O, Obach V, Toni D, Reverter JC, Cervera A, Torres F, Dávalos A, and RAPID Investigators. The Rapid Anticoagulation Prevents Ischemic Damage study in acute stroke - final results from the Writing Committee. *Cerebravascular Diseases* 2005; 19: 402-4.

159. Wong KS, Chen C, Ng PW, Tsoi TH, Li H-L, Fong WC, Yeung J, Wong CK, Yip KK, Gao H, Wong HB, and the FISS-tris Study Investigators. Low-molecular-weight heparin compared with aspirin for the treatment of acute ischaemic stroke in Asian patients with large artery occlusive disease: a randomised study. *Lancet* 2007; 6: 407-13.

160. Diener HC, Alkhedr A, Busse O, Hacke W, Zingmark PH, Jonsson N, *et al.* Treatment of acute ischaemic stroke with the low-affinity, use-dependent NMDA antagonist AR-R15896AR: a safety and tolerability study. *J Neurol* 2002; 249: 518-28.

161. Bath PM, Lindenstrom E, Boysen G, De Deyn P, Friis P, Leys D, Marttila R, Olsson J, O'Neill D, Orgogozo J, Ringelstein B, van der Sande J, Turpie AG. Tinzaparin in Acute Ischaemic Stroke (TAIST): a randomised aspirin-controlled trial. *Lancet* 2001; 358: 683-4.

162. The Stroke Prevention in Reversible Ischemia Trial (SPIRIT) Study Group. A randomized trial of anticoagulants versus aspirin after cerebral ischemia of presumed arterial origin. *Ann Neurol* 1997; 42: 857-65.

163. Chimowitz MI, Lynn MJ, Howlett-Smith H, Stern BJ, Hertzberg VS, Frankel MR, Levine SR, Chaturvedi S, Kasner SE, Benesch CG, Sila CA, Jovin TG, Romano JG, and the Warfarin-Aspirin Symptomatic Intracranial Disease Trial. Comparison of warfarin and aspirin for symptomatic intracranial arterial stenosis. *N Engl J Med* 2005; 352: 1305-16.

164. The SPAF III Writing Committee for the Stroke Prevention in Atrial Fibrillation Patients with nonvalvular atrial fibrillation at low risk of stroke during treatment with aspirin: Stroke Prevention in Atrial Fibrillation III Study. Investigators. *JAMA* 1998; 279: 1273-7.

165. Ezekowitz MD, Bridgers SL, James KE, Carliner NH, Colling CL, Gornick CC, Krause-Steinrauf H, Kurtzke JF, Nazarian SM, Radford MJ. Warfarin in the prevention of stroke associated with nonrheumatic atrial fibrillation. Veterans Affairs Stroke Prevention in Nonrheumatic Atrial Fibrillation Investigators. *N Engl J Med* 1992; 327: 1406-12.

166. Hellemons BS, Langenberg M, Lodder J, Vermeer F, Schouten HJ, Lemmens T, van Ree JW, Knottnerus JA. Primary prevention of arterial thromboembolism in non-rheumatic atrial fibrillation in primary care: randomized controlled trial comparing two intensities of coumarin with aspirin. *BMJ* 1999; 319: 958-64.

167. Pengo V, Zasso A, Barbero F, Banzato A, Nante G, Parissenti L, John Noventa F, Dalla VS. Effectiveness of fixed minidose warfarin in the prevention of thromboembolism and vascular death in nonrheumatic atrial fibrillation. *Am J Cardio* 1998; 82: 433-7.

Chapter 5

Interventions for acute ischemic stroke

Gabriel A. Smith BS, Medical Student
Temple University School of Medicine, Philadelphia, USA

Zakaria Hakma MD, Chief Neurosurgical Resident, Department
of Neurosurgery, Temple University Hospital, Philadelphia, USA

Christopher M. Loftus MD Dr. h.c. FACS, Professor and Chairman of the Department
of Neurosurgery, Temple University Hospital; Chairman of the AANS International
Outreach Committee; WFNS Assistant Treasurer; and Assistant Dean for
International Affiliations, Temple University School of Medicine, Philadelphia, USA

Introduction

The World Health Organization (WHO) estimates 15 million people suffer new strokes every year, and 55 million people globally have had a stroke in their lifetime with or without residual disability [1, 2]. In 2005, it was estimated 5.8 million people died worldwide, and strokes accounted for nearly 10% of all deaths second only to heart disease [1]. Stroke is also a leading cause of serious long-term disability in the world [2]. The 1-year mortality rate of stroke victims age >40 in 2010 was estimated at 20-25% with the median survival time of 6.8-7.4 years [3, 4]. Moderate-severe disability at discharge was 30% in the United States based on stroke registries, and at 6 months >20% of all patients were still disabled in an analysis of patients in the Framingham Heart Study [3-5]. There is no doubt that improvements in prevention, access to care, interventional techniques, management, and rehabilitation are worthwhile clinical goals.

Clinical and radiographic assessment

A thorough and focused evaluation must be conducted on all potential stroke victims. The National Institute of Neurological Disorders and Stroke (NINDS) study group and the AHA recommend time-sensitive guidelines in the evaluation of stroke victims [6-9]. The single most important piece of history is the time of symptom onset and duration since the patient was at their baseline [9, 10]. In the NINDS trial, poor outcomes defined as a modified Rankin Scale (mRS) >3 (Table 1) at 24 hours were most likely for stroke victims with NIHSS scores >22 or >17 plus atrial fibrillation with a positive predictive value (PPV) of 98%; 95% CI, 93-100% and PPV 96%; 95% CI, 88-100%, respectively [11, 12].

Table 1. The modified Rankin Scale (mRS). *Adapted from the NINDS Study Group* [6].	
0	No residual symptoms. Able to carry out all independent activities required for daily living (IADLS)
1	No significant disability. Can carry out IADLS, despite some symptoms
2	Slight disability. Unable to carry out all previous activities, can perform most IADLS
3	Moderate disability. Requires assistance with IADLS, but able to walk unassisted
4	Moderate-severe disability. Unable to attend to own bodily needs without assistance, and unable to walk
5	Severe disability. Requires constant nursing care and attention
6	Death

Non-contrast CT and multimodal CT imaging

Radiographic imaging plays an ever-increasing role in the evaluation of stroke victims. Findings including infarct size, location, vascular distribution, and coexisting hemorrhage affect both short and long-term treatment [13-15]. A non-contrast CT (NCCT) is the initial rapid study of choice to differentiate intracranial pathology such as tumors, intracerebral hemorrhage (ICH), subarachnoid hemorrhage (SAH), and ischemia. With enhancements in CT imaging, quantification of ischemia or hyperattenuation suggestive of arterial occlusion have now become possible within 6 hours of symptom onset in the anterior circulation, and are associated with poor outcomes [16-19]. However, up to 40% of stroke patients have a normal scan within the first few hours, and subtle signs of ischemia can be missed on NCCT imaging [20, 21].

Recent advancements allow for multimodal CT imaging, including NCCT, perfusion CT (CTP), and CT angiography (CTA) studies. Whole-brain CTP provides subtle signs delineating irreversible and reversible ischemia in the cerebral vasculature map with a high degree of sensitivity and specificity [22-25]. Bordering salvageable zones of the central infarcted core may show autoregulation with normal or increased cerebral blood volume (CBV) [15, 26, 27]. However, when cerebral blood flow (CBF) drops below a critical level of <20%, autoregulation begins to fail with a decline in CBV, transitioning to irreversible ischemia [28-30]. No cut-offs exist delineating salvageable tissue, but a marked decline in CBF with CBV, reduced time to peak perfusion (TTP), and mean transit time (MTT) >6 seconds indicate irreversible ischemia [28-32].

Helical CTA can provide information about the presence of proximal vessel occlusions, stenosis, and dictate potential local intra-arterial therapeutics [25, 33]. Thus, in <15 minutes multimodal CT imaging may predict salvageable tissue areas, elucidate which therapies the patient could benefit from, and is the most cost-effective imaging available.

Multimodal MRI imaging

In comparison with CT, multimodal MRI imaging including diffusion-weighted imaging (DWI), perfusion-weighted imaging (PWI), MR angiography (MRA), and gradient echo sequences allows visualization of ischemic regions within 20 minutes of symptom onset, predicts hemodynamic status of proximal and distal vessels with a sensitivity of 70-100%, assesses volumes of chronic infarcts, and has a sensitivity of 88-100% and specificity of 95-100% for strokes including smaller subcortical and posterior fossa infarcts [34-41]. MRI gradient sequences demonstrate hyperacute intraparenchymal hemorrhage within 6 hours of symptom onset, and are more accurate than multimodal CT when confounded with chronic hemorrhage, all factors supporting the utility of MRI evaluation of ischemia alone once SAH is ruled out [42, 43]. When considering the choice of ideal imaging options for stroke, we must consider that MRI has better localization of smaller infarcts, is equivalent in ruling out ICH, and can predict salvageable tissue volumes [24, 40, 44, 45]. The limitations of MRI in the acute setting include cost, contraindications such as pacemakers, and relative limited availability.

Anterior circulation ischemic strokes

Intravenous (IV) rt-PA

Ischemic stroke is a devastating disease. Until 2004, the only FDA-approved treatment was intravenous thrombolytics within 3 hours of symptom onset **(Ia/A)** [7, 46-53]. Recent data suggest that this window may be extended to 4.5 hours or longer but with a decline in functional recovery rates **(Ia/A)** [54-56]. In the NINDS rt-PA stroke trial, patients treated <3 hours from symptom onset had a 31-50% versus 20-38% improvement in >4 points on the NIHSS or complete recovery at 3-month and 1-year follow-up [6, 49, 50, 57]. The major risk of treatment is ICH with an increased risk of 5.8%; however, follow-up data suggest no effect on mortality at 3 months [6, 11]. The NINDS investigators also reported a time-to-treatment recommendation to improve functional outcomes (Table 2).

Patients receiving treatment within 90 minutes of symptom onset had an odds ratio (OR) of 2.11 (CI 95%, 1.33-3.55), and 90-180 minutes an OR of 1.69 (95% CI, 1.09-2.62), for favorable outcomes at 3 months defined by an >4 point decline on the NIHSS [6]. The ECASS trials in Europe had similar results in post hoc analysis for patients receiving rt-PA within 4.5 hours [7, 47, 48, 54, 55]. Thus, current recommendations are for time-sensitive treatment protocols for early rt-PA therapy **(Ia/A)**.

Table 2. Time targets for organized triage of acute stroke patients. *Adapted from the NINDS Study Group* [6].	
0-10 min	Door-to-doctor
10-25 min	Door-to-CT completed
25-45 min	Door-to-CT read
45-60 min	Door-to-thrombolytic therapy
1-2 hours	Neurosurgical consult
1-3 hours	Admission to monitored bed

Beyond IV rt-PA – intra-arterial (IA) rt-PA and combination therapy

A recent meta-analysis by Rha *et al*, suggests that recanalization alone is associated with a 4- to 5-fold increase in odds of good functional outcome and a 4- to 5-fold reduction in death [58] **(Ib/A)**. However, only 19-60% of stroke patients present within 3 hours, and moreover, only 14-32% arrive within 2 hours of symptom onset [9]. In Canada, in a retrospective cohort of 1806 patients admitted for stroke, only 4.7% received IV rt-PA due to time window constraints and exclusion criteria [59]. Thus, new research into alternatives to IV rt-PA such as intra-arterial recanalization/reperfusion strategies and combination therapies are under investigation to improve vessel patency, and hopefully, functional outcomes.

Numerous studies point out recanalization/reperfusion correlates with functional outcome in IA thrombolytic therapy response [60-62] **(IIa/B)**. In the multicenter, randomized controlled trial, Prolyse in Acute Cerebral Thromboembolism (PROACT) trials, 40% of patients receiving IA thrombolysis versus 24% of control patients receiving IV heparin had a mRS score of 0-2 at 90 days when administered <6 hours of symptom onset [63-65]. Moreover, >66% of patients had recanalization of occluded vessels in comparison to IV rt-PA estimations of 31-35% seen in M1 occlusions {275 del Zoppo GJ 1998; 222 Furlan A. 1999; 453 Ng PP 2004; 451 Demchuk AM 2001; 452 Demchuk AM 2001} **(IIa/B)**. Another retrospective cohort from Japan's Multicenter Stroke Investigators' Collaboration (J-MUSIC) showed 91 patients receiving intra-arterial urokinase (IA UK) within 4.5 hours with an NIHSS score of 5-22 on admission compared to a 182 patient control group with similar NIHSS scores had favorable outcomes more frequently, 50.5% to 34.1% (p=0.0124) [66]. These studies support the safety and efficacy of IA rt-PA for acute ischemic stroke treatment within a 6-hour window from symptom onset in patients ineligible for IV rt-PA **(IIa/B)**.

Moreover, studies show IA rt-PA establishes recanalization in comparison to IV rt-PA more effectively in situations where the clot burden is extremely high such as in carotid 'T' emboli, M1 occlusions, or complete acute carotid occlusions [61, 67-69] **(IIb/B)**. In conclusion, IA rt-PA is an alternative with good recanalization rates, functional outcome, expands the treatment window, and may benefit patients with radiologic evidence of a large clot burden **(IIa/B)**.

Combination therapy – IV rt-PA and IA rt-PA

Although IA rt-PA is effective, it remains time-to-treatment sensitive like IV rt-PA. The time delay required for cerebral angiography, microcatheter position, and long infusion times, have made IA rt-PA administration difficult within the proven greatest therapeutic window of <3 hours. Thus, combination therapy with IV rt-PA, allowing immediate initiation of thrombolysis followed by local IA rt-PA or clot retrieval is under investigation. Zaidat *et al*, in an IV/IA rt-PA versus IA rt-PA controlled trial showed 96 patients had recanalization in 69% versus 55%, and had good outcome versus all others with an OR of 3.9 (95% CI, 1.4-11.2; p=0.007) [61]. The complication rate of ICH with recanalization was 13.3% versus 7.6% and mortality rates were 33.3% versus 19.7%. In subgroup analysis, the degree of recanalization was directly related to time to therapy and associated with good clinical outcome. The Emergency Management of Stroke Bridging Trial initially showed no differences when combination IV/IA rt-PA was administered even though 70% of patients receiving IV rt-PA alone still had angiographically confirmed residual thrombus [70]. However, the recent Interventional Management of Stroke (IMS) trials have proven otherwise [71-73]. Eighty patients who were administered IV rt-PA within 3 hours of deficit onset and IA rt-PA over the subsequent 2 hours with a median NIHSS score of 18 compared to the NINDS trial placebo arm had better outcomes, 56% to 20-38%, respectively, with similar rates of ICH complication, 6% versus 6.6% [71, 72]. Although underpowered, these data suggest improved functional outcomes with combination therapy and no increased complication or mortality rates **(IIb/B)**.

Mechanical thrombolysis

Evidence for mechanical endovascular devices as an adjuvant or alternative to chemical thrombolysis is emerging. Mechanical disruption of a clot increases the working surface area of thrombolytic agents, can allow for partial removal of clot, and lessens the amount of thrombolytic agent needed for thrombolysis, lowering risk of ICH [74, 75]. The MERCI® device was FDA approved in 2004 for endovascular clot removal in acute ischemic stroke after results from the MERCI trial showed recanalization in 46% (69/151) of patients, comparable rates of ICH to the NINDS rt-PA study group, 7.8% versus 6.6%, respectively, and good functional outcomes of a mRS score 0-2 at 90 days in 46% of recanalized patients versus 10% in the historical PROACT II control arm **(IIb/B)** [76, 77]. Smith *et al*, in the Multi-MERCI trial, showed the MERCI® device had a combined 68.8% recanalization rate in patients receiving clot retrieval alone or as adjuvant therapy for refractory occlusion after IV rt-PA treatment [77, 78]. Favorable outcomes defined by mRS of 0-2 occurred in 49% and mortality was 25% versus 52% in the PROACT II control arm at 90 days. Symptomatic ICH occurred in 9.8% of patients with a 5.5% procedural complication rate [77, 78]. These results suggest the MERCI® device is efficacious in establishing reperfusion alone, as adjuvant therapy, or in patients with failed IV rt-PA therapy, with a good outcome and minimal complication rates

(IIb/B). Other devices that work similarly to the Merci® device include the Neuronet™ device (Guidant, Santa Clara, CA), the Phenox™ clot retriever (Phenox, Bochum, Germany), the Catch™ thrombectomy device (Balt Extrusion, Montmorency, France), and the Alligator™ retrieval device (Chestnut Medical Technologies, Menlo Park, CA) [75]. In a recent study, the efficacy of the MERCI®, Phenox, and Catch devices presented equal results with clot retrieval [79]. However, these devices have not been FDA approved and remain recommended only in clinical trials.

The Penumbra system™ was approved by the FDA in 2008 for mechanical thrombolysis in stroke. The device removes clots via clot aspiration, mechanical disruption, and extraction [80]. In a phase I multicenter, prospective, single-arm trial, the primary endpoint of vessel patency (defined by an adapted thrombolysis in myocardial infarction [TIMI] score of 2 or 3 [Table 3]) was achieved in 87% (21/23), and a secondary endpoint of a mRS score of 0-2 or improvement in the baseline NIHSS score by >4 was achieved in 45% of patients [80]. In phase II of the Penumbra Pivotal Stroke Trial, 125 patients received treatment within 8 hours of symptom onset with NIHSS scores >8 and large intracranial vessel occlusion with a TIMI score of 0-181. Post-procedure, 81.6% of treated vessels were revascularized to TIMI 2 or 3, and at 90 days, 25% of the patients had a mRS of 0-2. Rates of ICH and all-cause mortality were 11.2% and 32.8%, respectively [81]. Preliminary data suggest the benefits outweigh the risks of using the Penumbra system up to 8 hours after symptom onset **(IIb/B)**. Large multicenter studies are necessary to analyze time-to-treatment breakdown to effects on functional outcome before it is implemented into mainstream treatment options.

Table 3. Adapted thrombolytics in myocardial infarction vessel patency score for cerebrovasculature.	
Grade 0 (no perfusion)	There is no anterograde flow beyond the point of occlusion
Grade 1 (penetration without perfusion)	Contrast material fails to opacify the entire coronary bed distal to the obstruction for the entire duration of the imaging sequence
Grade 2 (partial perfusion)	Contrast passes through obstruction and opacifies the bed, but the rate of contrast entry and clearance is delayed relative to other arterial beds
Grade 3 (complete perfusion)	Rate of antegrade flow and clearance is equal distal and proximal to the occlusion, and relative to other arterial beds

Ultrasound-enhanced thrombolysis

Ultrasound-enhanced thrombolysis (UET) is a new therapeutic approach to monitor revascularization and augment other treatment modalities [82-84]. A recent meta-analysis of 224 patients from six randomized trials and 192 patients from three non-randomized trials done by Tsivgoulis et al, showed higher rates of complete recanalization with transcranial Doppler ultrasound (TCD) plus rt-PA versus rt-PA alone (37.2% vs. 17.2%) [85]. In eight of the trials, high-frequency UET was found to increase the likelihood of recanalization (a-OR 2.99; 95% CI, 1.70-5.25; p=0.0001), functional independence at 90 days (a-OR 2.09; 95% CI, 1.17-3.71; p=0.01), and had no statistically significant increased risk of hemorrhage (a-OR 1.26; 95% CI, 0.44-3.60; p=0.67) [84, 85]. Another emerging device aimed at augmenting treatment called the MicroLysUS™ infusion catheter (EKOS, Bothell, WA) uses monographic vibration thrombolysis [75]. Initial studies using the device in anterior or posterior strokes treated within 3-6 and 4-13 hours after symptom onset, respectively, show no additional complications or increased mortality rates, and a mean mRS score of 2 and 3 at 90-day follow-up [86]. These data suggest UET and the MicroLysUS™ system to augment fibrinolysis are emerging adjuvants to rt-PA, and further large multicenter studies are warranted **(IIb/B)**.

Angioplasty and stent placement

Concerns still remain about the limited treatment windows for IV rt-PA and low recanalization rates. Moreover, new treatment innovations are being galvanized by data suggesting that improved outcomes correlate with revascularization [47, 48, 54, 58]. The evolution of angioplasty and stenting for acute occlusive vessel disease has origins in the coronary vasculature, and emerging evidence supports stenting and angioplasty in carefully selected anterior circulation ischemic strokes. Nakano et al conducted a study on 70 patients presenting with radiologic evidence of large intracranial occlusive disease. Thirty-four patients received percutaneous transluminal angioplasty (PTA) followed by IA rt-PA if needed for distal embolization and 36 IA rt-PA alone [87]. Partial or complete recanalization in the PTA group was 91.2%, compared to 63.9% (p<0.01) with IA rt-PA alone. The complication rate of symptomatic ICH was 2.9% with PTA compared to 19.4% with IA rt-PA. There was no significant difference in favorable outcome between PTA and IA rt-PA groups measured by a mRS of 0-2 (52.9% vs. 41.7%, respectively). These results suggest PTA may be safe and efficacious in recanalization, but further clinical trials are needed **(IIb/B)**.

Preliminary results using balloon-mounted coronary stents found a 79% recanalization rate in 19 patients, but only four patients had a mRS <4 at 90 days, and mortality and symptomatic ICH rates were high at 39% [88]. Henkes et al found that higher radial force causing less endothelial damage make self-expanding stents (SES) a safer alternative for treatment [89]. Moreover, in a canine model, Levy et al found self-expanding stents (SES) to have higher recanalization rates and lower rates of complications such as vasospasm or side-branch occlusions [90].

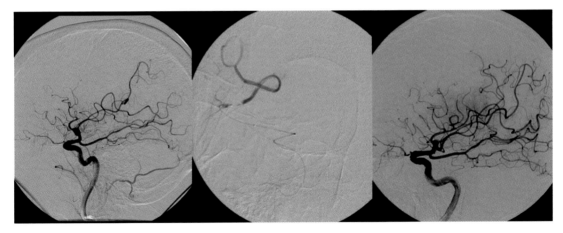

Figure 1. An 82-year-old patient with atrial fibrillation, who presents with acute-onset left-sided weakness and dysarthria. She was outside the 3-hour window, The patient's CT angiogram and CT perfusion studies demonstrated evidence of ischemia in the right frontotemporal region with occlusion of the superior M2 trunk of the right MCA. a) Complete occlusion of the mid-to-distal aspect of the superior M2 trunk of the right MCA. b) The microcatheter was advanced well beyond the thrombus into the distal M2 region. Selective injection from here via the microcatheter demonstrated evidence of a long segment of clot involving the M2 superior trunk, A total of 10mg of ReoPro®, as well as 8mg of rt-PA was slowly infused through the microcatheter. c) Final check angiogram demonstrated good opacification of the entire right MCA territory with no capillary perfusion defects on the angiogram.

Five intracranial SES are currently available: Neuroform™ (Boston Scientific, Natick, Massachusetts, USA), Enterprise™ (Codman Neurovascular, Raynham, Massachusetts, USA), Leo™ (Balt Extrusion, Montmorency, France), Solitaire/Solo™ (Ev3, Inc., Irvine, California, USA), and Wingspan™ (Boston Scientific). The first four are marketed for stent-assisted coil embolization of wide-necked aneurysms, whereas the Wingspan™ is approved for treatment of symptomatic intracranial atherosclerotic disease [75]. Early trials with the Wingspan™ and Neuroform™ stents have shown recanalization rates from 67-92%, but with restenosis rates of 11% [91-93]. Brekenfeld *et al* reported the use of Wingspan™ stents as rescue therapy following mechanical thrombectomy or thrombolytics in 12 patients with recanalization in 11/12 (92%) [93]. Sauvageau *et al*, in a subsequent retrospective study on rescue intracranial stenting after failure with Merci® retrieval, found that 9/10 (90%) patients with a mean NIHSS score of 16.4 experienced recanalization [94]. They also found a 40% mortality rate, with 60% of patients experiencing hemorrhage of any kind, and a 6-point improvement in NIHSS score at discharge although only one patient had a mRS score of <2 [94]. These results suggest rescue therapy with intracranial stenting warrants further investigation (III/B).

In 2009, the FDA approved the first prospective trial for the Wingspan™ stent in acute stroke [95]. Twenty patients were selected with a mean NIHSS score of 14, intracerebral occlusion of the MCA (16) or basilar artery (3) <15mm, an initial TIMI score of 0 (85%) or 1 (15%) with contraindication to IV rt-PA or no improvement 1 hour after administration of IV rt-PA. Twelve patients did receive multimodal endovascular therapy including IA rt-PA (8), IV rt-PA (2), and IA eptifibatide (10) along with intracranial Wingspan™ or Enterprise™ SES. Nineteen patients had successful stent placement and recanalization within 6 hours from symptom onset with TIMI scores of 2 (60%) or 3 (40%) with only 1 symptomatic ICH. At 1-month follow-up, researchers found mRS scores of <2 in 45% of patients, and an all-cause mortality of 25% [95]. SES do have limitations such as with large clots >15mm, distal occluded vessels, and require aggressive antiplatelet therapy for 3-6 months [88, 90, 95]. These results support SES as alternatives after failure of other therapy, in patients where IV rt-PA is contraindicated, or in carefully selected patients **(IIb/B)**. The data are still small and focused on safety and efficacy, and larger trials are needed aimed at improving outcomes.

Adjuvant glycoprotein IIb/IIIa antibody therapy

Thrombolytic administration induces clot lysis and at the same time activates platelets and thrombin. Platelet glycoprotein IIb/IIIa receptor activation is an important part of the cascade, and adjuvant therapeutics against this receptor are under investigation. Lee *et al*, in a small controlled study with the adjuvant IV abciximab, demonstrated a recanalization rate of 90% compared to 44% with urokinase alone, with no significant differences in the rates of hemorrhage and a trend towards better outcomes (80% to 50%) [96]. Qureshi *et al*, in a prospective open trial evaluating the safety and efficacy of adjuvant IV abciximab, found ICH of 5% with a recanalization rate of 65% [97]. Thus, exploratory combinations of a fibrinolytic plus either an anticoagulant or antiplatelet agent offer considerable potential at improving arterial patency and maintenance once achieved; definitive efficacy remains far on the horizon **(III/B)**.

Internal carotid artery

Occlusions of the extra- and intracranial portion of the internal carotid artery (ICA) can cause devastating neurological deficits in patients with poor collateral anastomoses. Distal ICA distribution involving the M1 and A1 segments and poor neurologic presentation are negative prognostic indicators in this type of stroke [98]. Linfante *et al*, in a retrospective analysis, compared acute MCA versus distal ICA occlusion response to IV rt-PA [99]. Controlling for all comorbidities and enrolling patients with similar initial NIHSS scores, they found recanalization rates of 88% versus 31%, respectively, with lower NIHSS scores at follow-up in ICA victims [99]. These results suggest that IV rt-PA in ICA occlusions may not be efficacious **(III/B)**. Arnold *et al*, in a prospective case series of 24 patients treated with IA UK, achieved partial revascularization in 63% of patients with distal ICA occlusion [100]. However, outcomes were still dismal, (only 16% good functional outcome and a 42% mortality rate at 3 months [100]), but still, in comparison to IV rt-PA, IA therapy almost doubled the rate of recanalization.

Carotid artery stenting (CAS) in acute ICA occlusion is also under investigation. Nikas *et al*, in a case series of 18 patients with proximal ICA occlusion, achieved successful recanalization in 83.3% of patients with 30-day mortality rates at 11.1% and a median mRS score of 1 at 30-day follow-up [101]. Thus, while still underpowered, these preliminary data show that CAS for extracranial ICA strokes merits consideration and study (III/B). Furthermore, in a 25-patient series, Jovin *et al* demonstrated revascularization in 92% of patients following IA thrombolysis with stenting in patients with ICA strokes [102]. These results suggest that combination therapy with stenting may improve recanalization rates (III/B).

Mechanical thrombectomy for distal ICA occlusions is another treatment option. Flint *et al* report an 80-patient series with distal ICA occlusions in the MERCI and Multi MERCI trials that received mechanical thrombectomy with or without adjuvant IA thrombolysis [103]. Recanalization rates were 53% with mechanical thrombectomy alone and 63% with adjuvant therapy. Favorable outcomes with a mRS of 0-2 at 90 days occurred in 39% of patients with ICA recanalization compared to 3% without [103]. Therefore, mechanical thrombectomy with or without adjuvant therapy has a high success rate and has favorable outcomes compared to alternative treatment (IIb/B).

Posterior circulation

Acute basilar artery occlusion (BAO) is a severe life-threatening event with mortality ranging from 86-100% attributable to destruction of the midbrain, pons, and medulla [104-106]. Fortunately, BAO only accounts for less than 10% of strokes [107]. Studies have demonstrated DWI-PWI mismatch on MRI in the posterior circulation well beyond 6 hours after onset of symptoms [108-111]. These results support a concept that denser collateral vascular flow dictates slower evolution of irreversible damage, thus potentially extending the time window for therapy. Macleod *et al*, in a randomized controlled trial of IA UK in 16 patients presenting within 24 hours of onset, had good outcomes in four of eight patients who received IA UK compared with one of eight patients in the control group [111]. Nagel *et al* evaluated the efficacy of combining IV abciximab with IA rt-PA or IA rt-PA alone in 75 patients with acute BAO, and found better recanalization rates (83.7% vs. 62.5%; p=0.03), higher survival rates (58.1% vs. 25%; p=0.01), an increase in favorable outcomes defined by a mRS score of 0-3 (34.9% vs. 12.5%; p=0.01), and no increase in symptomatic ICH (14% vs. 18.8%; p=0.41) [112] with the combination strategy. These results, still perhaps underpowered to make concrete clinical recommendations, do suggest increased favorable outcomes in patients treated within 24 hours after symptom onset with IA UK administration (IIb/B) and suggest that adjuvant therapy with IV glycoprotein IIa/IIIb inhibitors is efficacious, safe, and may augment results (IIb/B).

Research has looked into other treatment alternatives for patients with BAO including the FDA-approved IV rt-PA for anterior circulation strokes [104, 113]. In the Basilar Artery International Cooperation Study (BASICS), a prospective observational registry analysis, 619 patients were analyzed who received either anticoagulation alone, IV rt-PA with or without subsequent IA rt-PA, or IA therapies including mechanical thrombectomy, stenting, rt-PA, or IA combination therapy. Results showed a lower risk of severe deficit following thrombolytic therapy of any kind, and no difference in outcomes between IA and IV rt-PA treatment (a-risk ratio 1.06; 95% CI, 0.91-1.22) [104, 114]. Moreover, Pfefferkorn *et al* are investigating the use of IV rt-PA with subsequent early mechanical thrombectomy in BAO strokes in <6 hours from symptom onset. Results of 16 patients showed a 93% recanalization rate, a 75% 6-month survival rate, and 58% of survivors had a mRS of 0-2 [115]. These results are promising showing early recanalization is of paramount importance with thrombolytic therapy of any kind (IIb/B).

Neurosurgical intervention – hemicraniectomy

Malignant cerebral edema following ischemic supratentorial strokes occurs in 1-10% of patients [116, 117]. In space-occupying MCA infarctions, the prognosis is poor with mortality rates nearing 80% [118, 119]. Early CT hypodensity of >50% of the MCA territory or hyperdensity of the proximal MCA predicts malignant transformation [120]. Recently, three multicenter randomized trials were conducted to evaluate decompressive surgery in malignant MCA strokes: HAMLET, DECIMAL, and DESTINY [121-123]. Vahedi et al, in a pooled analysis of these trials, found patients receiving additional decompressive surgery within 48 hours compared to optimal medical management alone enjoyed increased survival (78% vs. 29%) and favorable outcomes defined by a mRS score <4 (43% vs. 21%) [124]. Further investigation into the therapeutic window in the HAMLET trial, found no improvement in outcome when surgery was performed up to 96 hours after symptom onset [121]. A limitation of the data from these trials was the age cut-off of 60. Arac et al, in a meta-analysis of 19 case series, stratified patients by age of up to 60 years old or >60 years old [125]. Pooled analysis of 230 patients at follow-up of 6-12 months found patients >60 years old to have higher rates of poor outcomes, 82% versus 33%, respectively [125]. Age may be an important prognostic indicator in patients receiving decompressive surgery; however, pre-stroke functional status, pre-existing comorbidities, and subgroup analysis of time-to-treatment warrant further investigation. Thus, current recommendations are for patients up to 60 years of age with predicted malignant transformation to receive decompressive hemicraniectomy within 48 hours (Ia/A).

Conclusions

Endovascular therapy is a rapidly expanding and continuously evolving area in the management of patients with stroke.

The prompt and aggressive management of acute stroke has been shown to directly affect clinical outcomes. Newer endovascular technologies have greatly expanded the treatment armamentarium of stroke clinicians with catheter-based thrombolytic and antiplatelet administration, mechanical embolectomy, and angioplasty with stent placement.

Multimodal intra-arterial thrombolysis will likely be the treatment of choice for many acute stroke patients, but safety and efficacy will have to be studied further in the setting of prospective randomized trials.

Key points	Evidence level
◆ Intra-arterial thrombolysis is indicated for treatment of selected patients with major stroke of ~6 hours' duration due to an occlusion of the middle cerebral artery.	Ia/A
◆ Intra-arterial thrombolysis may be reasonable for patients who have contraindications to the use of intravenous thrombolysis, such as recent surgery.	IIa/B
◆ The availability of intra-arterial thrombolysis should generally not preclude the intravenous administration of rt-PA in otherwise eligible patients.	Ia/A
◆ IV rt-PA is less effective at establishing recanalization in high clot burden cases such as carotid T emboli and M1 occlusions, and IA rt-PA with or without mechanical thrombectomy is more likely to establish recanalization in these circumstances.	III/B
◆ In selected cases, angioplasty and stenting is an additional option in multimodal reperfusion therapy and can be an independent predictor of recanalization.	III/B
◆ Decompressive hemicraniectomy may improve survival and functional outcomes in patients with malignant MCA infarcts.	Ia/A

References

1. Tunstall-Pedoe H. Preventing Chronic Diseases. A Vital Investment: WHO Global Report. Geneva: World Health Organization, 2005: 200. ISBN 92 4 1563001. Also published on http://www.who.int/chp/chronic_disease_report /en/. *Int J Epidemiol* 2006; Jul 19.

2. Morabia A, Abel T. The WHO report 'Preventing chronic diseases: a vital investment' and us. *Soz Praventivmed* 2006; 51(2): 74.

3. Writing Group Members, Lloyd-Jones D, Adams RJ, Brown TM, Carnethon M, Dai S, *et al.* Heart disease and stroke statistics - 2010 update: a report from the American Heart Association. *Circulation* 2010; 121(7): e46-e215.

4. Writing Group Members, Lloyd-Jones D, Adams RJ, Brown TM, Carnethon M, Dai S, *et al.* Executive summary: heart disease and stroke statistics - 2010 update: a report from the American Heart Association. *Circulation* 2010; 121(7): 948-54.

5. Wang TJ, Massaro JM, Levy D, Vasan RS, Wolf PA, D'Agostino RB, *et al.* A risk score for predicting stroke or death in individuals with new-onset atrial fibrillation in the community: the Framingham Heart Study. *JAMA* 2003; 290(8): 1049-56.

6. Marler JR, Tilley BC, Lu M, Brott TG, Lyden PC, Grotta JC, *et al.* Early stroke treatment associated with better outcome: the NINDS rt-PA stroke study. *Neurology* 2000; 55(11): 1649-55.

7. Steiner T, Bluhmki E, Kaste M, Toni D, Trouillas P, von Kummer R, *et al.* The ECASS 3-hour cohort. Secondary analysis of ECASS data by time stratification. ECASS Study Group. European Cooperative Acute Stroke Study. *Cerebrovasc Dis* 1998; 8(4): 198-203.

8. Marler J, Jones P, Emr M. Proceedings of a national symposium on rapid identification and treatment of acute stroke, December 12-13, 1996.

9. Adams HP, Jr, del Zoppo G, Alberts MJ, Bhatt DL, Brass L, Furlan A, *et al.* Guidelines for the Early Management of Adults with Ischemic Stroke: a Guideline from the American Heart Association/American Stroke Association Stroke Council, Clinical Cardiology Council, Cardiovascular Radiology and Intervention

Council, and the Atherosclerotic Peripheral Vascular Disease and Quality of Care Outcomes in Research Interdisciplinary Working Groups: The American Academy of Neurology affirms the value of this guideline as an educational tool for neurologists. *Circulation* 2007; 115(20): e478-534.

10. Adams HP, Jr, del Zoppo G, Alberts MJ, Bhatt DL, Brass L, Furlan A, *et al.* Guidelines for the Early Management of Adults with Ischemic Stroke: a Guideline from the American Heart Association/American Stroke Association Stroke Council, Clinical Cardiology Council, Cardiovascular Radiology and Intervention Council, and the Atherosclerotic Peripheral Vascular Disease and Quality of Care Outcomes in Research Interdisciplinary Working Groups: the American Academy of Neurology affirms the value of this guideline as an educational tool for neurologists. *Stroke* 2007; 38(5): 1655-711.

11. Frankel MR, Morgenstern LB, Kwiatkowski T, Lu M, Tilley BC, Broderick JP, *et al.* Predicting prognosis after stroke: a placebo group analysis from the National Institute of Neurological Disorders and Stroke rt-PA Stroke Trial. *Neurology* 2000; 55(7): 952-9.

12. Kothari R, Barsan W, Brott T, Broderick J, Ashbrock S. Frequency and accuracy of prehospital diagnosis of acute stroke. *Stroke* 1995; 26(6): 937-941.

13. Sorensen AG, Heiss WD. Advances in imaging 2009. *Stroke* 2010; 41(2): e91-2.

14. Kidwell CS, Villablanca JP, Saver JL. Advances in neuroimaging of acute stroke. *Curr Atheroscler Rep* 2000; 2(2): 126-35.

15. Khandelwal N. CT perfusion in acute stroke. *Indian J Radiol Imaging* 2008; 18(4): 281-6.

16. Moulin T, Cattin F, Crepin-Leblond T, Tatu L, Chavot D, Piotin M, *et al.* Early CT signs in acute middle cerebral artery infarction: predictive value for subsequent infarct locations and outcome. *Neurology* 1996; 47(2): 366-75.

17. Moulin T, Tatu L, Vuillier F, Cattin F. Brain CT scan for acute cerebral infarction: early signs of ischemia. *Rev Neurol* (Paris) 1999; 155(9): 649-55.

18. Mullins ME, Schaefer PW, Sorensen AG, Halpern EF, Ay H, He J, *et al.* CT and conventional and diffusion-weighted MR imaging in acute stroke: study in 691 patients at presentation to the emergency department. *Radiology* 2002; 224(2): 353-60.

19. Tambasco N, Corea F, Luccioli R, Ciorba E, Parnetti L, Gallai V. Brain CT scan in acute ischemic stroke: early signs and functional outcome. *Clin Exp Hypertens* 2002; 24(7-8): 687-96.

20. von Kummer R, Nolte PN, Schnittger H, Thron A, Ringelstein EB. Detectability of cerebral hemisphere ischaemic infarcts by CT within 6 h of stroke. *Neuroradiology* 1996; 38(1): 31-3.

21. von Kummer R, Bourquain H, Bastianello S, Bozzao L, Manelfe C, Meier D, *et al.* Early prediction of irreversible brain damage after ischemic stroke at CT. *Radiology* 2001; 219(1): 95-100.

22. Ezzeddine MA, Lev MH, McDonald CT, Rordorf G, Oliveira-Filho J, Aksoy FG, *et al.* CT angiography with whole brain perfused blood volume imaging: added clinical value in the assessment of acute stroke. *Stroke* 2002; 33(4): 959-66.

23. Wintermark M. Brain perfusion-CT in acute stroke patients. *Eur Radiol* 2005; 15 Suppl 4: D28-31.

24. Schramm P, Schellinger PD, Klotz E, Kallenberg K, Fiebach JB, Kulkens S, *et al.* Comparison of perfusion computed tomography and computed tomography angiography source images with perfusion-weighted imaging and diffusion-weighted imaging in patients with acute stroke of less than 6 hours' duration. *Stroke* 2004; 35(7): 1652-8.

25. Tan JC, Dillon WP, Liu S, Adler F, Smith WS, Wintermark M. Systematic comparison of perfusion-CT and CT-angiography in acute stroke patients. *Ann Neurol* 2007; 61(6): 533-43.

26. Popiela T, Pera J, Chrzan R, Strojny J, Urbanik A, Slowik A. Perfusion computed tomography and clinical status of patients with acute ischaemic stroke. *Neurol Neurochir Pol* 2008; 42(5): 396-401.

27. Wu O, Koroshetz WJ, Ostergaard L, Buonanno FS, Copen WA, Gonzalez RG, *et al.* Predicting tissue outcome in acute human cerebral ischemia using combined diffusion- and perfusion-weighted MR imaging. *Stroke* 2001; 32(4): 933-42.

28. Tomandl BF, Klotz E, Handschu R, Stemper B, Reinhardt F, Huk WJ, *et al.* Comprehensive imaging of ischemic stroke with multisection CT. *Radiographics* 2003; 23(3): 565-92.

29. Srinivasan A, Goyal M, Al Azri F, Lum C. State-of-the-art imaging of acute stroke. *Radiographics* 2006; 26 Suppl 1: S75-95.

30. Ledezma CJ, Fiebach JB, Wintermark M. Modern imaging of the infarct core and the ischemic penumbra in acute stroke patients: CT versus MRI. *Expert Rev Cardiovasc Ther* 2009; 7(4): 395-403.

31. Sparacia G, Iaia A, Assadi B, Lagalla R. Perfusion CT in acute stroke: predictive value of perfusion parameters in assessing tissue viability versus infarction. *Radiol Med* 2007; 112(1): 113-22.

32. Klotz E, Konig M. Perfusion measurements of the brain: using dynamic CT for the quantitative assessment of cerebral ischemia in acute stroke. *Eur J Radiol* 1999; 30(3): 170-84.

33. Camargo EC, Furie KL, Singhal AB, Roccatagliata L, Cunnane ME, Halpern EF, et al. Acute brain infarct: detection and delineation with CT angiographic source images versus nonenhanced CT scans. *Radiology* 2007; 244(2): 541-8.

34. Warach S, Chien D, Li W, Ronthal M, Edelman RR. Fast magnetic resonance diffusion-weighted imaging of acute human stroke. *Neurology* 1992; 42(9): 1717-23.

35. Warach S, Gaa J, Siewert B, Wielopolski P, Edelman RR. Acute human stroke studied by whole brain echo planar diffusion-weighted magnetic resonance imaging. *Ann Neurol* 1995; 37(2): 231-41.

36. Lutsep HL, Albers GW, DeCrespigny A, Kamat GN, Marks MP, Moseley ME. Clinical utility of diffusion-weighted magnetic resonance imaging in the assessment of ischemic stroke. *Ann Neurol* 1997; 41(5): 574-80.

37. Lovblad KO, Baird AE, Schlaug G, Benfield A, Siewert B, Voetsch B, et al. Ischemic lesion volumes in acute stroke by diffusion-weighted magnetic resonance imaging correlate with clinical outcome. *Ann Neurol* 1997; 42(2): 164-70.

38. Lovblad KO, Laubach HJ, Baird AE, Curtin F, Schlaug G, Edelman RR, et al. Clinical experience with diffusion-weighted MR in patients with acute stroke. *AJNR Am J Neuroradiol* 1998; 19(6): 1061-6.

39. Mascalchi M, Filippi M, Floris R, Fonda C, Gasparotti R, Villari N. Diffusion-weighted MR of the brain: methodology and clinical application. *Radiol Med* 2005; 109(3): 155-97.

40. Brazzelli M, Sandercock PA, Chappell FM, Celani MG, Righetti E, Arestis N, et al. Magnetic resonance imaging versus computed tomography for detection of acute vascular lesions in patients presenting with stroke symptoms. *Cochrane Database Syst Rev* 2009; 4(4): CD007424.

41. Kumar G, Kalita J, Kumar B, Bansal V, Jain SK, Misra U. Magnetic resonance angiography findings in patients with ischemic stroke from North India. *J Stroke Cerebrovasc Dis* 2010; 19(2): 146-52.

42. Kidwell CS, Chalela JA, Saver JL, Starkman S, Hill MD, Demchuk AM, et al. Comparison of MRI and CT for detection of acute intracerebral hemorrhage. *JAMA* 2004; 292(15): 1823-30.

43. Fiebach JB, Schellinger PD, Gass A, Kucinski T, Siebler M, Villringer A, et al. Stroke magnetic resonance imaging is accurate in hyperacute intracerebral hemorrhage: a multicenter study on the validity of stroke imaging. *Stroke* 2004; 35(2): 502-6.

44. Barber PA, Darby DG, Desmond PM, Gerraty RP, Yang Q, Li T, et al. Identification of major ischemic change. Diffusion-weighted imaging versus computed tomography. *Stroke* 1999; 30(10): 2059-65.

45. Gonzalez RG, Schaefer PW, Buonanno FS, Schwamm LH, Budzik RF, Rordorf G, et al. Diffusion-weighted MR imaging: diagnostic accuracy in patients imaged within 6 hours of stroke symptom onset. *Radiology* 1999; 210(1): 155-62.

46. Yamaguchi T, Mori E, Minematsu K, Nakagawara J, Hashi K, Saito I, et al. Alteplase at 0.6mg/kg for acute ischemic stroke within 3 hours of onset: Japan Alteplase Clinical Trial (J-ACT). *Stroke* 2006; 37(7): 1810-15.

47. Hacke W, Kaste M, Fieschi C, von Kummer R, Dávalos A, Meier D, et al. Randomised double-blind placebo-controlled trial of thrombolytic therapy with intravenous alteplase in acute ischaemic stroke (ECASS II). Second European-Australasian Acute Stroke Study Investigators. *Lancet* 1998; 352(9136): 1245-51.

48. Hacke W, Bluhmki E, Steiner T, Tatlisumak T, Mahagne MH, Sacchetti ML, et al. Dichotomized efficacy endpoints and global endpoint analysis applied to the ECASS intention-to-treat data set: post hoc analysis of ECASS I. *Stroke* 1998; 29(10): 2073-5.

49. Kwiatkowski TG, Libman RB, Frankel M, Tilley BC, Morgenstern LB, Lu M, et al. Effects of tissue plasminogen activator for acute ischemic stroke at one year. National Institute of Neurological Disorders and Stroke Recombinant Tissue Plasminogen Activator Stroke Study Group. *N Engl J Med* 1999; 340(23): 1781-7.

50. Tissue plasminogen activator for acute ischemic stroke. The National Institute of Neurological Disorders and Stroke rt-PA Stroke Study Group. *N Engl J Med* 1995; 333(24): 1581-7.

51. National Institute of Neurological Disorders Stroke rt-PA Stroke Study Group. Recombinant tissue plasminogen activator for minor strokes: the National Institute of Neurological Disorders and Stroke rt-PA Stroke Study experience. *Ann Emerg Med* 2005; 46(3): 243-52.

52. Donnan GA, Hommel M, Davis SM, McNeil JJ. Streptokinase in acute ischaemic stroke. Steering Committees of the ASK and MAST-E trials. Australian Streptokinase Trial. *Lancet* 1995; 346(8966): 56.

53. Wolpert SM, Bruckmann H, Greenlee R, Wechsler L, Pessin MS, del Zoppo GJ. Neuroradiologic evaluation of patients with acute stroke treated with recombinant tissue plasminogen activator. The rt-PA Acute Stroke Study Group. *AJNR Am J Neuroradiol* 1993; 14(1): 3-13.

54. Bluhmki E, Chamorro A, Dávalos A, Machnig T, Sauce C, Wahlgren N, *et al.* Stroke treatment with alteplase given 3.0-4.5 h after onset of acute ischaemic stroke (ECASS III): additional outcomes and subgroup analysis of a randomised controlled trial. *Lancet Neurol* 2009; 8(12): 1095-102.

55. Hacke W, Kaste M, Bluhmki E, Brozman M, Dávalos A, Guidetti D, *et al.* Thrombolysis with alteplase 3 to 4.5 hours after acute ischemic stroke. *N Engl J Med* 2008; 359(13): 1317-29.

56. Davis SM, Donnan GA, Parsons MW, Levi C, Butcher KS, Peeters A, *et al.* Effects of alteplase beyond 3 h after stroke in the Echoplanar Imaging Thrombolytic Evaluation Trial (EPITHET): a placebo-controlled randomised trial. *Lancet Neurol* 2008; 7(4): 299-309.

57. Spilker J, Kongable G, Barch C, Braimah J, Brattina P, Daley S, *et al.* Using the NIH Stroke Scale to assess stroke patients. The NINDS rt-PA Stroke Study Group. *J Neurosci Nurs* 1997; 29(6): 384-92.

58. Rha JH, Saver JL. The impact of recanalization on ischemic stroke outcome: a meta-analysis. *Stroke* 2007; 38(3): 967-73.

59. Barber PA, Zhang J, Demchuk AM, Hill MD, Buchan AM. Why are stroke patients excluded from TPA therapy? An analysis of patient eligibility. *Neurology* 2001; 56(8): 1015-20.

60. Mishra NK, Albers GW, Davis SM, Donnan GA, Furlan AJ, Hacke W, *et al.* Mismatch-based delayed thrombolysis: a meta-analysis. *Stroke* 2010; 41(1): e25-33.

61. Zaidat OO, Suarez JI, Sunshine JL, Tarr RW, Alexander MJ, Smith TP, *et al.* Thrombolytic therapy of acute ischemic stroke: correlation of angiographic recanalization with clinical outcome. *AJNR Am J Neuroradiol* 2005; 26(4): 880-4.

62. Bourekas EC, Slivka A, Shah R, Mohammad Y, Slone HW, Kehagias DT, *et al.* Intra-arterial thrombolysis within three hours of stroke onset in middle cerebral artery strokes. *Neurocrit Care* 2009; 11(2): 217-22.

63. Furlan AJ, Abou-Chebl A. The role of recombinant pro-urokinase (r-pro-UK) and intra-arterial thrombolysis in acute ischaemic stroke: the PROACT trials. Prolyse in Acute Cerebral Thromboembolism. *Curr Med Res Opin* 2002; 18 Suppl 2: s44-7.

64. Furlan A, Higashida R, Wechsler L, Gent M, Rowley H, Kase C, *et al.* Intra-arterial prourokinase for acute ischemic stroke. The PROACT II study: a randomized controlled trial. Prolyse in Acute Cerebral Thromboembolism. *JAMA* 1999; 282(21): 2003-11.

65. del Zoppo GJ, Higashida RT, Furlan AJ, Pessin MS, Rowley HA, Gent M. PROACT: a phase II randomized trial of recombinant pro-urokinase by direct arterial delivery in acute middle cerebral artery stroke. PROACT Investigators. Prolyse in Acute Cerebral Thromboembolism. *Stroke* 1998; 29(1): 4-11.

66. Inoue T, Kimura K, Minematsu K, Yamaguchi T, Japan Multicenter Stroke Investigators' Collaboration. A case-control analysis of intra-arterial urokinase thrombolysis in acute cardioembolic stroke. *Cerebrovasc Dis* 2005; 19(4): 225-8.

67. Trouillas P, Nighoghossian N, Getenet JC, Riche G, Neuschwander P, Froment JC, *et al.* Open trial of intravenous tissue plasminogen activator in acute carotid territory stroke. Correlations of outcome with clinical and radiological data. *Stroke* 1996; 27(5): 882-90.

68. Tomsick T, Brott T, Barsan W, Broderick J, Haley EC, Spilker J, *et al.* Prognostic value of the hyperdense middle cerebral artery sign and stroke scale score before ultra-early thrombolytic therapy. *AJNR Am J Neuroradiol* 1996; 17(1): 79-85.

69. Suarez JI, Zaidat OO, Sunshine JL, Tarr R, Selman WR, Landis DM. Endovascular administration after intravenous infusion of thrombolytic agents for the treatment of patients with acute ischemic strokes. *Neurosurgery* 2002; 50(2): 251-9; discussion 259-60.

70. Lewandowski CA, Frankel M, Tomsick TA, Broderick J, Frey J, Clark W, *et al.* Combined intravenous and intra-arterial r-TPA versus intra-arterial therapy of acute ischemic stroke: Emergency Management of Stroke (EMS) Bridging Trial. *Stroke* 1999; 30(12): 2598-605.

71. IMS Study Investigators. Combined intravenous and intra-arterial recanalization for acute ischemic stroke: the Interventional Management of Stroke Study. *Stroke* 2004; 35(4): 904-11.

72. IMS II Trial Investigators. The Interventional Management of Stroke (IMS) II Study. *Stroke* 2007; 38(7): 2127-35.

73. Khatri P, Hill MD, Palesch YY, Spilker J, Jauch EC, Carrozzella JA, *et al.* Methodology of the Interventional Management of Stroke III Trial. *Int J Stroke* 2008; 3(2):130-7.

74. Nogueira RG, Yoo AJ, Buonanno FS, Hirsch JA. Endovascular approaches to acute stroke, part 2: a comprehensive review of studies and trials. *AJNR Am J Neuroradiol* 2009; 30(5): 859-75.

75. Nogueira RG, Schwamm LH, Hirsch JA. Endovascular approaches to acute stroke, part 1: drugs, devices, and data. *AJNR Am J Neuroradiol* 2009; 30(4): 649-61.

76. Smith WS, Sung G, Starkman S, Saver JL, Kidwell CS, Gobin YP, *et al.* Safety and efficacy of mechanical embolectomy in acute ischemic stroke: results of the MERCI trial. *Stroke* 2005; 36(7): 1432-8.

77. Smith WS. Safety of mechanical thrombectomy and intravenous tissue plasminogen activator in acute ischemic stroke. Results of the multi Mechanical Embolus Removal in Cerebral Ischemia (MERCI) trial, part I. *AJNR Am J Neuroradiol* 2006; 27(6): 1177-82.

78. Smith WS, Sung G, Saver J, Budzik R, Duckwiler G, Liebeskind DS, *et al.* Mechanical thrombectomy for acute ischemic stroke: final results of the Multi MERCI trial. *Stroke* 2008; 39(4): 1205-12.

79. Liebig T, Reinartz J, Hannes R, Miloslavski E, Henkes H. Comparative *in vitro* study of five mechanical embolectomy systems: effectiveness of clot removal and risk of distal embolization. *Neuroradiology* 2008; 50(1): 43-52.

80. Bose A, Henkes H, Alfke K, Reith W, Mayer TE, Berlis A, *et al.* The Penumbra System: a mechanical device for the treatment of acute stroke due to thromboembolism. *AJNR Am J Neuroradiol* 2008; 29(7): 1409-13.

81. Penumbra Pivotal Stroke Trial Investigators. The Penumbra Pivotal Stroke Trial: safety and effectiveness of a new generation of mechanical devices for clot removal in intracranial large vessel occlusive disease. *Stroke* 2009; 40(8): 2761-8.

82. Alexandrov AV, Molina CA, Grotta JC, Garami Z, Ford SR, Alvarez-Sabin J, *et al.* Ultrasound-enhanced systemic thrombolysis for acute ischemic stroke. *N Engl J Med* 2004; 351(21): 2170-8.

83. Alexandrov AV. Ultrasound identification and lysis of clots. *Stroke* 2004; 35(11 Suppl 1): 2722-5.

84. Tsivgoulis G, Alexandrov AV. Ultrasound-enhanced thrombolysis: applications in acute cerebral ischemia. *J Clin Neurol* 2007; 3(1): 1-8.

85. Tsivgoulis G, Eggers J, Ribo M, Perren F, Saqqur M, Rubiera M, *et al.* Safety and efficacy of ultrasound-enhanced thrombolysis: a comprehensive review and meta-analysis of randomized and nonrandomized studies. *Stroke* 2010; 41(2): 280-7.

86. Mahon BR, Nesbit GM, Barnwell SL, Clark W, Marotta TR, Weill A, *et al.* North American clinical experience with the EKOS MicroLysUS infusion catheter for the treatment of embolic stroke. *AJNR Am J Neuroradiol* 2003; 24(3): 534-8.

87. Nakano S, Iseda T, Yoneyama T, Kawano H, Wakisaka S. Direct percutaneous transluminal angioplasty for acute middle cerebral artery trunk occlusion: an alternative option to intra-arterial thrombolysis. *Stroke* 2002; 33(12): 2872-6.

88. Levy EI, Ecker RD, Horowitz MB, Gupta R, Hanel RA, Sauvageau E, *et al.* Stent-assisted intracranial recanalization for acute stroke: early results. *Neurosurgery* 2006; 58(3): 458-63; discussion 458-63.

89. Henkes H, Miloslavski E, Lowens S, Reinartz J, Liebig T, Kuhne D. Treatment of intracranial atherosclerotic stenoses with balloon dilatation and self-expanding stent deployment (WingSpan). *Neuroradiology* 2005; 47(3): 222-8.

90. Levy EI, Sauvageau E, Hanel RA, Parikh R, Hopkins LN. Self-expanding versus balloon-mounted stents for vessel recanalization following embolic occlusion in the canine model: technical feasibility study. *AJNR Am J Neuroradiol* 2006; 27(10): 2069-72.

91. Zaidat OO, Wolfe T, Hussain SI, Lynch JR, Gupta R, Delap J, *et al.* Interventional acute ischemic stroke therapy with intracranial self-expanding stent. *Stroke* 2008; 39(8): 2392-5.

92. Levy EI, Mehta R, Gupta R, Hanel RA, Chamczuk AJ, Fiorella D, *et al.* Self-expanding stents for recanalization of acute cerebrovascular occlusions. *AJNR Am J Neuroradiol* 2007; 28(5): 816-22.

93. Brekenfeld C, Remonda L, Nedeltchev K, Bredow F, Ozdoba C, Wiest R, *et al.* Endovascular neuroradiological treatment of acute ischemic stroke: techniques and results in 350 patients. *Neurol Res* 2005; 27 Suppl 1: S29-35.

94. Sauvageau E, Samuelson RM, Levy EI, Jeziorski AM, Mehta RA, Hopkins LN. Middle cerebral artery stenting for acute ischemic stroke after unsuccessful Merci retrieval. *Neurosurgery* 2007; 60(4): 701-6; discussion 706.

95. Levy EI, Siddiqui AH, Crumlish A, Snyder KV, Hauck EF, Fiorella DJ, *et al.* First Food and Drug Administration-approved prospective trial of primary intracranial stenting for acute stroke: SARIS (stent-assisted recanalization in acute ischemic stroke). *Stroke* 2009; 40(11): 3552-6.

96. Lee DH, Jo KD, Kim HG, Choi SJ, Jung SM, Ryu DS, *et al.* Local intraarterial urokinase thrombolysis of acute ischemic stroke with or without intravenous abciximab: a pilot study. *J Vasc Interv Radiol* 2002; 13(8): 769-74.

97. Qureshi AI, Harris-Lane P, Kirmani JF, Janjua N, Divani AA, Mohammad YM, *et al.* Intra-arterial reteplase and intravenous abciximab in patients with acute ischemic stroke: an open-label, dose-ranging, phase I study. *Neurosurgery* 2006; 59(4): 789-96; discussion 796-7.

98. Meier P, Knapp G, Tamhane U, Chaturvedi S, Gurm HS. Short-term and intermediate-term comparison of endarterectomy versus stenting for carotid artery stenosis: systematic review and meta-analysis of randomised controlled clinical trials. *BMJ* 2010; 340: c467.

99. Linfante I, Llinas RH, Selim M, Chaves C, Kumar S, Parker RA, *et al.* Clinical and vascular outcome in internal carotid artery versus middle cerebral artery occlusions after intravenous tissue plasminogen activator. *Stroke* 2002; 33(8): 2066-71.

100. Arnold M, Nedeltchev K, Mattle HP, Loher TJ, Stepper F, Schroth G, *et al.* Intra-arterial thrombolysis in 24 consecutive patients with internal carotid artery T occlusions. *J Neurol Neurosurg Psychiatry* 2003; 74(6): 739-42.

101. Nikas D, Reimers B, Elisabetta M, Sacca S, Cernetti C, Pasquetto G, *et al.* Percutaneous interventions in patients with acute ischemic stroke related to obstructive atherosclerotic disease or dissection of the extracranial carotid artery. *J Endovasc Ther* 2007; 14(3): 279-88.

102. Jovin TG, Gupta R, Uchino K, Jungreis CA, Wechsler LR, Hammer MD, *et al.* Emergent stenting of extracranial internal carotid artery occlusion in acute stroke has a high revascularization rate. *Stroke* 2005; 36(11): 2426-30.

103. Flint AC, Duckwiler GR, Budzik RF, Liebeskind DS, Smith WS, MERCI and Multi MERCI Writing Committee. Mechanical thrombectomy of intracranial internal carotid occlusion: pooled results of the MERCI and Multi MERCI Part I trials. *Stroke* 2007; 38(4): 1274-80.

104. Schonewille WJ, Wijman CA, Michel P, Algra A, Kappelle LJ, BASICS Study Group. The Basilar Artery International Cooperation Study (BASICS). *Int J Stroke* 2007; 2(3): 220-3.

105. Levy EI, Firlik AD, Wisniewski S, Rubin G, Jungreis CA, Wechsler LR, *et al.* Factors affecting survival rates for acute vertebrobasilar artery occlusions treated with intra-arterial thrombolytic therapy: a meta-analytical approach. *Neurosurgery* 1999; 45(3): 539-45; discussion 545-8.

106. Arnold M, Nedeltchev K, Schroth G, Baumgartner RW, Remonda L, Loher TJ, *et al.* Clinical and radiological predictors of recanalisation and outcome of 40 patients with acute basilar artery occlusion treated with intra-arterial thrombolysis. *J Neurol Neurosurg Psychiatry* 2004; 75(6): 857-62.

107. Tjoumakaris SI, Jabbour PM, Rosenwasser RH. Neuroendovascular management of acute ischemic stroke. *Neurosurg Clin N Am* 2009; 20(4): 419-29.

108. Ostrem JL, Saver JL, Alger JR, Starkman S, Leary MC, Duckwiler G, *et al.* Acute basilar artery occlusion: diffusion-perfusion MRI characterization of tissue salvage in patients receiving intra-arterial stroke therapies. *Stroke* 2004; 35(2): e30-4.

109. Brandt T, von Kummer R, Muller-Kuppers M, Hacke W. Thrombolytic therapy of acute basilar artery occlusion. Variables affecting recanalization and outcome. *Stroke* 1996; 27(5): 875-81.

110. Becker KJ, Monsein LH, Ulatowski J, Mirski M, Williams M, Hanley DF. Intraarterial thrombolysis in vertebrobasilar occlusion. *AJNR Am J Neuroradiol* 1996; 17(2): 255-62.

111. Macleod MR, Davis SM, Mitchell PJ, Gerraty RP, Fitt G, Hankey GJ, *et al.* Results of a multicentre, randomised controlled trial of intra-arterial urokinase in the treatment of acute posterior circulation ischaemic stroke. *Cerebrovasc Dis* 2005; 20(1): 12-7.

112. Nagel S, Schellinger PD, Hartmann M, Juettler E, Huttner HB, Ringleb P, *et al.* Therapy of acute basilar artery occlusion: intra-arterial thrombolysis alone vs. bridging therapy. *Stroke* 2009; 40(1): 140-6.

113. Lindsberg PJ, Mattle HP. Therapy of basilar artery occlusion: a systematic analysis comparing intra-arterial and intravenous thrombolysis. *Stroke* 2006; 37(3): 922-8.

114. Schonewille WJ, Wijman CA, Michel P, Rueckert CM, Weimar C, Mattle HP, *et al.* Treatment and outcomes of acute basilar artery occlusion in the Basilar Artery International Cooperation Study (BASICS): a prospective registry study. *Lancet Neurol* 2009; 8(8): 724-30.

115. Pfefferkorn T, Mayer TE, Opherk C, Peters N, Straube A, Pfister HW, *et al.* Staged escalation therapy in acute basilar artery occlusion: intravenous thrombolysis and on-demand consecutive endovascular mechanical thrombectomy: preliminary experience in 16 patients. *Stroke* 2008; 39(5): 1496-500.

116. Hatashita S, Hoff JT. The effect of craniectomy on the biomechanics of normal brain. *J Neurosurg* 1987; 67(4): 573-8.
117. Rieke K, Schwab S, Krieger D, von Kummer R, Aschoff A, Schuchardt V, *et al.* Decompressive surgery in space-occupying hemispheric infarction: results of an open, prospective trial. *Crit Care Med* 1995; 23(9): 1576-87.
118. Berrouschot J, Sterker M, Bettin S, Koster J, Schneider D. Mortality of space-occupying ('malignant') middle cerebral artery infarction under conservative intensive care. *Intensive Care Med* 1998; 24(6): 620-3.
119. Hacke W, Schwab S, Horn M, Spranger M, De Georgia M, von Kummer R. 'Malignant' middle cerebral artery territory infarction: clinical course and prognostic signs. *Arch Neurol* 1996; 53(4): 309-15.
120. Barber PA, Demchuk AM, Zhang J, Kasner SE, Hill MD, Berrouschot J, *et al.* Computed tomographic parameters predicting fatal outcome in large middle cerebral artery infarction. *Cerebrovasc Dis* 2003; 16(3): 230-5.
121. Hofmeijer J, Kappelle LJ, Algra A, Amelink GJ, van Gijn J, van der Worp HB, *et al.* Surgical decompression for space-occupying cerebral infarction (the Hemicraniectomy After Middle Cerebral Artery infarction with Life-threatening Edema Trial [HAMLET]): a multicentre, open, randomised trial. *Lancet Neurol* 2009; 8(4): 326-33.
122. Vahedi K, Vicaut E, Mateo J, Kurtz A, Orabi M, Guichard JP, *et al.* Sequential-design, multicenter, randomized, controlled trial of early Decompressive Craniectomy in Malignant Middle Cerebral Artery Infarction (DECIMAL Trial). *Stroke* 2007; 38(9): 2506-17.
123. Juttler E, Schwab S, Schmiedek P, Unterberg A, Hennerici M, Woitzik J, *et al.* Decompressive Surgery for the Treatment of Malignant Infarction of the Middle Cerebral Artery (DESTINY): a randomized, controlled trial. *Stroke* 2007; 38(9): 2518-25.
124. Vahedi K, Hofmeijer J, Juettler E, Vicaut E, George B, Algra A, *et al.* Early decompressive surgery in malignant infarction of the middle cerebral artery: a pooled analysis of three randomised controlled trials. *Lancet Neurol* 2007; 6(3): 215-22.
125. Arac A, Blanchard V, Lee M, Steinberg GK. Assessment of outcome following decompressive craniectomy for malignant middle cerebral artery infarction in patients older than 60 years of age. *Neurosurg Focus* 2009; 26(6): E3.

Chapter 6

Interventions for carotid artery disease and intracranial stenosis

Gabriel A. Smith BS, Medical Student
Temple University School of Medicine, Philadelphia, USA

Zakaria Hakma MD, Chief Neurosurgical Resident, Department
of Neurosurgery, Temple University Hospital, Philadelphia, USA

Christopher M. Loftus MD Dr. h.c. FACS, Professor and Chairman of the Department
of Neurosurgery, Temple University Hospital; Chairman of the AANS International
Outreach Committee; WFNS Assistant Treasurer; and Assistant Dean for
International Affiliations, Temple University School of Medicine, Philadelphia, USA

Introduction

The World Health Organization (WHO) estimates 15 million people suffer new strokes every year, and 55 million people globally have had a stroke in their lifetime with or without residual disability [1, 2]. In 2005, it was estimated 5.8 million people died worldwide, and strokes accounted for nearly 10% of all deaths second only to heart disease [1]. Stroke is also a leading cause of serious long-term disability in the world. The 1-year mortality rate of stroke victims age >40 in 2010 was estimated at 20-25% with the median survival time of 6.8-7.4 years [3, 4]. Moderate-severe disability at discharge was 30% in the United States based on stroke registries, and at 6 months, >20% of all patients were still disabled in an analysis of patients in the Framingham Heart Study [3-5]. There is no doubt that improvements in prevention, access to care, interventional techniques, management, and rehabilitation are worthwhile clinical goals.

Carotid vascular disease is devastating and can lead to serious neurological impairment. The timing of carotid endarterectomy (CEA) and carotid artery stenting (CAS) post-stroke remains a controversial area. Based on reports of hemorrhage and increased stroke rates with early surgery [6-10], most authorities advocated waiting at least 2 to 6 weeks after stroke before performing a CEA. More recently, prospective studies, meta-analyses of existing data, and review of the North American Symptomatic Carotid Endarterectomy Trial and European Carotid Surgery Trial have challenged these recommendations (Table 1) [11-13]. This chapter reviews the current literature recommendations regarding CEA after acute stroke, TIAs, within evolving strokes, and current literature regarding neuroradiologic imaging findings and their implications in decision-making regarding CEA post-stroke. Moreover, we will assess emerging data including the recently released CREST trial on CAS and the current recommendations for endovascular management of carotid artery disease.

Table 1. Summary of study findings for CEA.			
Stenosis	Studies	Recommendations	Risk reduction
Symptomatic stenosis			
70-99%	NASCET	CEA, level A	16.5% @ 2 yrs
>60%	ECST	CEA, level A	11.6% @ 3 yrs
50-69%	NASCET	CEA, level A	10.1% @ 5 yrs
Asymptomatic stenosis			
>60%	ACAS, ACST	CEA, level A	6.3% @ 5 yrs

Imaging findings and their relationship to the timing of surgery

Can imaging data predict patients at risk for postoperative complications and allow choosing of the best surgical candidates? After the introduction of readily available CT scanning, a great deal of effort has gone into using this technology to risk stratify patients and, ultimately, predict which patients benefit from early versus delayed surgery. Dosick and colleagues [14] found that in patients who have neurologic deficits lasting longer than 24 hours and appropriate carotid lesions at angiography, serial pre-operative CT scans negative for acute hemorrhage were predictive of 0% mortality and 0.9% (1/110) morbidity (III/B). In the group of patients who had positive CT scans, 9.5% (7/74) had at least one event while waiting for delayed surgery at 4-6 weeks; angiography revealed significant lesions in 69% (51/74) of this subgroup, and all patients who had additional neurologic events had positive angiograms. The postoperative stroke rate was 2% (1/51).

Little and coworkers [15] analyzed a subgroup of CEA patients who had surgery within 30 days of onset of their neurologic symptoms. They concluded that patients who have negative CT scans and minimal residual neurologic symptoms are at low risk for early surgery, perhaps even approaching the risk of patients presenting with TIAs alone; of the 22 patients in this subgroup, none experienced new postoperative permanent neurologic deficits. Patients who had positive scans and moderate, stable neurologic deficits were at intermediate risk. In addition, two patients who had repeat TIAs and normal CT scans had an uncomplicated postoperative course. The high-risk category comprised patients who had deteriorating neurologic examinations and positive CT scans. Two of three patients in this subgroup had postoperative extension of their infarctions and one patient died, representing 66% morbidity and 33% mortality rates.

Despite Little and colleagues [15] having advocated early surgery only in the presence of normal cranial imaging findings, most series looking at brain CT stroke-related imaging findings fail to note a substantial correlation in relation to outcomes of patients undergoing CEA post-stroke [16-18] **(IIb/B)**.

Timing of CEA in patients who have stable, non-disabling, or mildly disabling strokes (Table 2)

Most of the early literature regarding CEA after a stroke recommended performing CEA in a delayed manner. In 1963, before the advent of CT scanning, Bruetman and colleagues [8] published a series of 900 patients undergoing CEA, six of whom had postoperative cerebral hemorrhage; this was confirmed at autopsy (5) or surgery for removal of a suspected clot (1). The intracerebral hemorrhages (ICHs) occurred in a delayed fashion 3-6 days after surgery and all patients were improving neurologically, even ambulatory, at the time of their acute deterioration. Wylie *et al* [6] described their experience with nine patients who had acute stroke undergoing CEA. They noted a 56% (5/9) fatal ICH rate in this group of patients, although their overall mortality rate after surgery for transient ischemic attacks (TIAs) or chronic cerebral insufficiency was 5%. Four of the patients were operated 3-10 days after a probable cerebral infarction, and the fifth was 22 days out from the initial stroke. No single patient was symptomatic from the ICH immediately after the operation; the time to symptom onset ranged from 2 hours to 3 days. These historical studies suggest a critical period following large cerebral infarction associated with carotid vascular occlusion where fatal intracranial hemorrhage could occur near the infarcted zones.

Data from the Joint Study of Extracranial Arterial Occlusion [19] seemed to support the practice of delayed surgery after stroke. In one subgroup of patients who had acute stroke and altered mental status, the postoperative mortality was twice that of the medically treated group (42% vs. 20%, respectively) when surgery was performed within 2 weeks of the onset of neurologic symptoms. The investigators noted that CEA performed 14 days after stroke was associated with better outcomes (17% mortality) than the medically treated group, but also noted that the groups were not really comparable because many of the patients in the medically treated group had expired before 14 days had passed **(III/B)**.

Despite aforementioned concerns in years past that, to reduce complications, a waiting period post-stroke of at least 4-6 weeks is optimal before performing CEA, the vast majority of studies in the past 20 years have demonstrated no increased risk of stroke for early CEA after a recent stroke and, rather, suggest a distinct benefit (in terms of preventing recurrent stroke during medical observation) to quick surgical intervention. The early reports detailing high mortality rates from ICH described heterogeneous groups of patients, many of whom had severe neurologic deficits and probable hemorrhagic complications pre-operatively. The lack of brain imaging techniques at the time of many of the reports makes it impossible to determine with any accuracy the extent of pre-existing infarction or hemorrhage [20]. Compelling evidence now exists to suggest that patients may benefit from endarterectomy performed shortly after symptoms have stabilized (in the subacute phase), in patients who have non-disabling or mildly disabling strokes **(IIa/B)**.

Current evidence suggests that surgical delay, and any arbitrarily assigned waiting before consideration of CEA after stroke, seems to leave patients at great risk for recurrent cerebral ischemia. Dosick and colleagues [14] report a 9.5% stroke rate (new dense neurologic deficit) in surgical candidate patients undergoing a 6-week waiting period post-stroke. Similarly, in the North American Symptomatic Carotid Endarterectomy Trial, 4.9% of the 103 medically treated patients diagnosed with stroke and severe internal carotid artery stenosis experienced a recurrent ipsilateral stroke within 30 days of trial entry [21] **(III/B)**.

Whittemore *et al* [22] confirm the feasibility of performing CEA within 4 weeks of stroke in 28 patients sustaining small fixed, neurologic deficits. They reported a mean time from onset of stroke to surgery of 11 days and also that 53% of patients were operated on within 7 days of onset of symptoms. Postoperatively, there was one death resulting from pulmonary embolism and no patient sustained a new stroke **(IIb/B)**. Rosenthal and coworkers [23] noted a seemingly protective effect of CEA against stroke when performed on patients sustaining a reversible ischemic neurologic deficit or stroke. Twenty-nine of their patients who had limited stable strokes and abnormal CT scans underwent CEA within 3 weeks of their event, whereas 75 patients who had strokes and significant infarction on a CT scan underwent surgery greater than 3 weeks after their events. Of these, those undergoing surgery less than 3 weeks from onset of stroke had a 3% recurrent stroke rate, whereas those undergoing surgery greater than 3 weeks from stroke had a recurrent stroke rate of 5.3%. In the 10-year follow-up, the cumulative incidence of recurrent stroke was 7% in the endarterectomy group versus 18% in a non-operative control group **(IIb/B)**. In a retrospective study of 129 patients experiencing stroke, Piotrowski and colleagues [24] note no significant difference in cerebrovascular events or death between patients operated on within 6 weeks and more than 6 weeks after stroke. For the group operated with early surgery, the investigators waited until neurologic recovery reached a plateau, as determined clinically by a neurologist (76% of these patients had surgery within 4 weeks of their event). They conclude that early CEA could be performed without an increase in morbidity or mortality after stroke as long as neurologic recovery has reached such equilibrium **(IIb/B)**.

In a retrospective analysis of 100 patients entered into the North American Symptomatic Carotid Endarterectomy Trial who had severe (70-99%) angiographically defined carotid artery stenosis, Gasecki and coworkers [21] studied patients who were operated on within 30 days of stroke versus those operated beyond 30 days. They noted the baseline clinical characteristics of the groups to be comparable and they noted similar postoperative complication rates, with the group undergoing early CEA having a slightly lower complication rate (4.8% in the early group and 5.2% in the delayed group). Thus, conclusions were to not

Table 2. Literature review of studies of early vs. late CEA.

Study	Type of study	Number of patients	Recurrent stroke rates (early vs. late CEA)	Recommendations	Level of evidence
Blaisdell et al [9]	Prospective	1927	N/A	After 2 weeks post-stroke	IIb/B
Gasecki et al [17]	Retrospective case series	100	4.8% vs. 5.2%	Within 2 weeks – patients at higher risk of recurrent stroke if delayed	III/B
Whittemore et al [22]	Prospective trial	28	0%	Early CEA is safe and efficacious	IIb/B
Rosenthal et al [23]	Prospective trial	29	3% vs. 5.3%	Early CEA lowered recurrent stroke rate	IIb/B
Piotrowski et al [24]	Retrospective case series	129	N/A	No significant difference in morbidity or mortality of early CEA	III/B
Hoffman and Robbs [25]	Retrospective case series	207	N/A	No differences in morbidity between late or early CEA	III/B
Ballotta et al [26]	Prospective randomized trial	86	2% vs. 2%	No differences in early or late CEA	Ib/A
Bond et al [12]	Meta-analysis of 11 trials	4218	5.04% vs. 4.26%	No differences in morbidity or mortality with early CEA	Ia/A
Rothwell et al [13]	Meta-analysis	5893	N/A	Absolute risk reduction of 23% in recurrent stroke with CEA <2 weeks from patient's symptoms with >70% stenosis	Ia/A

delay the procedure by 30 days for patients with symptomatic high-grade stenosis because of risk of recurrent stroke, which may be avoidable by earlier surgery (III/B).

Hoffman and Robbs [25] performed a retrospective study in which they compared 86 patients who underwent early CEA (<6 weeks) for stable strokes with minor deficits or crescendo TIAs with stroke to 121 patients who had strokes and underwent delayed CEA. There were no statistical differences regarding baseline medical comorbidities, neurologic deficits, or degree of carotid stenosis. No significant differences were seen between groups in postoperative morbidity (defined as myocardial infarction and stroke) or mortality. The investigators thus advocated reconsideration and abandonment of the dogmatic 6-week waiting period for CEA post-stroke (III/B).

In an important Mantel-Haenszel meta-analysis performed by Bond et al [12], from pooled studies performed between 1980 and 2000, they noted 11 studies comparing early (<3-6 weeks) versus late (>3-6 weeks) CEA in patients who had stable symptoms post-stroke. Using their methodology, 794 patients were studied in the early group and 3424 patients were studied in the late group. Stroke or death rates compared between early surgery versus late surgery were not statistically significant, 5.04% versus 4.26 (OR 1.13; p=0.62) (Ia/A). Ballotta et al [26] performed a prospective randomized trial in which patients underwent CEA within 30 days (n=45) or more than 30 days (n=41) after non-disabling ischemic stroke with similar mean ipsilateral stenosis rates of 85% versus 83%, respectively. The presence of an ulcerated plaque was noted in 33% of those patients undergoing early operation and in 27% of patients undergoing delayed operation. Both groups were noted to have 2% peri-operative stroke rates and similar 3-year survival rates. These results suggest early CEA has no increased risks and can be performed safely with peri-operative mortality and stroke rates comparable with those of delayed CEA in non-disabling ischemic stroke patients with stable symptoms (Ib/A).

Patients who have stroke of carotid origin are at highest risk for recurrent ischemia within the first 2 weeks. Perhaps the largest data pool regarding the timing of CEA after stable stroke was analyzed by Rothwell and coworkers in their analysis of data from the European Carotid Surgery Trial and North American Symptomatic Carotid Endarterectomy Trial [13]. A total of 5893 patients with 33,000 patient-years of follow-up were studied with patients randomized to medical treatment or surgery at intervals of less than 2 weeks (20.1%), 2-4 weeks (17.9%), 4-12 weeks (39.2%), and greater than 12 weeks (22.8%) from patients' last symptoms. Entry neurologic events included ocular symptoms only (19.8%), TIAs (35.8%), and non-disabling ischemic strokes (44%). A total of 3157 patients underwent surgery. In patients who had greater than or equal to 70% carotid stenosis, absolute risk reduction (ARR) of ipsilateral ischemic stroke was greatest over 5 years in those who had experienced prior stroke (ARR 17.7%) and least in those experiencing ocular symptoms alone (ARR 5.5%) (Ia/A).

The 5-year risk reduction for ipsilateral ischemic carotid stroke seen in the surgical arm was greatest in patients randomized within 2 weeks of symptoms (23%) and tapered off with increasing time for the other groups (reductions of 15.9%, 7.9%, and 7.4%, respectively).

The cumulative 5-year absolute risk reduction for ipsilateral stroke, any stroke or death within 30 days of surgery, for those patients who had greater than or equal to 70% stenosis (but not nearly occluded) was 30.2% for the group randomized within 2 weeks of symptoms, 17.6% for the group randomized within 2-4 weeks of symptoms, 11.4% for those randomized within 4 weeks after symptoms, and 8.9% for those randomized 12 weeks after symptoms. The fall-off in benefit of CEA seen with time was highly significant (p=0.009). Thus, these results support CEA being performed within 2 weeks of the patient's last symptoms **(Ia/A)**.

Surgery in patients who have crescendo transient ischemic attacks or stroke in evolution

The indications for urgent or emergency CEA are controversial. Given that the risk of CEA is significantly higher in patients who are neurologically unstable versus patients who are neurologically stable [27], emergency surgery should be indicated only if it offers improved outcomes over medical treatment [28]. Regarding crescendo TIAs, there are reports of patients doing well with emergency surgery [29-31]. Equally compelling reports exist with good results in patients undergoing anticoagulation followed by delayed CEA [32, 33]. Given the lack of a direct comparison of emergency surgery versus anticoagulation initially and the lack of compelling evidence of the superiority of emergency CEA over initial anticoagulation followed by CEA, current recommendations are treatment of crescendo TIAs with anticoagulation and delayed CEA with emergent CEA indicated only for those who have progressive symptoms despite anticoagulation [28] **(III/B)**.

The authors' policy on CEA slightly differs from this: crescendo TIAs are treated urgently, once they have been heparinized, and operations are within 24 hours on patients who are fully heparinized. The only exception is when a propagating intraluminal thrombus beyond the reach of the surgical field is identified. These patients have a very high surgical risk (from operative carotid manipulation and dislodgement) and the preference is to anticoagulate them for 6 weeks and return for delayed routine CEA at that time [34, 35], following repeat angiography which invariably demonstrates thrombus resolution, in our experience **(III/B)**.

CEA for acute stroke and stroke in evolution also is controversial. In general, the severity of acute neurologic deficit at the time of surgery is the greatest risk factor for poor outcomes [28]. Acute stroke with associated debilitating fixed deficits or changes in level of consciousness generally are considered contraindications to CEA; patients undergoing emergent CEA for stroke with profound deficits are reported to have mortalities ranging between 20% and 37% [36, 37]. Nevertheless, Meyer and colleagues [36], in their series of patients undergoing emergent CEA for carotid occlusion presenting with severe neurologic deficits, note 38% of their patients made a dramatic recovery. These results suggest emergent CEA may be indicated in carefully selected patients with acute internal carotid artery occlusion with profound neurological deficits **(IIb/B)**.

The overall data, however, may not support a general policy of emergent CEA for unselected patients who have stroke in evolution or crescendo TIAs. In their meta-analysis looking at 13 studies reporting results for patients undergoing emergency CEA for crescendo TIAs, stroke in evolution, or 'urgent' CEA, Bond et al [12] calculated an overall OR of 4.9 (95% CI, 3.4-7.1) of stroke or death over stable stroke patients undergoing CEA. Given that the overall risk of stroke and death, based on their calculations, was approximately 20%, this suggests the data do not support a blanket policy of urgent CEA (Ia/A).

Some investigators advocate urgent surgery in highly selected patients for acute stroke and stroke in evolution [38-42], arguing surgery can reduce the risk of further progression of symptoms by removing a source of further emboli and increasing flow to the ischemic penumbra [43]. Schneider et al [39] report a 1-month mortality, ranging from 0-9.5% with no statistical difference in outcomes at 90-day follow-up in patients undergoing emergent CEA versus elective CEA with >70% stenosis (IIb/B). Similarly, Gay et al [42] report good results in 21 patients who underwent carotid artery repair <24 hours after diagnostic work-up for crescendo TIAs (5), fluctuating neurologic deficits (11), and stroke in evolution (5). Survival rates at 1 and 5 years were 90% and 62% with neurologic deficit-free rates at 1 and 5 years of 95% and 76%, respectively. Thus, the decision to proceed with urgent CEA should be made on a case-by-case basis and patients experiencing a frank stroke with severe symptoms or disturbances in consciousness most likely may not benefit from CEA (IIb/B).

Neuroendovascular interventions for acute internal carotid artery occlusion

Occlusions of the extra- and intra-cranial portion of the internal carotid artery (ICA) can cause devastating neurological deficits in patients with poor collateral anastomoses. Intracranial ICA distribution involving the M1 and A1 segments and poor neurologic presentation are negative prognostic indicators in this type of stroke [44]. Linfante et al, in a retrospective analysis, compared acute MCA versus intracranial ICA occlusion response to IV rt-PA [45]. Controlling for all comorbidities and enrolling patients with similar initial NIHSS scores, they found recanalization rates of 88% versus 31%, respectively, with lower NIHSS scores at follow-up in ICA victims [45]. These results suggest that IV rt-PA in intracranial ICA occlusions may not be efficacious (III/B). Arnold et al, in a prospective case series of 24 patients treated with IA urokinase, achieved partial revascularization in 63% of patients with distal ICA occlusion [46]. However, outcomes were still dismal with only 16% good functional outcome and a 42% mortality rate at 3 months, but still, in comparison to IV rt-PA, IA therapy almost doubled the rate of recanalization (IIb/B).

Mechanical thrombectomy for intracranial ICA occlusions is another treatment option. Flint et al report an 80-patient series with intracranial ICA occlusions in the MERCI and Multi MERCI trials that received mechanical thrombectomy with or without adjuvant IA thrombolysis [47]. Recanalization rates were 53% with mechanical thrombectomy alone and 63% with adjuvant therapy. Favorable outcomes with a mRS of 0-2 at 90 days occurred in

39% of patients with ICA recanalization compared to 3% without [47]. Therefore, mechanical thrombectomy with or without adjuvant therapy has a high success rate and has favorable outcomes compared to alternative treatment **(IIb/B)**.

Carotid artery stenting (CAS) in acute cervical ICA occlusion is under investigation. Nikas *et al*, in a case series of 18 patients with proximal ICA occlusion, achieved successful recanalization in 83.3% of patients with 30-day mortality rates at 11.1% and a median mRS score of 1 at 30-day follow-up [48]. Thus, while still underpowered, this preliminary data show that CAS for extracranial ICA strokes merits consideration and study **(III/B)**. Furthermore, in a 25-patient series, Jovin *et al* demonstrated revascularization in 92% of patients following IA thrombolysis with stenting in patients with extracranial ICA strokes [49]. These results suggest that combination therapy with stenting may improve recanalization rates in the setting of acute occlusion **(III/B)**.

Carotid artery stenting for chronic carotid occlusive disease

Carotid artery stenting, protected (CAS-P) for chronic occlusive disease remains the subject of much debate. Original data suggested CAS-P was safe and effective; however, more recent randomized trials comparing CAS-P with CEA have shown ambiguous results.

Recently, the CREST trial was completed, which randomly assigned 2502 patients with asymptomatic or symptomatic carotid stenosis to undergo CAS-P or CEA. The primary composite endpoint was composed of stroke, myocardial infarction, or death during the periprocedural period or within 4 years after randomization. Over a median follow-up time of 2.5 years, there was no significant difference in the primary composite endpoint between CAS-P or CEA patients or between symptomatic or asymptomatic patients receiving treatment, respectively. Periprocedural rates of endpoints did vary with CEA patients at higher risk for myocardial infarction (2.3% vs. 1.1%; p=0.03) and CAS-P patients at higher risk for ipsilateral stroke (2.3% vs. 4.1%; p=0.01). Patients who had an MI reported a better quality of life after recovery than patients who had a stroke. CREST thus showed that CAS-P had a statistically higher stroke rate at 30 days than CEA. It is difficult for us, based on these data, to consider the safety of CAS-P to be the equal of CEA.

In a recent meta-analysis evaluating CEA versus CAS, Meier *et al* found 11 randomized controlled trials reporting short-term outcomes (n=4790), and nine trials on intermediate outcomes (1-4 years) in patients with TIAs or asymptomatic stenosis [44]. They found CEA to have a lower periprocedural risk of mortality or stroke (OR 0.67; 95% CI, 0.47-0.95; p=0.025). Moreover, CEA had a composite decreased risk of stroke (OR 0.65; 95% CI, 0.43-1.00; p=0.049). CAS did have lower odds of periprocedural MI (OR 2.69; 95% CI, 1.06-6.79; p=0.036), and did not present risk to cranial nerve injury. In the intermediate outcome evaluation, the two treatments did not differ significantly.

These results suggest CAS-P is effective and durable but without the same short-term safety profile as CEA. CAS-P does carry an increased risk of peri-operative stroke, but affords a lower risk for myocardial infarction. Thus, current recommendations are careful patient selection and medical clearance to specifically assess the risks before undergoing either procedure (Ia/A). To our thinking, no study has yet shown that CAS-P is superior to CEA by any evaluation, and most contemporary randomized trials suggest that it is probably not even equivalent in terms of safety.

Neuroendovascular interventions for intracranial stenosis

With the advent of neuroendovascular techniques, there has been widespread adoption of treatment for patients with symptomatic and asymptomatic intracranial stenosis of 50-99%. Patients with intracranial stenosis have an annual risk of recurrent TIAs or ischemic events in excess of 30-60% [50-53]. The WASID study comparing aspirin and warfarin therapy for intracranial stenosis >50% showed a total stroke or death rate of 22.5% over 15-19 months of follow-up [53]. Studies have shown favorable results at reducing these rates with balloon angioplasty combined with self-expanding stent placement [53-59].

In 2004, the multicentre randomized study, Stenting of Symptomatic Atherosclerotic Lesions in the Vertebral or Intracranial Arteries (SSYLVIA), evaluated the balloon-mounted NEUROLINK™ stent system for treatment of symptomatic intracranial stenosis [59]. Forty-three patients with intracranial stenosis >50% (15 ICA, 5 MCA, 1 PCA, 17 basilar, 5 vertebral) had a composite endpoint of stroke and death of 6.6% at 30 days and 7.3% from 30 days to 1 year with restenosis in 32.4% found on 6-month angiogram. However, 61% of these patients were asymptomatic. Thus, the authors concluded the benefits outweighed the risks of using the NEUROLINK™ system and decreased stroke rates in the first year after deployment of the balloon mounted stent [59]. Comparing these results with the WASID trial, the FDA approved the NEUROLINK™ system and current recommendations are for treatment of atherosclerotic disease refractory to medical therapy ranging from 2.5 to 4.5mm in diameter with >50% stenosis (IIb/B).

Other neuroendovascular techniques have been under investigation in recent years. In 2005, Henkes, et al [58], in a case series using combination balloon angioplasty with the Wingspan™ self-expanding stent system in 15 patients reduced the mean intracranial stenosis from 72% to 38%. Recurrent TIA did not occur in any patient and all patients were stable or improved 4 weeks after treatment [58]. Bose et al [54], in an international prospective multicenter single-arm study, investigated combination therapy with balloon angioplasty and subsequent Wingspan™ self-expanding stent placement. Intracranial lesions in 45 patients were reduced from a mean of 74.9% to 31.9% immediately post-stenting. The composite ipsilateral stroke/death rate at 6 months was 7% with all-cause mortality of 2.3% [54]. Moreover, Fiorella et al [56], in a multicenter prospective study using the Wingspan™ stent, reported a 98.8% stenting success rate on 78 patients with mean intracranial stenosis of

74.6% (32 ICA, 22 MCA, 14 vertebral, 14 basilar). There was a 6.4% stroke rate following stent placement and a 5% mortality rate. These prospective studies prove that combination balloon angioplasty with self-expanding stent placement is safe, maintains vessel patency, and decreases TIA and stroke rates compared to the WASID study rates of total stroke or death. Thus, the combination of balloon angioplasty and Wingspan™ self-expanding stent system received FDA approval and current recommendations are for use in intracranial stenosis >50% in patients refractory to medical management **(IIb/B)**.

Conclusions

Despite the earlier accepted notion that CEA should be delayed 4-6 weeks after a stroke, current evidence suggests that CEA may be performed safely earlier in most patients with mild to moderate deficits once symptoms stabilize. Current evidence on CEA shows surgery to be advantageous within 2 weeks to avoid recurrent stroke in patients with high-grade stenosis.

However, gray areas exist as outlined. Crescendo TIAs are urgent cases in the authors' practice; others advocate a more moderate delayed approach in such cases, but nearly everyone agrees that propagating (extending too far up the ICA to cross-clamp above it) intraluminal thrombus (with the possible exception being the simpler 'bullet' type localized to the region of maximal stenosis itself, which can be isolated with the cross-clamps at surgery) is treated best with a moderate-delayed approach that allows the thrombus to resolve first with anticoagulants. Acute carotid occlusion must be assessed on an individual basis: cases that occlude under observation should be explored immediately; cases that come from the field with profound deficits have dismal outcomes, but intervention may be effective in salvaging a small group of good functional survivors. Surgery for stroke in evolution is associated with higher morbidity and mortality rates, but carefully selected patients may benefit from emergency surgery.

CAS and intracranial stenting are emerging neuroendovascular approaches to treating atherosclerotic disease that has been shown to be effective in treating symptomatic and asymptomatic stenosis in long-term studies, although still not (for CAS) with the same safety profile as operative CEA. Furthermore, CAS and intracranial stenting as possible treatment options in the setting of acute occlusion are under current investigation. Nevertheless, both interventions carry risks including peri-operative stroke. Therefore, further studies are warranted to evaluate proper patient selection to limit these risks.

A final thought is that for patients who have routine TIA or small stroke, with minimal imaging evidence of infarction or mass effect, a stable deficit, and a normal level of consciousness, there is no reason to empirically delay vessel reconstruction, and patients are served best by a fast-track approach to aggressive interventional treatment.

Key points	Evidence level
◆ CEA is established as effective for recently symptomatic (within previous 6 months) patients with 70-99% ICA angiographic stenosis.	Ia/A
◆ CEA may be considered for patients with 50-69% symptomatic stenosis but the clinician should consider additional clinical and angiographic variables.	Ia/A
◆ It is recommended that the patient has at least a 5-year life expectancy and that the peri-operative stroke/death rate should be <6% for symptomatic patients.	Ia/A
◆ CEA should not be considered for symptomatic patients with <50% stenosis.	Ia/A
◆ Medical management is preferred to CEA for symptomatic patients with <50% stenosis.	Ia/A
◆ It is reasonable to consider CEA for patients between the ages of 40 and 75 years and with asymptomatic stenosis of 60-99% if the patient has an expected 5-year life expectancy and if the surgical stroke or death frequency can be reliably documented to be <3%. The 5-year life expectancy is important since peri-operative strokes pose an upfront risk to the patient and the benefit from CEA emerges only after a number of years.	Ia/A
◆ Patients with hemispheric TIA/stroke have greater benefit from CEA than patients with retinal ischemic events.	Ib/A
◆ For patients with severe stenosis and a recent TIA or non-disabling stroke, CEA should be performed without delay, preferably within 2 weeks of the patient's last symptomatic event.	Ib/A
◆ There is insufficient evidence to support or refute the performance of CEA within 4-6 weeks of a recent moderate to severe stroke.	

References

1. Tunstall-Pedoe H. Preventing Chronic Diseases. A Vital Investment: WHO Global Report. Geneva: World Health Organization, 2005: 200. ISBN 92 4 1563001. Also published on http://www.who.int/chp/chronic_disease_report/en/. *Int J Epidemiol* 2006; Jul 19.

2. Morabia A, Abel T. The WHO report 'Preventing chronic diseases: a vital investment' and us. *Soz Praventivmed* 2006; 51(2): 74.

3. Writing Group Members, Lloyd-Jones D, Adams RJ, Brown TM, Carnethon M, Dai S, *et al.* Executive summary: heart disease and stroke statistics - 2010 update: a report from the American Heart Association. *Circulation* 2010; 121(7): 948-54.

4. Writing Group Members, Lloyd-Jones D, Adams RJ, Brown TM, Carnethon M, Dai S, *et al.* Heart disease and stroke statistics - 2010 update: a report from the American Heart Association. *Circulation* 2010; 121(7): e46-215.

5.   Wang TJ, Massaro JM, Levy D, Vasan RS, Wolf PA, D'Agostino RB, *et al.* A risk score for predicting stroke or death in individuals with new-onset atrial fibrillation in the community: the Framingham Heart Study. *JAMA* 2003; 290(8): 1049-56.

6.   Wylie EJ, Hein MF, Adama JE. Intracranial hemorrhage following surgical revascularization for treatment of acute strokes. *J Neurosurg* 1964; 21: 212-5.

7.   Giordano JM, Trout HH, 3rd, Kozloff L, DePalma RG. Timing of carotid artery endarterectomy after stroke. *J Vasc Surg* 1985; 2(2): 250-5.

8.   Bruetman ME, Fields WS, Crawford ES, Debakey ME. Cerebral hemorrhage in carotid artery surgery. *Arch Neurol* 1963; 9: 458-67.

9.   Blaisdell WF, Clauss RH, Galbraith JG, Imparato AM, Wylie EJ. Joint study of extracranial arterial occlusion. IV. A review of surgical considerations. *JAMA* 1969; 209(12): 1889-95.

10.   Thompson JE, Talkington CM. Carotid endarterectomy. *Ann Surg* 1976; 184(1): 1-15.

11.   Rothwell PM, Gutnikov SA, Warlow CP, European Carotid Surgery Trialists' Collaboration. Reanalysis of the final results of the European Carotid Surgery Trial. *Stroke* 2003; 34(2): 514-23.

12.   Bond R, Rerkasem K, Rothwell PM. Systematic review of the risks of carotid endarterectomy in relation to the clinical indication for and timing of surgery. *Stroke* 2003; 34(9): 2290-301.

13.   Rothwell PM, Eliasziw M, Gutnikov SA, Warlow CP, Barnett HJ, Carotid Endarterectomy Trialists' Collaboration. Endarterectomy for symptomatic carotid stenosis in relation to clinical subgroups and timing of surgery. *Lancet* 2004; 363(9413): 915-24.

14.   Dosick SM, Whalen RC, Gale SS, Brown OW. Carotid endarterectomy in the stroke patient: computerized axial tomography to determine timing. *J Vasc Surg* 1985; 2(1): 214-9.

15.   Little JR, Moufarrij NA, Furlan AJ. Early carotid endarterectomy after cerebral infarction. *Neurosurgery* 1989; 24(3): 334-8.

16.   Paty PS, Darling RC, 3rd, Woratyla S, Chang BB, Kreienberg PB, Shah DM. Timing of carotid endarterectomy in patients with recent stroke. *Surgery* 1997; 122(4): 850-4; discussion 854-5.

17.   Gasecki AP, Eliasziw M, Ferguson GG, Hachinski V, Barnett HJ. Long-term prognosis and effect of endarterectomy in patients with symptomatic severe carotid stenosis and contralateral carotid stenosis or occlusion: results from NASCET. North American Symptomatic Carotid Endarterectomy Trial (NASCET) Group. *J.Neurosurg* 1995; 83(5): 778-82.

18.   Wolfle KD, Pfadenhauer K, Bruijnen H, Becker T, Engelhardt M, Wachenfeld-Wahl C, *et al.* Early carotid endarterectomy in patients with a nondisabling ischemic stroke: results of a retrospective analysis. *Vasa* 2004; 33(1): 30-5.

19.   Fields WS, Lemak NA. Joint Study of Extracranial Arterial Occlusion. Internal carotid artery occlusion. *JAMA* 1976; 235(25): 2734-8.

20.   Estes JM, Whittemore AD. Subacute carotid surgery in recent stroke patients. In: *Carotid Artery Surgery.* Loftus CM, Kresowik TF, Eds. New York, USA: Thieme, 2000: 209-13.

21.   Gasecki AP, Ferguson GG, Eliasziw M, Clagett GP, Fox AJ, Hachinski V, *et al.* Early endarterectomy for severe carotid artery stenosis after a nondisabling stroke: results from the North American Symptomatic Carotid Endarterectomy Trial. *J Vasc Surg* 1994; 20(2): 288-95.

22.   Whittemore AD, Ruby ST, Couch NP, Mannick JA. Early carotid endarterectomy in patients with small, fixed neurologic deficits. *J Vasc Surg* 1984; 1(6): 795-9.

23.   Rosenthal D, Borrero E, Clark MD, Lamis PA, Daniel WW. Carotid endarterectomy after reversible ischemic neurologic deficit or stroke: is it of value? *J Vasc Surg* 1988; 8(4): 527-34.

24.   Piotrowski JJ, Bernhard VM, Rubin JR, McIntyre KE, Malone JM, Parent FN, 3rd, *et al.* Timing of carotid endarterectomy after acute stroke. *J Vasc Surg* 1990; 11(1): 45-51; discussion 51-2.

25.   Hoffmann M, Robbs J. Carotid endarterectomy after recent cerebral infarction. *Eur J Vasc Endovasc Surg* 1999; 18(1): 6-10.

26.   Ballotta E, Da Giau G, Baracchini C, Abbruzzese E, Saladini M, Meneghetti G. Early versus delayed carotid endarterectomy after a nondisabling ischemic stroke: a prospective randomized study. *Surgery* 2002; 131(3): 287-93.

27.   Sundt TM, Sandok BA, Whisnant JP. Carotid endarterectomy. Complications and preoperative assessment of risk. *Mayo Clin Proc* 1975; 50(6): 301-6.

28.   Amin-Hanjani S, Ogilvy CS. Indications and techniques for emergent carotid exploration. In: *Carotid Artery Surgery.* Loftus CM, Kresowik TF, Eds. New York, USA: Thieme, 2000: 303-13.

29. Mentzer RM, Jr, Finkelmeier BA, Crosby IK, Wellons HA, Jr. Emergency carotid endarterectomy for fluctuating neurologic deficits. *Surgery* 1981; 89(1): 60-6.

30. Najafi H, Javid H, Dye WS, Hunter JA, Wideman FE, Julian OC. Emergency carotid thromboendarterectomy. Surgical indications and results. *Arch Surg* 1971; 103(5): 610-4.

31. Walters BB, Ojemann RG, Heros RC. Emergency carotid endarterectomy. *J Neurosurg* 1987; 66(6): 817-23.

32. Nehler MR, Moneta GL, McConnell DB, Edwards JM, Taylor LM, Jr, Yeager RA, *et al.* Anticoagulation followed by elective carotid surgery in patients with repetitive transient ischemic attacks and high-grade carotid stenosis. *Arch Surg* 1993; 128(10): 1117-21; discussion 1121-3.

33. Putman SF, Adams HP, Jr. Usefulness of heparin in initial management of patients with recent transient ischemic attacks. *Arch Neurol* 1985; 42(10): 960-2.

34. Loftus CM. *Carotid Endarterectomy: Principles and Technique*, 2nd ed. Taylor and Francis, 2006.

35. Loftus CM. Propagating intraluminal carotid thrombus - surgery or anticoagulation? In: *Carotid Artery Surgery.* Loftus CM, Kresowik T, Eds. New Tork, USA: Thieme, 2000: 321-8.

36. Meyer FB, Sundt TM, Jr, Piepgras DG, Sandok BA, Forbes G. Emergency carotid endarterectomy for patients with acute carotid occlusion and profound neurological deficits. *Ann Surg* 1986; 203(1): 82-9.

37. DeWeese JA. Management of acute strokes. *Surg Clin North Am* 1982; 62(3): 467-72.

38. Van der Mieren G, Duchateau J, De Vleeschauwer P, De Leersnijder J. The case for urgent carotid endarterectomy. *Acta Chir Belg* 2005; 105(4): 403-6.

39. Schneider C, Johansen K, Konigstein R, Metzner C, Oettinger W. Emergency carotid thromboendarterectomy: safe and effective. *World J Surg* 1999; 23(11): 1163-7.

40. Peiper C, Nowack J, Ktenidis K, Hopstein S, Keresztury G, Horsch S. Prophylactic urgent revascularization of the internal carotid artery in the symptomatic patient. *Vasa* 2001; 30(4): 247-51.

41. Huber R, Muller BT, Seitz RJ, Siebler M, Modder U, Sandmann W. Carotid surgery in acute symptomatic patients. *Eur J Vasc Endovasc Surg* 2003; 25(1): 60-7.

42. Gay JL, Curtil A, Buffiere S, Favre JP, Barral X. Urgent carotid artery repair: retrospective study of 21 cases. *Ann Vasc Surg* 2002; 16(4): 401-6.

43. Mead GE, O'Neill PA, McCollum CN. Is there a role for carotid surgery in acute stroke? *Eur J Vasc Endovasc Surg* 1997; 13(2): 112-21.

44. Meier P, Knapp G, Tamhane U, Chaturvedi S, Gurm HS. Short term and intermediate term comparison of endarterectomy versus stenting for carotid artery stenosis: systematic review and meta-analysis of randomised controlled clinical trials. *BMJ* 2010; 340: c467.

45. Linfante I, Llinas RH, Selim M, Chaves C, Kumar S, Parker RA, *et al.* Clinical and vascular outcome in internal carotid artery versus middle cerebral artery occlusions after intravenous tissue plasminogen activator. *Stroke* 2002; 33(8): 2066-71.

46. Arnold M, Nedeltchev K, Mattle HP, Loher TJ, Stepper F, Schroth G, *et al.* Intra-arterial thrombolysis in 24 consecutive patients with internal carotid artery T occlusions. *J Neurol Neurosurg Psychiatry* 2003; 74(6): 739-42.

47. Flint AC, Duckwiler GR, Budzik RF, Liebeskind DS, Smith WS, MERCI and Multi MERCI Writing Committee. Mechanical thrombectomy of intracranial internal carotid occlusion: pooled results of the MERCI and Multi MERCI Part I trials. *Stroke* 2007; 38(4): 1274-80.

48. Nikas D, Reimers B, Elisabetta M, Sacca S, Cernetti C, Pasquetto G, *et al.* Percutaneous interventions in patients with acute ischemic stroke related to obstructive atherosclerotic disease or dissection of the extracranial carotid artery. *J Endovasc Ther* 2007; 14(3): 279-88.

49. Jovin TG, Gupta R, Uchino K, Jungreis CA, Wechsler LR, Hammer MD, *et al.* Emergent stenting of extracranial internal carotid artery occlusion in acute stroke has a high revascularization rate. *Stroke* 2005; 36(11): 2426-30.

50. Qureshi AI, Kirmani JF, Hussein HM, Harris-Lane P, Divani AA, Suri MF, *et al.* Early and intermediate-term outcomes with drug-eluting stents in high-risk patients with symptomatic intracranial stenosis. *Neurosurgery* 2006; 59(5): 1044-51; discussion 1051.

51. Qureshi AI, Hussein HM, El-Gengaihy A, Abdelmoula M, K Suri MF. Concurrent comparison of outcomes of primary angioplasty and of stent placement in high-risk patients with symptomatic intracranial stenosis. *Neurosurgery* 2008; 62(5): 1053-60; discussion 1060-2.

52. Mazighi M, Tanasescu R, Ducrocq X, Vicaut E, Bracard S, Houdart E, *et al.* Prospective study of symptomatic atherothrombotic intracranial stenoses: the GESICA study. *Neurology* 2006; 66(8): 1187-91.

53. Kasner SE, Chimowitz MI, Lynn MJ, Howlett-Smith H, Stern BJ, Hertzberg VS, *et al.* Predictors of ischemic stroke in the territory of a symptomatic intracranial arterial stenosis. *Circulation* 2006; 113(4): 555-63.

54. Bose A, Hartmann M, Henkes H, Liu HM, Teng MM, Szikora I, *et al.* A novel, self-expanding, nitinol stent in medically refractory intracranial atherosclerotic stenoses: the Wingspan study. *Stroke* 2007; 38(5): 1531-7.

55. Derdeyn CP, Grubb RL, Jr, Powers WJ. Indications for cerebral revascularization for patients with atherosclerotic carotid occlusion. *Skull Base* 2005; 15(1): 7-14.

56. Fiorella D, Levy EI, Turk AS, Albuquerque FC, Niemann DB, Aagaard-Kienitz B, *et al.* US multicenter experience with the Wingspan stent system for the treatment of intracranial atheromatous disease: periprocedural results. *Stroke* 2007; 38(3): 881-7.

57. Fiorella D, Chow MM, Anderson M, Woo H, Rasmussen PA, Masaryk TJ. A 7-year experience with balloon-mounted coronary stents for the treatment of symptomatic vertebrobasilar intracranial atheromatous disease. *Neurosurgery* 2007; 61(2): 236-42; discussion 242-3.

58. Henkes H, Miloslavski E, Lowens S, Reinartz J, Liebig T, Kuhne D. Treatment of intracranial atherosclerotic stenoses with balloon dilatation and self-expanding stent deployment (WingSpan). *Neuroradiology* 2005; 47(3): 222-8.

59. SSYLVIA Study Investigators. Stenting of Symptomatic Atherosclerotic Lesions in the Vertebral or Intracranial Arteries (SSYLVIA): study results. *Stroke* 2004; 35(6): 1388-92.

Chapter 7

Surgery for acute ischemic stroke

Katayoun Vahedi MD, Consultant Neurologist
Marie-Germaine Bousser MD, Professor in Neurology
Neurology Department, Lariboisière Hospital
Assistance Publique Hôpitaux de Paris
Paris, France

Introduction

Stroke is one of the leading causes of death and long-term disability worldwide. In the acute phase of brain hemispheric infarctions, neurological deterioration is the major cause of early death. Neurological deterioration may be the consequence of either hemorrhagic transformation or progression of brain ischemic edema. Both situations are the consequences of cerebral capillary dysfunction and progressive alteration in the permeability of the blood-brain barrier [1]. Brain edema has a progressive course during the first hours and days after a focal ischemia with a maximum on days 3-5 [2]. It causes mass effect with midline shift, raised intracranial pressure, damage to normal brain tissue and finally brain herniation and brain death in some cases of large middle cerebral artery (MCA) infarction (Figure 1). This type of stroke has been called malignant MCA infarction with a mortality ranging between 50-80% in observational studies and 70% in randomized trials that included patients less than 60 years of age [2, 3]. Almost all deaths are related to brain herniation and occur during the first days after stroke onset, particularly in younger patients. The underlying mechanism of malignant MCA infarction is either a carotid occlusion or a proximal MCA occlusion [2, 4]. In young patients, the most frequent etiologies are carotid dissection and a cardiac source of emboli, although in half of the patients, the stroke remains cryptogenic with no identified etiology [2, 5]. In patients older than 55 years, a cardiac source of emboli (particularly atrial fibrillation) may be more prevalent [6].

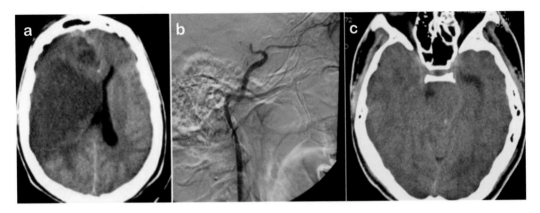

Figure 1. Brain imaging of a 22-year-old man showing: a) in an axial CT scan, right total middle cerebral artery and anterior cerebral artery acute infarction; b) in conventional angiography, internal carotid occlusion at the siphon; c) 5 days later at the time of clinical deterioration (coma and bilateral mydriasis) in an axial CT scan, temporal brain herniation.

Treatment of brain ischemic edema

Antiedema drugs include osmotic agents such as mannitol or glycerol, corticosteroids and diuretics. None of these agents have been shown in controlled trials or in observational studies to prevent brain herniation or to improve survival and outcome in cases of compressive brain ischemic edema, although some may temporarily reduce intracranial pressure. In addition, all of these drugs have potential serious side effects that limit their frequent use.

Malignant MCA infarction

Medical management versus surgery for malignant MCA infarction

The earliest studies on the relevance of decompressive surgery in malignant MCA infarction were observational studies (either retrospective or more recently prospective) that suggested that hemicraniectomy could be associated with higher survival and acceptable outcome [7]. This surgical procedure consists in removing ipsilateral to the stroke, a bone flap as large as possible including temporal, frontal, parietal and even partly occipital bones, but usually with no resection of swollen ischemic brain tissue (Figure 2). The dura is widely open to give more volume to the swollen brain. In general, duraplasty by implantation of various materials for dural expansion depends on the choice of the neurosurgeon. Hemicraniectomy aims at decreasing intracranial pressure by means of an increase in intracranial volume, therefore preventing brain temporal herniation and subsequent brain death.

Although it is essential to prevent brain death in this severe form of stroke, it is also of crucial importance to leave survivors with no extremely severe residual disability. Until

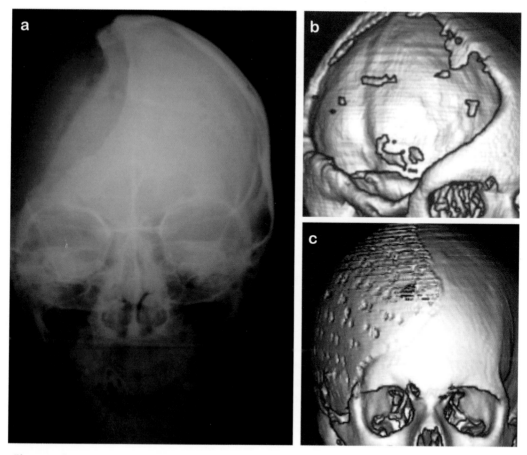

Figure 2. Extensive right hemicraniectomy: a) X-rays; b) CT scan 3D; c) followed by reconstructive cranioplasty 6 months later (CT scan 3D).

recently, data from randomized controlled trials were missing for non-biased comparison between surgery and no surgery. Thus, the decision to perform a hemicraniectomy was extremely controversial since questions regarding the outcome for patients were considered unanswered. Of particular concern was whether patients could have 'acceptable' residual disability and a good quality of life. In addition, because of the very sudden onset of a malignant MCA infarction, it is impossible to consider the preference of the patient at the time of decision.

Recently, the effect of early decompressive surgery on functional outcome in patients with malignant hemispheric infarction has been studied in three European randomised controlled trials: the French DECIMAL (DEcompressive Craniectomy In MALignant middle cerebral artery infarcts) trial, the German DESTINY (DEcompressive Surgery for the Treatment of malignant INfarction of the middle cerebral arterY) trial, and the Dutch HAMLET (Hemicraniectomy After Middle cerebral artery infarction with Life-threatening Edema Trial) [5, 8-9] **(Ia/A)**.

As no antiedema drug has proven to be effective in brain ischemic edema, 'standard medical management' has been used as reference treatment in all three randomized trials for comparison with the hemicraniectomy group. This was based on established stroke treatment guidelines [10, 11]. Standard medical management in the acute phase of a large hemispheric infarction aims to prevent general complications and neurological deterioration secondary to the stroke.

After about half of the calculated sample size was included in each of the three trials (between 2002 and 2007), they stopped prematurely for different reasons (difficulty with recruitment, results of interim analyses, ethical concerns). However, while the three trials were still recruiting and their final results were strictly unknown, the principal investigators decided on a novel protocol of prospective pooled analysis of the individual data from the three trials by an independent research group. This was possible as all three trials shared a common methodology with an identical primary hypothesis and primary outcome measure (i.e. significantly less patients alive with severe disability at 1 year in the surgery group). Importantly, this pooled analysis would allow the necessary statistical power by sharing individual data and thus reducing the number of patients needed in each therapeutic group.

Indeed the pooled analysis included a total of 93 patients and showed very significantly more patients alive with a moderate residual disability (modified Rankin score of 2 or 3 at 1-year follow-up) in the surgery group compared to the medical group, with an absolute risk reduction of 23% (5-41) [3] **(Ia/A)** (Tables 1 and 2). In total, mortality was reduced by 50% (33-67) by surgery. There were also more patients alive with a moderately severe residual

Table 1. Score description of the modified Rankin Scale (mRS).	
0	No symptoms at all
1	No significant disability despite symptoms; able to carry out all usual duties and activities
2	Slight disability; unable to carry out all previous activities, but able to look after own affairs without assistance
3	Moderate disability; requiring some help, but able to walk without assistance
4	Moderately severe disability; unable to walk without assistance and unable to attend to own bodily needs without assistance
5	Severe disability; bedridden, incontinent and requiring constant nursing care and attention
6	Dead

Table 2. Randomized controlled trials of decompressive hemicraniectomy versus standard medical treatment in malignant middle cerebral artery infarction.

Author	Surgical procedure	Number of patients	Follow-up	Absolute risk reduction% (95% CI) for mRS 4-6	Absolute risk reduction% (95% CI) for mRS 5-6	Absolute risk reduction% (95% CI) for death
Vahedi et al, 2007 [5]	Hemicraniectomy <30 hours	38	1 year	28 (-1 to 57)	53 (26 to 80)	53 (26 to 80)
Juettler et al, 2007 [8]	Hemicraniectomy <36 hours	32	1 year	20 (-12 to 53)	43 (12 to 74)	36 (5 to 67)
Hofmeijer et al 2009 [12]	Hemicraniectomy <99 hours	64	1 year	0 (-21 to 21)	19 (-5 to 43)	38 (15 to 60)
Prospective pooled analysis [3]	Hemicraniectomy <48 hours	91	1 year	23 (5 to 41)	51 (34 to 69)	50 (33 to 67)
Pooled analysis [12]	Hemicraniectomy <48 hours	109	1 year	16 (-0 to 33)	42 (25 to 59)	50 (34 to 66)

mRS = modified Rankin Scale

disability (Rankin 4) after surgery, whereas the number of patients with a severe residual disability was not increased and remained small (about 5%) [3] (Ia/A).

In the DECIMAL trial, which included younger patients than the two other trials, younger age was correlated with better outcome on the modified Rankin scores in the surgery group [4]. But without surgery the best predictor of bad outcome (death) was the volume of infarction measured on baseline diffusion-weighted imaging (DWI) within 24 hours of symptoms onset. No patients with a volume more than $210cm^3$ survived, whereas all patients screened but not included because of a DWI infarct volume less than $145cm^3$ survived [5] (Ia/A). In the surgery group, baseline infarct volume on DWI was also a prognostic factor with a non-significant trend toward better outcome with smaller infarct volume [5].

After the results of the pooled analysis, HAMLET was the only trial that continued patients' recruitment for those randomized after 48 hours (and before 96 hours) of stroke onset, but it finally had to completely stop inclusions as interim analyses suggested that the initial calculated sample size of 112 patients would lack statistical power to show significant differences between the two groups [12] (Ia/A). At the time of the premature end of the HAMLET trial, 64 patients were randomized. The final results showed no benefit of late surgery (<99 hours) over medical management for the functional outcome (survival with no severe disability), but significant benefit on survival with an absolute risk reduction of 38%, p=0.002.

It should be noted that in all three randomized trials any serious co-existent disorder that may interfere with the short- and long-term outcome after hemicraniectomy, as well as any significant pre-existing disability that may interfere with functional outcome and rehabilitation, were exclusion criteria. This should be considered whenever an individual decision of hemicraniectomy has to be taken.

Combined therapy

Moderate hypothermia (32-33°C) has been found to reduce intracranial pressure in malignant MCA infarction but during rewarming there is an increase of intracranial pressure [13]. There is yet no reported randomized trial comparing hypothermia to decompressive hemicraniectomy but combined hypothermia (35°C) and hemicraniectomy has been compared to hemicraniectomy alone in a small randomized clinical trial within the first 24 hours of a brain infarction involving more than two thirds of one hemisphere [14]. There was no statistical difference in overall mortality between the two therapeutic groups of patients.

Early clinical and radiological criteria of malignant MCA infarction

Impairment in level of consciousness during the first 24 hours of a hemispheric ischemic stroke is a powerful independent predictor of mortality [15]. Higher scores of NIHSS ($\geq$15) and an infarct volume on diffusion-weighted imaging $\geq$145cm^3 within the first 24 hours are other predictors of a malignant course of the infarction [5, 16]. On a CT scan, predictors of fatal outcome within 48 hours of stroke onset are midline shift $\geq$5mm, pineal shift $\geq$2mm, hydrocephalus, temporal lobe infarction, and involvement beyond the MCA territory [17].

In the DECIMAL and DESTINY trials, patients were included on the basis of either early large hypodensity on CT scans (>50% MCA territory) or large diffusion restriction on MRI ($\geq$145 cm^3) before signs of mass effect [5, 8].

The combination of both clinical and radiological signs can be an early predictor of a malignant course of a hemispheric infarction. They include early impairment in level of consciousness (<24 hours), a high baseline NIHSS score, severe hemiplegia and a large volume of ischemic lesions on CT or diffusion-weighted MRI. Clinical signs of brain herniation such as anisocoria, oculomotor nerve palsy, coma, decerebration, tachycardia, a mass effect on brain imaging were not selective criteria for the evaluation of early decompressive hemicraniectomy in randomised trials as they appear late in the course of the ischemic edema and may shortly precede brain herniation and death [3]. By comparison to DESTINY, death rate was much higher in the medical group of DECIMAL (78% vs. 53%). This suggests that MRI criteria (calculation of baseline infarct volume) are more powerful than CT criteria (early hypodensity >50% MCA territory) for the selection of patients who are at very high risk of herniation and will best benefit from decompressive surgery.

Specific complications related to hemicraniectomy

Reported complications related to the surgical procedure of hemicraniectomy are extradural or intracerebral hemorrhages, CSF collection under the scalp or within the brain, communicating hydrocephalus, local infection (empyema and cerebral abscess) and CSF hypotension (sinking skin flap syndrome). Sinking skin flap syndrome may be more prevalent than expected as shown in a prospective study of 27 patients followed until cranioplasty who had at 3-5 months post-hemicraniectomy either symptomatic or asymptomatic (1/4 of patients) scalp depression which progressed to a 'paradoxical' brain herniation in two patients as a consequence of atmospheric pressure exceeding intracranial pressure (Figure 3) [18].

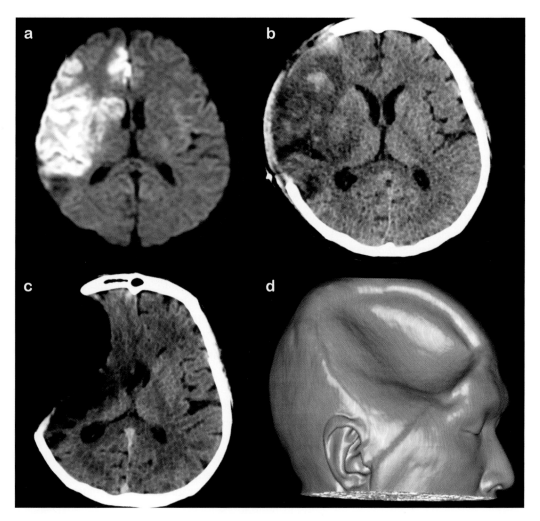

Figure 3. Brain imaging of a 45-year-old man showing: a) in axial DWI, a right total MCA and partial ACA infarction; b) 10 days later on axial CT scan, a right hemicraniectomy; c) 4 months after stroke and at the time of clinical symptoms of brain herniation (severe orthostatic headache with vomiting) on an axial CT scan, depressed and severe compression of the right hemispheric parenchyma and lateral ventricular and subfalcine herniation; d) CT scan 3D volume rendering profound depression of the skin through the craniectomy.

Orthostatic hemicrania and seizures were the two other main symptoms of sinking skin flap syndrome which was more prevalent in older patients and those who had a smaller surface of craniectomy [18]. It can be prevented by early cranioplasty for restoration of normalization of cerebral hemodynamics and intracranial pressure. It is also crucial for psychological, esthetic and rehabilitation concerns to perform cranioplasty as soon as possible during the 2-3 months post-stroke. Different procedures are used for the closure of the cranial defect including autologous bone and different types of synthetic resins and titanium. Some implants like titanium may need costly high-tech equipment. In all three European randomized trials, cranioplasty was left to the decision of the neurosurgeon and no recommendations for timing, material, procedure and specific evaluation of side effects of cranioplasty were pre-specified.

Patients with malignant MCA infarction and who have hemicraniectomy are at high risk of deep venous thrombosis and should have all evidence-based prophylactic measures that decrease the risk of venous thrombosis including early mobilization and sub-cutaneous low-molecular-weight heparin [10, 11].

Quality of life and long-term outcome after hemicraniectomy for a malignant MCA infarction

Although the results of randomized trials are very significant toward an increase of probability of survival without increasing the number of very severely disabled survivors, the decision to perform decompressive hemicraniectomy should be made on an individual basis in every patient [3]. Indeed a favorable outcome after a malignant hemispheric infarction doesn't mean complete recovery but recovery with disability. It is still a debate about what is an 'acceptable' disability and who should decide, the patient him or herself, the relatives or the physicians? Is a modified Rankin 4 (moderately severe disability) an 'acceptable' disability [19]? This will depend on many individual and subjective factors that can hardly be evaluated in randomized trials. In addition, quantitative measurements of quality of life are lacking validation in severe stroke patients. Residual neuropsychological disability including aphasia, hemineglect and frontal executive dysfunction may over or underestimate health-related quality of life in such patients.

In malignant MCA infarction, it is not easy to predict outcome in all cases and it is often impossible to consider the preferences of the patient except if it has been expressed in advance. Therefore, when deciding on surgery, prognostic factors such as young age, the absence of pre-existing disability or severe comorbid disease, as well as pragmatic predictive factors such as strong family support, should be considered at each time. Ideally, the decision should be made with the family informed about overall prognosis of the patient without surgery and with surgery in the presence of neurologists, neurosurgeons and intensivists.

More studies on patients' and family members' perception of surviving with a substantial disability would improve patient management and follow-up.

Rehabilitation after hemicraniectomy for malignant MCA infarction

Surviving after a malignant MCA infarction means early and long duration rehabilitation by a multidisciplinary team with expertise in severe stroke [10, 11]. The interventions should include speech therapy, physiotherapy, occupational therapy, and nursing. Assistive devices and orthoses are usually needed to help gait and walking ability. Spasticity in the chronic phase needs posture and movement therapy as well as botulinium toxin or neurotomy to improve range of movements, balance and gait. In this specific form of severe stroke, it is crucial to maintain rehabilitation for a long period of time (at least 5-10 years after stroke).

Depression has been reported in up to 50% of malignant hemispheric infarctions and may even be more prevalent. Antidepressant drugs such as selective serotonin reuptake inhibitors can improve post-stroke depression [10, 11]. Their primary administration has also been proven to reduce the incidence of 1-year post-stroke depression [20] **(Ib/A)**. Their early and systematic use should be recommended and depressive mood should be repeatedly evaluated after a malignant MCA infarction.

In a retrospective study of young patients (mean age 43 ± 10 years) who had hemicraniectomy for malignant MCA infarction, the length of hospitalisation in the rehabilitation ward after the acute phase was 194 ± 119 days with direct home discharge for 58% (7/12 patients) [21]. Ten out of 12 patients needed antidepressant therapy and the authors reported important psychological impact of the skull deformity, particularly in cases where the bone flap was temporarily preserved in the abdominal subcutaneous tissue of the patient [21].

There are no data on the incidence of mood disorders in close relatives or carers of patients with hemicraniectomy and no evidence-based specific prophylactic recommendations for prevention of such disorders. However, psychotherapy may help relatives including children to better understand and support the severe stroke in the patient.

Space-occupying edematous cerebellar infarction

Although rare, space-occupying edematous cerebellar infarction is a very serious condition that may lead to death or severe disability by edematous brainstem compression, obstructive hydrocephalus and brain transforaminal or transtentorial herniation. Some patients may deteriorate as late as 10 days after stroke onset. There has been no specific controlled trial of efficacy of antiedematous drugs such as mannitol in edematous cerebellar infarction. However, as in hemispheric infarction, their efficacy seems limited in reducing efficiently and durably cerebellar ischemic edema.

According to case series, mainly of retrospective design, decompressive surgery by means of suboccipital craniectomy and external ventricular drainage improves survival [22]. In two recent clinical retrospective studies, bilateral suboccipital craniectomy at the time of neurological deterioration due to edematous compression or hydrocephalus, showed 40% death and 35-40% of patients alive with good functional outcome (mRS 0-2) at follow-up [23, 24]. However, there are several limitations to these studies as regards the heterogeneity of the surgical procedures (suboccipital craniectomy only, external ventricular drainage only or both, with or without evacuation of necrotic tissue), the timing of surgery from stroke onset and the clinical presentation at the time of decision of surgery. Overall, surgery was performed late at the time of deterioration, whereas earlier prophylactic surgery may be much more effective as it has been shown in malignant hemispheric infarction. By comparison with hemispheric infarction, clinical outcome after cerebellar decompressive surgery may even be better with a higher proportion of patients alive with mild residual disability.

Predictive factors of good outcome after suboccipital craniectomy in space-occupying or malignant edematous cerebellar infarction may be younger age, lower delay to surgery, the absence of clinical signs of brainstem compression, and a normal level of consciousness, but in the absence of confirming data from controlled trials none of these factors can be accepted as definitely predictive or their absence be source of rejection of surgery.

Conclusions

The evidence suggests that early (<48 hours) decompressive hemicraniectomy in malignant MCA infarction:

- is remarkably life-saving;
- allows more patients (<60 years) to survive with a good functional outcome (moderate disability) at 1 year;
- is less effective when delayed up to 99 hours.

The evidence suggests also that decompressive suboccipital craniectomy may be life-saving in space-occupying edematous cerebellar infarction, with a substantially high number of surviving patients with good functional outcome.

Key points	Evidence level
◆ No anti-edematous drug has proven its efficacy to reduce efficiently and durably brain ischemic edema and improve patient's outcome.	IIa/B
◆ In malignant middle cerebral artery infarction, decompressive hemicraniectomy is a life-saving emergency treatment.	Ia/A
◆ In malignant middle cerebral artery infarction, early decompressive hemicraniectomy (<48 hours) in patients younger than 60 years allows more patients to survive with a slight to moderate disability (modified Rankin score of 2 or 3).	Ia/A
◆ Late decompressive hemicraniectomy (<99 hours) improves survival but not significantly functional outcome.	Ib/A
◆ Age is the best predictor of outcome after decompressive hemicraniectomy.	Ia/A
◆ There is no evidence for the benefit of decompressive hemicraniectomy in older patients (>60 years).	III/B
◆ Decompressive surgery may be life-saving in space-ocupying edematous cerebellar infarction.	III/B
◆ The best procedure of decompressive surgery (suboccipital craniectomy only, external ventricular drainage only or both, with or without evacuation of necrotic tissue) is still a matter of debate.	III/B

References

1. Simard JM, Kent TA, Chen M, *et al*. Brain oedema in focal ischaemia: molecular pathophysiology and theoretical implications. *Lancet Neurol* 2007; 6: 258-68.
2. Hacke W, Schwab S, Horn M, *et al*. 'Malignant' middle cerebral artery territory infarction: clinical course and prognostic signs. *Arch Neurol* 1996; 53: 309-15.
3. Vahedi K, Hofmeijer J, Juettler E, *et al*. Early decompressive surgery in malignant infarction of the middle cerebral artery: a pooled analysis of three randomised controlled trials. *Lancet Neurol* 2007; 6: 215-22.
4. Jaramillo A, Góngora-Rivera F, Labreuche J, *et al*. Predictors for malignant middle cerebral artery infarctions: a postmortem analysis. *Neurology* 2006; 66: 815-20.
5. Vahedi K, Vicaut E, Mateo J, *et al*. Sequential-design, multicenter, randomized, controlled trial of early Decompressive Craniectomy in Malignant Middle Cerebral Artery Infarction (DECIMAL Trial). *Stroke* 2007; 38: 2506-17.
6. Holtkamp M, Buchheim K, Unterberg A, *et al*. Hemicraniectomy in elderly patients with space occupying media infarction: improved survival but poor functional outcome. *J Neurol Neurosurg Psychiatry* 2001; 70: 226-8.
7. Schwab S, Steiner T, Aschoff A, *et al*. Early hemicraniectomy in patients with complete middle cerebral artery infarction. *Stroke* 1998; 29: 1888-93.
8. Jüttler E, Schwab S, Schmiedek P, *et al*. Decompressive Surgery for the Treatment of Malignant Infarction of the Middle Cerebral Artery (DESTINY): a randomized, controlled trial. *Stroke* 2007; 38: 2518-25.
9. Hofmeijer J, Amelink GJ, Algra A, *et al*. Hemicraniectomy After Middle Cerebral Artery Infarction with Life-threatening Edema Trial (HAMLET). Protocol for a randomised controlled trial of decompressive surgery in space-occupying hemispheric infarction. *Trials* 2006; 7: 29.

10. Adams HP, Jr, del Zoppo G, Alberts MJ, *et al.* Guidelines for the early management of adults with ischemic stroke. *Circulation* 2007;115: e478-534.

11. European Stroke Organisation (ESO) Executive Committee; ESO Writing Committee. Guidelines for management of ischaemic stroke and transient ischaemic attack 2008. *Cerebrovasc Dis* 2008; 25: 457-507.

12. Hofmeijer J, Kappelle LJ, Algra A, *et al.* Surgical decompression for space-occupying cerebral infarction (the Hemicraniectomy After Middle Cerebral Artery infarction with Life-threatening Edema Trial [HAMLET]): a multicentre, open, randomised trial. *Lancet Neurol* 2009; 8: 326-33.

13. Schwab S, Schwarz S, Spranger M, *et al.* Moderate hypothermia in the treatment of patients with severe middle cerebral artery infarction. *Stroke* 1998; 29: 2461-6.

14. Els T, Oehm E, Voigt S, *et al.* Safety and therapeutical benefit of hemicraniectomy combined with mild hypothermia in comparison with hemicraniectomy alone in patients with malignant ischemic stroke. *Cerebrovasc Dis* 2006; 21: 79-85.

15. Cucchiara BL, Kasner SE, Wolk DA, *et al.* Early impairment in consciousness predicts mortality after hemispheric ischemic stroke. *Crit Care Med* 2004; 32: 241-5.

16. Oppenheim C, Samson Y, Manai R, *et al.* Prediction of malignant middle cerebral artery infarction by diffusion-weighted imaging. *Stroke* 2000; 31: 2175-81.

17. Barber PA, Demchuk AM, Zhang J, *et al.* Computed tomographic parameters predicting fatal outcome in large middle cerebral artery infarction. *Cerebrovasc Dis* 2003; 16: 230-5.

18. Sarov M, Guichard JP, Chibarro S, *et al.* Sinking skin flap syndrome and paradoxical herniation after hemicraniectomy for malignant hemispheric infarction. *Stroke* 2010; 41: 560-2.

19. Puetz V, Campos CR, Eliasziw M, Hill MD, Demchuk AM; Calgary Stroke Program. Assessing the benefits of hemicraniectomy: what is a favourable outcome? *Lancet Neurol* 2007; 6: 580; author reply 580-1.

20. Robinson RG, Jorge RE, Moser DJ, *et al.* Escitalopram and problem-solving therapy for prevention of post-stroke depression: a randomized controlled trial. *JAMA* 2008; 299: 2391-400.

21. Mandon L, Bradaï N, Guettard E, Bonan I, Vahedi K, Bousser MG, Yelnik A. Do patients have any special medical or rehabilitation difficulties after a craniectomy for malignant cerebral infarction during their hospitalization in a physical medicine and rehabilitation department? *Ann Phys Rehabil Med* 2010; 53: 86-95.

22. Jauss M, Krieger D, Hornig C, Schramm J, Busse O, for the GASCIS study centers. Surgical and medical management of patients with massive cerebellar infarctions: results of the German-Austrian cerebellar infarction study. *J Neurol* 1999; 249: 257-64.

23. Jüttler E, Schweickert S, Ringleb PA, *et al.* Long-term outcome after surgical treatment for space-occupying cerebellar infarction: experience in 56 patients. *Stroke* 2009; 40: 3060-6.

24. Pfefferkorn T, Eppinger U, Linn J, *et al.* Long-term outcome after suboccipital decompressive craniectomy for malignant cerebellar infarction. *Stroke* 2009; 40: 3045-50.

Chapter 8

Management of ruptured cerebral aneurysms and aneurysmal subarachnoid hemorrhage

Stephen F. Shafizadeh MD PhD DC [1], Resident Physician, PGY-6 and infolded
Cerebrovascular and Skull Base Fellow
Rudy J. Rahme MD [1], Post-Doctoral Research Fellow
Christopher S. Eddleman MD PhD [2], Cerebrovascular Fellow
Bernard R. Bendok MD [1], Associate Professor of Neurosurgery and Radiology
H. Hunt Batjer MD [1], Michael J. Marchese Professor and Chair
1 Department of Neurosurgery, Feinberg School of Medicine
Northwestern University, Chicago, Illinois, USA
2 Department of Neurosurgery and Radiology, UT Southwestern Medical Center
Dallas, Texas, USA

Introduction

Epidemiology

Aneurysmal subarachnoid hemorrhage (aSAH) is a common and often pernicious etiology of acute neurological and multisystem demise. aSAH affects approximately 30,000 Americans each year accounting for nearly 5% of all strokes [1, 2]. Ingall *et al*, in a multinational World Health Organization comparison, report a ten-fold variance between countries in incidence of aSAH from 2 per 100,000 population in China to greater than 22 in Finland and Japan [3]. The estimated annual rate of aSAH in most western populations is 6-8 per 100,000 population, not accounting for a significant number of persons with aSAH who are misdiagnosed or do not receive prompt medical assessment and diagnosis [4, 5]. The peak age for aSAH is 55-60 years with, however, one fifth of cases occurring between the ages of 15 and 45 years [6-8]. As a whole, aSAH is approximately 1.6 times greater in women than in men [1, 7, 8]. This increased risk of aSAH in women is reduced amongst premenopausal women and amongst women of older age at the onset of menarche or birth of their first child, implying a possible relationship between hormonal status and aSAH [1, 9, 10].

The prevalence of cerebral aneurysms has historically been highly variable, ranging from 0.2-7.9% with recent investigations suggesting a prevalence of 5% in the general population [11]. Thus, it is evident comparing incidence of aSAH with prevalence rates that, as a whole, the vast majority of cerebral aneurysms do not rupture. The science and art of aneurysmal rupture risk is maturing but is not yet predictive for the individual patient. As such, current management strategies weigh presumptive population-based risk-benefit ratios of watchful waiting against open and endovascular surgical interventions and attempt to maximize short and long-term outcome once aSAH has occurred.

Etiology

Trauma is the leading cause of SAH overall, with aSAH accounting for approximately 80% of non-traumatic (spontaneous) subarachnoid hemorrhage (ntSAH) [12-14]. The remaining etiologies are spread amongst arteriovenous malformations (AVMs), perimesencephalic hemorrhage, cerebral artery dissection, venous thrombosis, autoimmune/allergic reactions, angiopathies, coagulopathies, primary and metastatic brain tumors, pituitary apoplexy, rupture of superficial cortical artery, spinal AVM/fistula, and miscellaneous sources such as eclampsia, meningitis, cocaine, sickle cell disease, and electrolyte abnormalities [15, 16]. Of note, approximately 10-25% of ntSAH have no known initial etiology and are negative on the primary angiogram [17-20]. Potential causes of angiogram-negative SAH include thrombosis of aneurysmal neck, radiographic obliteration of the aneurysm by intraparenchymal hemorrhage, lack of filling secondary to vasospasm, incomplete imaging especially of the posterior circulation, angiographically occult vascular malformation, and perimesencephalic/pretruncal non-aneurysmal SAH.

The pathophysiological forces and mechanisms driving aneurysm formation are still developing. Histological analysis of cerebral vasculature demonstrates several potential contributing factors. Compared to extracranial vasculature, cerebral blood vessels have a thinner adventitia with less elastic proteins, a tunica media which is less elastic and has less muscle, and a less prominent external elastic lamina [21, 22]. In addition, the extracranial vasculature is supported by extensive supportive soft tissue, dampening the transmural pressure transmitted with each cardiac cycle. However, cerebral vasculature most commonly associated with aneurysm formation is bathed in cerebrospinal fluid of the subarachnoid space surrounded by little supportive tissue, thus leading to less dampening of the pressure wave transmitted by the cardiac cycle and heightened transmural pressure [23, 24]. The tendency of cerebral aneurysm formation to occur at or near natural turning points of the parent artery or in the crotch between the parent artery and a significant branch and the propensity to align in the imaginary vector of the parent artery if it would have continued without branching, support the hypothesis based on transmural pressures, vectors, and focal hemodynamic stress [24-27].

Risk factors for aneurysmal SAH and aneurysm formation

Hypertension, smoking, and heavy alcohol consumption have shown to be independent risk factors in multivariate models for aSAH [28-32] (IIa/B). Expectantly, sympathomimetic agents have been implicated as a cause of aSAH and include cocaine [33, 34]. Diurnal variations in blood pressure, increasing age, during CSF diversion or cerebral angiography in patients with known cerebral aneurysm, pregnancy and parturition have also been associated with aSAH [35-37]. There is considerable overlap between risk factors for aSAH and the formation of saccular cerebral aneurysms themselves. Hypertension, smoking, female gender, postmenopausal state, and history of cerebrovascular disease are associated with increased risk for development of multiple aneurysms [38-40] **(IIa/B)**.

Additionally, certain conditions and genetic syndromes have been associated with an increased tendency for cerebral aneurysm formation. These include adult polycystic kidney disease (APKD), arteriovenous malformation, Osler-Weber-Rendu syndrome (hereditary hemorrhagic telangiectasia), moyamoya disease, fibromuscular dysplasia (FMD), alpha-1 antitrypsin deficiency, neurofibromatosis type-1, connective tissue disorders such as Ehlers-Danlos type IV, coarctation of the aorta, and familial intracranial aneurysm syndrome (FIA) **(III/B)**. The prevalence of cerebral aneurysms in APKD varies from 10-30% [41, 42]. The proclivity to form cerebral aneurysms in APKD is made more insidious by the increased risk of rupture in these patients and thus APKD may carry a 10-20-fold cumulative increased risk of aSAH compared to the general population [16, 43, 44]. Of patients with AVMs, the overall incidence of cerebral aneurysms is between 2.7-23% [45-47]. Cerebral aneurysms associated with AVMs can be divided into several categories based on location: proximal aneurysms on major feeding artery, pedicle aneurysms along AVM arteriole feeders, intra-nidal aneurysms, unassociated aneurysms directly unrelated to the AVM, and venous aneurysms. The reported incidence of cerebral aneurysms in patients with FMD varies widely between 7 to greater than 50% [48].

Family history has been shown to be an independent risk factor for aSAH **(IIa/B)**. In a multivariate analysis, a family history of aSAH was found to be an independent risk factor for aSAH [49]. Additionally, nearly one third of asymptomatic siblings were shown to have a cerebral aneurysm by angiography in a review of published sibships with aSAH [50]. In FIA syndrome, where two or more third degree relatives or closer harbor a radiographically evident aneurysm, family members have an 8% risk of also harboring a cerebral aneurysm [51]. In FIA, siblings and mother-daughter pairings were associated with aSAH at a younger age and higher incidence of multiple intracranial aneurysms [1, 52, 53]. Of note, patients who have been treated for a ruptured aneurysm still carry a 1-2% rate of new aneurysm formation per year [54, 55].

Natural history of aneurysmal SAH and cerebral aneurysms

The natural history of aSAH is incomplete without bridging these discussions with the natural history of unruptured intracranial aneurysms. The natural history of unruptured intracranial aneurysms is a study in progress and currently a debated one. This conversation is well needed and detailed in another chapter. In brief, however, until recently, the majority of investigations into the natural history of unruptured intracranial aneurysms stemmed from case series studies at single institutions [11, 56, 57]. These and similar studies determined a fairly consistent annual risk of hemorrhage of 1.3-2.3% per year. In an attempt to better elucidate the risk of rupture of unruptured intracranial aneurysms, the International Study of Unruptured Intracranial Aneurysms (ISUIA) was spawned. In the first part of this study, a total of 2621 patients in 53 centers in the US, Canada, and Europe were enrolled [58]. This study included a retrospective and prospective component. In the retrospective component, the natural history of unruptured intracranial aneurysms was assessed in 1449 patients with 1937 aneurysms. There was no distinction made between symptomatic and asymptomatic patients.

Patients with mycotic, fusiform, traumatic, or aneurysms <2mm were excluded. The retrospective cohort was subdivided into 727 patients with no history of aSAH (Group 1) and 722 patients with a history of aSAH from a different and successfully treated aneurysm than the one(s) being studied (Group 2). The cumulative rate of rupture in Group 1 of aneurysms <10mm was less than 0.05% per year versus 0.5% in Group 2, nearly 11 times greater rupture rate, but both still significantly lower than historical comparisons. The rupture rate of aneurysms 10mm or greater in diameter was 1% per year in both groups. Aneurysms 25mm in diameter had a rupture rate of 6% in the first year in Group 1. Aneurysm size and location were cited as being independent predictors of rupture. Compared to historical data, the findings of the ISUIA were unexpected with respect to such low annual rupture rates of unruptured intracranial aneurysms. This initiated debate and controversy.

In the year 2000, the American Heart Association published recommendations for the management of patients with unruptured intracranial aneurysms driven by literature review, including the retrospective component of ISUIA [59]. These recommendations regarding the management of unruptured intracranial aneurysms included **(IIa/B)**:

- treatment could not be advocated over observation in aneurysms <10mm in diameter in patients without previous SAH given the apparent low risk of rupture. In this group of patients, the authors do comment on special considerations for treatment in young patients, aneurysms with a daughter sac or approaching 10mm, aneurysms with increasing size, or in patients with a family history of aneurysms or aSAH;
- asymptomatic aneurysms 10mm in diameter warrant strong consideration for treatment if meeting safe treatment thresholds with regards to patient age, overall medical and neurological status, and relative risk of chosen treatment;
- coexisting or remaining aneurysms of any size in patients with a history of aSAH from another treated aneurysm warrant consideration for treatment if meeting safe treatment thresholds with regards to patient age, overall medical and neurological status, and relative risk of chosen treatment;
- symptomatic intradural aneurysms of any size should be considered for treatment with relative urgency of acutely symptomatic intradural aneurysms;
- small intracavernous internal carotid artery aneurysms generally need no treatment while the treatment of large symptomatic aneurysms in this location is individualized on the basis of patient age, progression and severity of symptoms, and treatment options.

In the second part of ISUIA published in 2003, a prospective assessment of the natural history of unruptured aneurysms was undertaken including clinical outcomes and risks of endovascular and surgical treatment [60]. There were 1692 patients followed prospectively without treatment with 2686 aneurysms, of which 1077 had no history of aSAH (Group 1) and 615 patients with a history of aSAH from another aneurysm (Group 2). There were 51 patients (3%) in this prospective cohort of 1692 patients who had a confirmed aSAH over the mean 4.1 years of follow-up (49/51 ruptures occurred within 5 years of diagnosis). In Group 1 there were a total of 41 aSAHs with two ruptures in aneurysms <7mm and five ruptures in aneurysms 7-9mm diameter. In Group 2 there were ten aSAHs with seven ruptures in aneurysms 2-6mm and one rupture in an aneurysm 7-9mm. Of note, in the 51 patients who had unruptured aneurysms at baseline but had subsequent hemorrhage in the untreated arm (Group 1 and 2), 33 (65%) died. The authors of the second part of ISUIA concurred with investigators of the 1998 ISUIA study that treatment of small aneurysms in patients without previous aSAH could not be advocated over the natural history of these lesions. The 2003 ISUIA investigation differed from the 1998 study in that it did lower the size of the aneurysm from <10mm to <7mm for this recommendation.

Much deliberation and controversy was generated given the difference between historical comparisons and expertise versus the suggestions of part 1 and 2 of ISUIA in terms of the 'natural history' of unruptured aneurysms. This debate was strengthened by the many limitations of the ISUIA investigation which included:

◆ lack of randomization into observational and treatment arms;
◆ short observational period with approximately only 20% of patients being followed for 4 years or more. This is important since the knowledge gained by this investigation is meaningful when applied to individual patients. In the clinical setting it is these same patients with relatively long life expectancy that would be considered for treatment, hence the lack of an appropriate and longer observational period limits the translation of this investigation to the individualized patient;
◆ the inclusion of cavernous carotid aneurysms, which comprised nearly 17% and >12% of all aneurysms studied in ISUIA part 1 and 2, respectively, by default lowered the overall risk of rupture given that these aneurysms are known to possess very low rates of rupture;
◆ the inclusion of posterior communicating artery aneurysms (13.9% and 14.5% in ISUIA part 1 and 2, respectively) into the posterior circulation subgroup artificially lowered the rupture rate of aneurysms in the anterior circulation;
◆ the inclusion of treated patients (410 had surgery and 124 endovascular treatment) and patients who died from unrelated causes (193) in the 'non-ruptured' denominator up to the point of removal from the study synthetically favors low rupture rates and the more benign natural course of unruptured aneurysms;
◆ lack of evaluation of aneurysm morphology and rate of growth dealt with aneurysms as static but yet conclusions were made in a prospective fashion;
◆ the unexplained discrepancy in ISUIA between the reported very low rupture rates of asymptomatic aneurysms <7mm and the fact that the majority of ruptured aneurysms evaluated were in this same category.

The importance of the need to better understand the natural history of unruptured intracranial aneurysms is underscored by the devastating consequences once there is an aSAH. The 30-day mortality amongst all patients after aSAH is >45% with 10-15% of all patients dying prior to reaching medical attention [61, 62]. In the 1966 Cooperative Study on Intracranial Aneurysms, the mortality rate at 29 days post-aSAH was approximately 50% [63]. There are an approximate 6700 in-hospital deaths annually from aSAH in the US [64]. Of survivors, approximately 30% suffer from moderate to severe disability and approximately two thirds of patients successfully treated after aSAH never return to the same quality of life [65, 66]. Currently, the most treatable cause of mortality and poor outcome after aSAH is prevention of rehemorrhage. There are approximately 3000 deaths per year in North America attributable to rebleeding of ruptured intracranial aneurysms [67]. Recurrent hemorrhage after initial aSAH carries a 70% mortality rate [68]. The risk of rehemorrhage is approximately 20% within 2 weeks after initial aSAH. The greatest probability for recurrent hemorrhage after initial aSAH is within the first 24 hours at a likelihood of 4% and then 1.5% daily for the next 13 days [65, 69] (Ib/A). Within the first 6 months after aSAH, 50% of aneurysms will rehemorrhage and thereafter the risk is approximately 3% per year [69-71]. Given that the initial aSAH and, to a much greater extent, rehemorrhage, carries such a high morbidity and mortality, early diagnosis is of paramount importance.

Diagnosis of aneurysmal SAH

Headache and other presenting symptoms

The sine qua non of aSAH in the conscious sufferer is "the worst headache of my life", present in approximately 80% of patients after aSAH. The quintessential headache of aneurysmal rupture is sudden in onset, severe, and without warning. Yet in approximately 20% of patients who will have aneurysmal rupture there is a warning or sentinel headache weeks prior to explicit aneurysm rupture and aSAH [1, 72]. This reported warning headache is associated with a minor aSAH or leak and is typically sudden in onset but milder, generally not associated with meningismus, and resolves in a few days [73-75]. However, sentinel headaches can occur without aSAH and may be a result of change in aneurysm size and morphology or hemorrhage confined to the wall of the aneurysm [76]. Sudden and severe headache is also associated with crash migraine or benign thunderclap headache. This form of headache is global, sudden, severe, and accompanied by emesis in approximately half of patients [77, 78]. Benign thunderclap headache is generally not associated with meningismus and there is no evidence of aSAH on CT or in the CSF. There are no clinical criteria that can dependably differentiate crash migraine from the headache associated with aSAH [78]. To compound the difficulties with differential diagnosis further, benign thunderclap headache is thought to be vascular in origin and patients may present with transient focal neurological symptoms and signs. The headache attributed to benign orgasmic cephalgia is also described as severe and 'explosive' but onset is near the time of orgasm and as in benign thunderclap headache, CT and lumbar puncture (LP) are negative for SAH.

Though headache is a very common chief complaint in the emergency department setting and aSAH is the most feared source, aSAH is the ascribed etiology in approximately only 1% of headache sufferers in the ED [79]. This compounds the existing aSAH misdiagnosis rate which is currently approximated at 12% [79-81]. In one retrospective review, nausea and emesis was observed in 77%, loss of consciousness in 53%, and meningismus in 35% of patients after aSAH [82]. Meningismus often arises within 6 to 24 hours after aSAH and can be clinically characterized by nuchal rigidity (especially to flexion) and Kerning's and Brudzinski's signs.

Loss of consciousness post-aSAH has been attributed to one or a combination of potential pathophysiological processes to include sudden increase in intracranial pressure, hydrocephalus, and diffuse reduced cerebral blood flow and ischemia as well as seizure [83].

Seizure has been reported in up to 20% of patients after aSAH, especially if associated with intraparenchymal hemorrhage [84, 85].

Ocular hemorrhage

There are three potential ocular hemorrhage syndromes that may occur after aSAH unaccompanied or in combination at an incidence of 20-40% [86-89]. These ocular hemorrhage syndromes post-aSAH are thought to be a result of sudden and elevated increases in intracranial pressure leading to compression of the central retinal vein and the retino-choroidal anastomoses causing venous disruption [87]. Pre-retinal hemorrhage is observed funduscopically as bright red blood at the optic disc, obscuring the normal retinal vasculature. Intra-retinal hemorrhage surrounds the fovea centralis. Terson's syndrome is hemorrhage within the vitreous humor. It is most often bilateral and symptoms can range from near normal visual acuity to only light perception. The degree of decline in vision is generally proportional to the amount of hemorrhage within the vitreous humor. Patients with ocular hemorrhage after aSAH should be followed for potential complications of retinal membrane formation, retinal folds, and retinal detachment. However, the long-term prognosis is good in approximately 80% of cases [90, 91].

Non-contrast high resolution head CT and lumbar puncture

The likelihood of detecting a hemorrhage on head CT is directly proportional to the degree of SAH and inversely proportional to the time past from aSAH and acquisition of the head CT **(Ib/A)**. If head CT is performed within the first 12 hours from onset of aSAH, the sensitivity of head CT for SAH is greater than 98%. This sensitivity is 95% if the head CT is completed within 48 hours of symptomatic aSAH. After 6 days from aSAH, the sensitivity of head CT declines significantly and is highly variable, from 57-85% [92-95]. In a more recent investigation by Cortnum *et al* in 2010 of nearly 500 patients with aSAH, head CT had a 100% sensitivity if performed within the first 5 days after aSAH [96]. As the resolution of computed tomography increases with each generation, it is expectant that so will the sensitivity of head CT for aSAH detection.

Given that the sensitivity of head CT for aSAH is not widely accepted to be 100%, small volume lumbar puncture is performed in patients with a compelling clinical presentation but negative head CT for aSAH **(Ib/A)**. Cerebrospinal fluid after aSAH needs to be differentiated from traumatic sources of blood in the CSF. Findings consistent with aSAH as the source of hemorrhage in the CSF include: non-clotting blood fluid, an RBC count >100,000/mm^3 with only small changes as CSF drains between sampling, and elevated opening pressure. The most sensitive marker of aSAH in the CSF is xanthochromia. Xanthochromia of the supernatant is rarely detected prior to 2 hours from onset of symptomatic aSAH, is present in >95% at 12 hours, and persists in 70% at 3 weeks [16, 97]. If both head CT and lumbar puncture are negative for aSAH detection and the patient presented within limits of detection of these studies, most clinicians advocate symptomatic relief and reassurance.

Magnetic resonance imaging

The use of MRI for the detection of aSAH in the emergency department setting is often not a practical and sometimes safe option in this patient population. However, the development of dedicated stroke centers, geographic localization of the MR modality in the ED, and more rapid sequencing have added some value in the detection of aSAH and is an evolving technology. The main technical limitation of MRI in the detection of aSAH is the inverse relation between the sensitivity of this modality and the acuity of the hemorrhage. The most sensitive of the imaging modalities of MRI are gradient echo (GRE) and fluid-attenuated inversion recovery (FLAIR). In a study by Mitchell in 2001, the sensitivity of GRE and FLAIR in the detection of SAH in the acute phase was 94% and 81%, respectively, while in the subacute phase there was 100% and 87% sensitivity for GRE and FLAIR, respectively [98]. In a similar report by da Rocha in 2006, FLAIR and GRE sequencing had a 100% and 37.5% respective sensitivity for detection of acute SAH and a sensitivity of 100% for FLAIR and 30% for GRE in the subacute phase [99]. Acute was defined as <4 days and subacute as between 4 and 15 days from the time of onset of symptoms in these investigations. These studies call attention to the strengths and weakness of current MRI sequencing modalities in the detection of aSAH. There is inherent variability in the detection of aSAH, both in terms of timing and sequences. Though the radiographic delineation of acute (<4 days) allows for comparable sensitivity of MRI to CT and LP in the detection of aSAH, this is not a practical clinical situation in that most patients present within hours and not days of their aSAH. However, in the setting of a sentinel hemorrhage or delayed presentation, MRI may be superior to both CT and LP since these studies lose while MRI gains sensitivity with time.

CT angiography and magnetic resonance angiography

CT angiography (CTA) is a rapid, common, and less invasive alternative to conventional catheter angiography (IIb/B). The sensitivity of CTA for aneurysm detection is largely based on aneurysm characteristics such as size, vascular location, and proximity of bony anatomy as well as timing of image acquisition to coincide with maximal intravenous contrast dose at the site of interest. In most investigations, aneurysm size has been the greatest predictor for the sensitivity and specificity of CTA for cerebral aneurysm detection. For cerebral aneurysms ≥5mm, the sensitivity of CTA is between 95-100% [100-103]. However, for aneurysms <5mm, sensitivity has been highly variable ranging from 19-100% [101, 104, 105]. It is evident that neuroradiologist and neurosurgeon experience play a critical role in the perceived sensitivity of CTA in the detection of small cerebral aneurysms. As mentioned before, it should be noted that it is not only size and interpreter experience that contribute to the sensitivity of CTA for aneurysm detection but also the location of the aneurysm. In the above and similar investigations, aneurysms leading to the lowest sensitivities for detection by CTA were small and located near bony structures, for example, ophthalmic artery aneurysms. Additionally, amongst aneurysms detected by CTA that later underwent surgery, there was a 100% correlation between CTA and catheter angiography [106, 107]. The information attained from CTA also has some independent advantages. CTA can better coordinate the anatomical relationship of the aneurysm to bony surgical landmarks and intraparenchymal hemorrhage.

CTA can also better depict intraluminal aneurysm thrombosis and wall calcification. Collectively, these properties of CTA have allowed many neurosurgeons to operate on unruptured and ruptured cerebral aneurysms on the basis of CTA alone – without catheter angiography. However, some intrinsic shortcomings of CTA include radiation, iodinated intravenous contrast, bony and metal artifact interference, and as of yet limited sensitivity for very small aneurysms. As such, the utilization of CTA should be individualized to the patient as sometimes a substitute for, in conjunction with, or inferior modality to catheter angiography. As the sensitivity of and comfort by neurosurgeons for CTA increases so will its increasing likelihood to be the sole imaging modality for aneurysm anatomic localization both for diagnosis as well as pre-operative planning.

Magnetic resonance angiography (MRA) in the diagnosis of cerebral aneurysms is an ever-evolving modality. The same inherent fundamental limitations of MRI also apply to MRA and hence render it impractical in the acute setting for the anatomic identification of the source of aSAH. However, the utilization of MRA in the diagnosis and interval monitoring of unruptured cerebral aneurysms appears to show promise. The reported sensitivities of MRA and time-of-flight MRA have been widely variable and, similar to CTA, largely dependent on aneurysm size. In addition, the direction and rate of blood flow, natural vascular branching patterns, and thrombosis or calcification of the aneurysm may interfere with accurate or complete image acquisition. For aneurysms ≥5mm, the sensitivity of MRA for aneurysm detection ranges between 85-100% but declines to <60% for smaller aneurysms [108-113] **(IIb/B)**. Given that image acquisition of time-of-flight MRA is dependent on a number of excitation pulses captured and this is inversely proportional to rate of blood flow, blood vessel morphology is recapitulated due to its limited number of excitation pulses as compared to the relatively stationary surrounding parenchyma. As this method is dependent on differences in rates and direction of blood flow, turbulence and aneurysm necks in plane with the parent vessel or at branching points diminish the precision of this modality. However, time-of-flight MRA does not require iodinated contrast or deliver ionizing radiation, thus becoming more commonly utilized in patient screening for and follow-up of previously well-characterized cerebral aneurysms by catheter or CT angiography.

Grading of aneurysmal SAH

There are two commonly utilized clinical and one radiographic grading scales to describe aSAH patients and their imaging characteristics by CT. In 1968, William E. Hunt and Robert M. Hess published their work on the clinical severity post-aSAH as a predictor of outcome (Table 1) [114]. This classification was later modified to include unruptured aneurysms (Grade 0) and patients with no acute meningeal reaction but with a fixed neurological deficit (Grade 1a) [115]. A serious systemic disease advances the patient to the next worst Hunt and Hess grade.

In 1987, the Executive Committee of the World Federation of Neurosurgical Societies approved the report from the World Federation of Neurological Surgeons (WFNS) Committee in the grading of aSAH. The WFNS Committee reviewed data from the

Table 1. Hunt and Hess aneurysmal SAH grading system.		
Grade	**Description**	**Survival (%)**
1	Asymptomatic or mild headache and slight nuchal rigidity	70
2	Moderate to severe headache or nuchal rigidity or cranial nerve palsy	60
3	Lethargy, confusion, or mild focal deficit	50
4	Stupor, moderate to severe hemiparesis, or early decerebrate rigidity	20
5	Deep coma, decerebrate rigidity, moribund appearance	10

International Cooperative Aneurysm Study to conclude that headache, nuchal rigidity, and major focal neurological deficit were not independent predictors of survival after aSAH. Level of consciousness was the major predictor of death and disability, whilst major focal neurological deficit was only a predictor of future disability in survivors [116]. Hence, the WFNS grading system (Table 2) was developed around the patient's Glasgow Coma Scale (GCS) as a familiar measure of level of consciousness and the presence or absence of aphasia, hemiplegia, or hemiparesis to forecast mortality and disability, respectively, after aSAH [117]. Like the Hunt and Hess system, Grade 0 was assigned to the unruptured aneurysm.

Table 2. WFNS aneurysmal SAH grading system.		
Grade	**GCS score**	**Major focal deficit**
1	15	-
2	13-14	-
3	13-14	+
4	7-12	+ or -
5	3-6	+ or -

Table 3. Fisher grading system.

| Grade | Amount of SAH on CT | n (total=47) | Angiographic vasospasm | | | Clinical vasospasm |
			None	Slight-Moderate	Severe	
1	None detected	11	7	2	2	0
2	Diffuse/vertical layers <1mm in thickness	7	4	3	0	0
3	Localized clot and/or vertical layers ≥1mm	24	0	1	23	23
4	Intracerebral/intraventricular clot with diffuse or no SAH	5	3	2	0	0

Note that these original and today commonly utilized grading systems to gauge clinical outcome after aSAH do not take into account commonly known factors that presently are known to also influence prognosis such as patient's age, the amount of subarachnoid hemorrhage, time passed from aSAH to admission, aneurysm location and size, intracerebral or intraventricular hemorrhage, and hydrocephalus.

In 1980, Fisher *et al* published on 47 cases of verified ruptured cerebral aneurysms and investigated the relationship of the amount and distribution of subarachnoid hemorrhage detected by CT to the later development of cerebral vasospasm [118]. Only patients who underwent CT within the first 5 days and had catheter angiography during the period when vasospasm is most likely to occur (days 7-17) after aSAH were included in the study. Virtually all patients (23 of 24) with subarachnoid clots larger than 5 x 3mm or vertical layers 1mm in fissures and vertical cisterns developed severe angiographic and clinical cerebral vasospasm (Table 3). The positive correlation of cerebral angiographic and clinical vasospasm with the amount of aSAH allowed clinicians to identify patients at highest risk and institute early potential prophylactic measures.

In an effort to advance the predictive risk stratification of patients with aSAH who then undergo microneurosurgical clipping of their cerebral aneurysm, a multivariate clinical and radiographic grading system was developed by Ogilvy and Carter [119]. In this investigation, it was determined that patient age, size of aneurysm, clinical condition based on Hunt and Hess grade, and degree of aSAH based on Fisher grade were each independent predictors of long-term outcome after microneurosurgical clipping. In addition, there was a trend of increased surgical risk with larger (≥25mm) posterior circulation aneurysms. Although each of these factors independently influenced outcome after microneurosurgical clipping, the combination of these variables was a much stronger predictor of outcome and, hence, leading to the proposed comprehensive grading system. In this system, there are five grades (0-4), with 1 point assigned for Hunt and Hess Grade IV or V, Fisher Grade III or IV, aneurysm size >10mm, aneurysm ≥25mm and of the posterior circulation, and if patient age is >50 years. In both the retrospective and prospective arms of this investigation, there was good correlation of this grading system with outcome **(IIa/B)**. This grading system was consistent with neurovascular experience in that multiple variables, demographic, clinical, and radiographic, influence individual patient management and, hence, outcome in both ruptured and unruptured intracranial aneurysms.

The goal of these and other grading systems is to minimize intra and inter-observer variability thereby standardizing assessment, facilitating triage, and prognosticating outcome and, thus, aiding in patient-specific treatment paradigms driven by similar outcome groups **(IIa/B)**.

Medical management after aneurysmal SAH

The initial management of a patient after aSAH must take into account several general and disease-specific concerns. Given that the first medical evaluation of the majority of patients who suffer aSAH is by mobile emergency medical personnel, education to include rapid neurological assessment is paramount. Fortunately, there has been much effort in recent years to expand the effective 'protocol' measures in the management of myocardial infarction to 'brain attack' as well. This has had direct and serendipitous effects on ischemic stroke which now needs to be better expanded to hemorrhagic stroke, specifically, aneurysmal subarachnoid hemorrhage. Fortuitously, many of the symptoms and neurological consequences of ischemic and hemorrhagic stroke can overlap with aSAH leading to rapid notice, 911 contact, and transport to the emergency department without unnecessary delays at the field of injury. Upon presentation to the emergency department the acuity and severity of headache, especially if coincident with altered level of consciousness or focal neurological signs, triggers a head CT (after assurance of and maintenance of an adequate airway, breathing, and circulation), even if aSAH is not the premier working diagnosis. Prior to the acquisition of imaging, an efficient current, past, and family medical history is obtained, if possible. Points to note include are time of onset of symptoms and presenting blood pressure as well as a personal history of smoking, hypertension, or sentinel headache. Likewise, a family history of cerebral aneurysms, aSAH, or unexplained early sudden death should be attained. A neurological and directed physical examination and one or more of the above grading systems allows for proper and translatable patient assessment and triage. Coagulation studies, platelet function assays, and a toxicology screen should be obtained in patients documented to have an aSAH in whom a clinical history cannot be obtained.

Initial disease-specific management concerns after aSAH include attenuation of rehemorrhage risk, seizures, and the development of cerebral vasospasm as well as management of hydrocephalus.

Medical measures to prevent rehemorrhage after aSAH

Rehemorrhage is the most feared acute concern after aSAH in that it carries a 70% mortality. It is estimated that approximately 3000 North Americans die each year from rehemorrhage of ruptured cerebral aneurysms [67]. This concern is heightened by the fact that the greatest likelihood of rehemorrhage is in the few days after initial aneurysmal rupture. The peak incidence of rehemorrhage is during the first 24 hours, 4% on day 1, followed by approximately 1.5% each day for the next 13 days. This yields an approximate 1 in 5 chance of rehemorrhage in the first 2 weeks post-aSAH without treatment, recalling a 70% mortality.

By 6 months post-aSAH, 50% of untreated ruptured cerebral aneurysms will have re-ruptured. Thereafter, the rehemorrhage rate approximates the initial yearly hemorrhage rate of unruptured cerebral aneurysms, in the order of 3% per year [69]. A higher Hunt and Hess grade at initial rupture is associated with higher rehemorrhage rates [120].

Bed rest and blood pressure control

Though common practice, bed rest is not a measure that independently diminishes the risk of rehemorrhage and as such is included with more definitive measures in a broader treatment protocol [71] **(IIb/B)**. Likewise though virtually universally practiced, blood pressure control has not been demonstrated in well-controlled studies to independently attenuate rehemorrhage post-aSAH. Most studies have been retrospective and confounding. Though Wijdicks *et al* in a retrospective investigation demonstrated that rebleeding after aSAH occurred less often in patients treated with antihypertensives, mean blood pressure was higher in the treatment group [121]. In another retrospective review, 17% of patients with aSAH admitted within 24 hours suffered a rehemorrhage associated with a systolic blood pressure of 150mm Hg [122]. Yet in another retrospective investigation, there was no relationship between blood pressure and the 6.9% rehemorrhage rate after admission with aSAH [123]. Alternatively, rehemorrhage after aSAH may be a consequence of variations in rather than absolute blood pressure [124]. The discrepancies between the above and similar studies in correlating blood pressure and risk of rehemorrhage after aSAH may be related to their retrospective review, intrinsic differences in starting blood pressure at the time of initial aSAH, inherent difficulty in randomization, variable and type of antihypertensives used, as well as controlling for confounding factors such as inconsistent time of observation, use of external ventricular drainage, treatment paradigms balancing cerebral perfusion pressure (CPP) and intracranial pressure (ICP). Due to the lack of randomized and well-controlled studies, the management of blood pressure after aSAH but prior to definitive treatment is controversial. However, it is commonplace to maintain blood pressure in the normotensive range, avoiding large fluctuations and hypotension, while respecting baseline blood pressure and balancing CPP and ICP **(Ib/A)**.

Antifibrinolytic therapy

Rehemorrhage after aSAH is thought to originate from clot dissolution at the site of original aneurysm rupture. At baseline, prothrombotic and antithrombotic factors are in equilibrium. At the time of vascular injury prothrombotic factors are favored while shortly thereafter clot stabilization and eventually dissolution is encouraged. As such, it is conceivable that if one could attenuate the antithrombotic effects of serum and subarachnoid factors, then clot stabilization could be protracted. Since many antifibrinolytic agents rapidly cross the blood-brain barrier and reduce fibrinolytic activity of factors, these agents were investigated as a means to reduce rehemorrhage after aSAH leading to decreased morbidity and mortality.

Antifibrinolytic therapy in the prevention of rerupture after aSAH is not a novel notion. In 1967, Gibbs et al published the first known report on antifibrinolytic therapy after aSAH [125]. Numerous investigations have since studied the role of antifibrinolytic agents in aSAH but most have been uncontrolled and not randomized. Common antifibrinolytic agents utilized include tranexamic acid and epsilon aminocaproic acid. Likewise, many individual studies have contraindicated one another. Torner et al, in a multicenter, randomized, double-blind, placebo-controlled study, demonstrated that tranexamic acid reduced rehemorrhage from aSAH by 60%. However, overall outcome was similar between groups given the increased rate of ischemic cerebral infarction in the treated group [126]. Kassell et al, correspondingly, in a controlled but not randomized investigation, demonstrated an approximate 40% reduction in rehemorrhage post-aSAH. Unfortunately, this was offset by a 43% increase in ischemic complications [127]. In an investigation by Hillman et al in 2002, there was a reported 80% reduction in mortality rate from early rerupture after aSAH with immediate and short-term use (<72 hours) of tranexamic acid. The prophylactic benefit of this antifibrinolytic was not associated with the previously noted increased occurrence of vasospasm or ischemic consequence [128]. Roos et al in a 2008 review of nine randomized trials could not support the routine use of antifibrinolytics for the prevention of rehemorrhage after aSAH. Despite the overall consensus by this review that there was a reduction in rehemorrhage rate in the antifibrinolytic arms, there was no demonstrative improvement in clinical outcome secondary to the deleterious effects of cerebral ischemia with antifibrinolytic therapy [129] (IIb/B). Of note in this review, all but one of the trials were performed prior to 1990 with a majority in the 1970s and early 80s – prior to the relatively widespread use of agents and measures to prevent and treat cerebral vasospasm after aSAH. In the single trial included in this review performed recently (Roos et al 2000), there was a significant reduction in rehemorrhage after initial rupture in the antifibrinolytic arm without a concurrent increase in occurrence of cerebral ischemia. Importantly, in this study all patients received anti-ischemic/spastic prophylaxis/treatment with nimodipine and hypervolemia [130].

The above confounding and often contradicting results may largely be driven by the heterogeneous clinical and study designs in the above investigations leading to statistical heterogeneity.

As evidenced by recent investigations by Roos et al in 2000 and Hillman et al in 2002, the effects of antifibrinolytic therapy in reducing the risk of rehemorrhage after aneurysmal rupture merits further investigation [128, 130]. These future studies will have to control for clinical and radiographic grade at baseline, use of agents and measures in the prevention and treatment of vasospasm, dosage and type of antifibrinolytic, administration paradigm and length of use of antifibrinolytic, as well as defined clinical and radiographic outcome assessments. These investigations may yield treatment guidelines in the use of antifibrinolytic agents that balance their prophylactic and adverse effects post-aSAH until definitive therapy can be implemented.

Definitive treatment

Timing

Though the aforementioned measures may temper the risk of rerupture after aSAH, as stated previously, a significant number of patients will still rehemorrhage and will most likely do so in the first few days after the initial rupture – thus mandating definitive treatment. Despite this fact, the timing of microsurgery for ruptured cerebral aneurysms has historically been controversial. The ill-defined treatment paradigms of early versus late microsurgery attempted to balance the difficult clinical circumstance of early reactive brain swelling accompanying the initial aSAH with the latter development of cerebral vasospasm and resultant ischemic consequence, while in the meantime absorbing the risk of rehemorrhage and the clinical stability of the patient.

The initial consensus in North America in the 1970s and 80s was that better outcomes would be obtained in delaying surgery until reactive brain swelling had abated and the patient had clinically stabilized or improved [131-133]. Others promoted early microsurgery with acceptable clinical outcome for the time, given the diminution of the patient from rehemorrhage during the waiting period [134, 135].

In an attempt to reconcile the above matter and improve surgical outcome after aSAH, the International Cooperative Study on the Timing of Aneurysm Surgery was organized [6, 136]. This was a multicenter, prospective, non-randomized investigation that included 68 neurosurgical centers in 14 countries comprising >3500 patients. Neurosurgeons were required to prospectively choose from one of several planned surgery time periods (0-3; 4-6; 7-10; 11-14; 15-32 days and no planned surgery). The data were accumulated in an intent-to-treat paradigm. Risk of pre-operative rehemorrhage was directly related to time to definitive treatment (5.7%, 0-3 days; 9.4%, 4-6 days; 12.7%, 7-10 days; 13.9%, 11-14 days; and 21.5%, 15-32 days). As a collective, there was no difference between early and delayed surgery in mortality and outcome in survivors.

However, in this same cohort of patients, results restricted to North American centers demonstrated a significant improvement in rates of good recovery in the early (0-3 days) versus patients planned for surgery between days 11 and 32. Overall mortality was similar between these two subgroups. Patients in the intent to treat interval of 7-10 days had nearly twice the mortality rate as compared to other subgroups, coinciding with the period of greatest risk for cerebral vasospasm. Results were best amongst patients who were actually treated in the 11-14-day interval, reflecting the selection bias and attrition which occurs prior to this time interval [137]. Similarly, in a population-based investigation of the impact of the timing of surgical treatment on the outcome after aSAH, there was no significant difference in survival between the early (0-7 days) and late (>8 days) groups. However, there was a significant increase in functional outcome and number of totally independent survivors between the early and late groups, 82 vs. 64% [138]. Of note, during the time period of later surgical intervention only 14% of aSAH patients were treated versus 46% in the early group.

In a prospective randomized study of 216 patients between Hunt and Hess grades I-III admitted within 72 hours from the time of aSAH, there was a direct correlation between delay in surgery and poor outcome, both in terms of mortality and functional capacity [139]. Patients were randomly divided into one of three subgroups dependent on time of operation: acute (0-3 days), intermediate (4-7 days), and late surgery (>7 days). The mortality rate in the acute surgery group was significantly better than the late surgery group, 5.6% versus 12.9%. At 3 months post-aSAH, there was a significant increase in number of patients classified as independent in the early surgically treated subgroup (91.5% of the acute versus 78.6% of the intermediate and 80% of the late).

Proponents of early surgery after aSAH advocate this approach because this virtually negates the risk of rehemorrhage, there is at least equivalent survival rates with a trend towards increased number of high functioning survivors, allows for dilution or lavage of potentially vasospasmogenic SAH and clot, and allows for the medical and endovascular treatment of cerebral vasospasm after securing of aneurysm **(IIb/B)**. Advocates in favor of late surgery point to the increased likelihood and severity of cerebral edema necessitating greater and more injurious brain retraction and lack of time for dissolution of subarachnoid clot with early surgery as well as corresponding mortality rates. Poor clinical grade (Hunt and Hess grades IV and V) is a controversial reason to delay surgery. The argument for early surgery in these poor grade patients argues that the risk of rehemorrhage (and its associated very high mortality rate) outweighs the added medical and surgical challenges [140]. Furthermore, patients who present in poor grade are not necessarily mandated into poor long-term outcome after definitive treatment. Le Roux et al demonstrated that over 50% of Hunt and Hess grade IV and nearly 25% of grade V had favorable outcome after microsurgical clipping [141]. In another retrospective review of 355 patients, there was no statistical difference in surgical complications between good and bad grade patients with ruptured anterior circulation aneurysms [142].

On balance, there has been an overall trend in recent years towards early surgery for ruptured cerebral aneurysms. However, this decision is directed by several factors that influence this verdict. Patient presentation shortly after aSAH, good medical condition and clinical grade, high Fisher grade, mass effect from large subarachnoid or intraparenchymal hematoma, and increasing aneurysm size or change in morphology favor early operative intervention **(IIb/B)**. Likewise if the patient presents during the peak vasospasm period or is in poor medical condition or clinical grade, then most would advocate delayed surgery after the time period of peak cerebral vasospasm (see below) **(IIb/B)**.

As mentioned previously, patients surgically treated between days 4 and 10 had the worst outcome both in terms of survival and functionality in the International Cooperative Study [6, 136, 137]. Given current presentation, diagnostic, and referral delays, it is not uncommon for patients to present at centers of excellence in delayed fashion and during the above worst outcome period. This period coincides with the interval of peak cerebral vasospasm. As such, it was suggested that patients who present during this period have microsurgery delayed until after day 10. Note that the above conversation was limited to the timing of microsurgery and not endovascular treatment. Since the publication of the International Cooperative Study, endovascular treatment has been a widely accepted alternative for the treatment of cerebral aneurysms in a selected group of patients. One such group of patients includes those who present during the peak vasospasm period and rather than delaying microsurgery until after day 10, endovascular treatment is a viable option **(IIb/B)**. In a review of 119 consecutive aSAH patients who underwent endovascular coiling at either 0-3 days or 4-10 days, there was no difference in mortality or poor clinical outcome [143].

Microsurgical and endovascular treatment of ruptured intracranial aneurysms

The decision between microsurgical and endovascular treatment of ruptured intracranial aneurysms should not be viewed as static or dogmatic but a dynamic choice which considers multiple variables and individualizes therapy to the patient and aneurysm at hand. Decisions are best made at centers where both cerebrovascular and endovascular expertise is present and decisions are made jointly. Variables that need consideration and assist in this decision process include patient age and overall medical status, pre-operative grade, time of presentation since aSAH, anatomy and morphology of the aneurysm, and cerebrovascular and endovascular expertise. The goal of both microsurgical and endovascular treatment is to exclude the aneurysm from the circulation while maintaining flow in the parent and branching vasculature.

In patients under the age of 70, in good clinical grade, and presenting shortly after aneurysmal rupture with either giant or very small aneurysms, wide necks (>5mm), or dome/fundus-to-neck ratio of <2, there is a general inclination towards microsurgery [144, 145].

In 1999, Vanninen *et al* published a prospective randomized study on 109 patients that presented within 72 hours of their hemorrhage who underwent either microsurgery (n=57) or endovascular coiling (n=52) [146]. In an intent-to-treat analysis, there was no significant difference in functional outcome at 3 months between the microsurgical and endovascular treatment arms. In a similar prospective randomized investigation, there was no significant difference in clinical, neuropsychological, or mortality outcomes between the endovascular and microsurgical groups at 1-year follow-up [147].

The largest prospective randomized trial comparing microsurgical clipping to endovascular coiling in ruptured cerebral aneurysms is the International Subarachnoid Aneurysm Trial (ISAT) [148-150]. ISAT was published in three sequential reviews between 2002 and 2009, each review was based on the same 2143 patients in the original cohort. Patients with known aSAH were included in the trial if the ruptured intracranial aneurysm was deemed suitable for treatment by both microsurgical clipping or endovascular coiling based on angiographic anatomy. In the first ISAT published in 2002, the authors report no significant difference in survival at 1 year. At 1 year, in the endovascular treatment group there was an absolute reduction in having a poor functional outcome of approximately 7% as compared to the microsurgical group (23.7% vs. 30.6%, respectively). In the follow-up ISAT review published in 2005, it is reported that this increased likelihood of independent survival at 1 year in the endovascular group is extended to at least 7 years. In the latest ISAT publication in 2009, the authors conclude a significant increase in number of rehemorrhages from the originally treated aneurysm in the endovascular versus the microsurgical treated group when comparing actual treatment but not in intent-to-treat analysis. The proportion of patients deemed independent at 5 years post-microsurgical or endovascular treatment was the same (82% vs. 83%, respectively). At 5 years, there was a significant difference in the fraction of patients who had died between the endovascular (11%) and microsurgical (14%) treated groups.

After the publication of the first ISAT in 2002, the authors report a shift in practice in the United Kingdom and other parts of Europe [149]. This enthusiasm for endovascular treatment may be tempered by the above findings in the more recent 2009 ISAT review, as well as the growing opinion towards the many methodological shortcomings of ISAT:

◆ the 2143 patients included in ISAT represent only 22% of the originally enrolled cohort (9559) of patients with aSAH;
◆ outcomes were not provided on non-randomized patients;
◆ more non-randomized patients underwent microsurgical clipping than endovascular treatment;
◆ 93% of the ruptured aneurysms were ≤10mm;
◆ 97% of the ruptured aneurysms were of the anterior circulation;
◆ 80% of the enrolled patients were of good grade (Hunt and Hess grade I or II);
◆ there is a statistical increase in number of rehemorrhages from the originally treated aneurysm in the endovascular versus the microsurgical treated group when comparing actual treatment;
◆ the proportion of patients deemed functionally independent at 5 years post-microsurgical or endovascular treatment was the same;
◆ despite the reported significant difference in fraction of patients who had died between the endovascular (11%) and microsurgical (14%) treated groups, the leading causes of death were cancer and cardiovascular;
◆ the findings of ISAT cannot be extrapolated to unruptured cerebral aneurysms.

Notwithstanding the above and other limitations of ISAT, this investigation laid the fundamental groundwork for weighing microsurgical and endovascular treatment options for ruptured cerebral aneurysms in a large prospective and randomized method. Independent of these shortcomings, the results from ISAT have demonstrated that endovascular therapy is an appropriate modality in the treatment of ruptured cerebral aneurysms (Ib/A). The discussion of microsurgical clipping and endovascular coiling should not be an argument of 'versus' but rather a consultation towards individualized efficacy. In this light, cerebrovascular and endovascular surgeons work in harmony as members of a vascular team and deliver the most efficacious treatment in the management of ruptured (and unruptured) cerebral aneurysms. As such we have finished where we began prior to ISAT; patient age and overall medical status, pre-operative grade, time of presentation since aSAH, anatomy and morphology of the aneurysm, and cerebrovascular and endovascular expertise should determine the individualized modality for that patient at hand (Ib/A).

Cerebral vasospasm

After aSAH, the mere presence of subarachnoid blood can initiate a sequence of neurological and visceral sequalae independent of aneurysm treatment. These consequences of aSAH can at the least prolong recovery but often aggravate inherent morbidity and mortality associated with subarachnoid blood as well as introducing novel complications.

Cerebral vasospasm is the delayed narrowing of cerebral vasculature after subarachnoid hemorrhage. It is most often after aSAH but can also less commonly occur after hemorrhage in other cerebral compartments, intraventricular and intraparenchymal, or from SAH from other etiologies. Cerebral vasospasm can be defined by clinical and angiographic endpoints. Angiographic vasospasm is defined by arterial narrowing after SAH as demonstrated by cerebral angiography. Since angiography exhibits primarily large-capacitance arteries so is the definition of cerebral vasospasm. After aSAH, the incidence of angiographic cerebral vasospasm ranges from 30-70% [151]. Clinical or symptomatic cerebral vasospasm is defined by a delayed ischemic neurologic deficit (DIND) following SAH. Though the incidence of angiographic cerebral vasospasm is as high as 70%, this translates to approximately a 20-30% incidence of symptomatic vasospasm [151]. DIND is often focal and can be attributed to the specific cerebral vasculature affected.

The development of new focal neurological deficits not attributable to aneurysmal rehemorrhage, hydrocephalus, seizure, hypoxia, fever, or hyponatremia is often the first clinical clue to the development of cerebral vasospasm after aSAH. Commonly symptoms develop gradually and fluctuate or progress. In the non-comatose patient, indications to the development of cerebral vasospasm include new or increasing headache, declining or fluctuating orientation and level of consciousness, and meningismus. Expectantly, signs of cerebral vasospasm of the middle cerebral artery (MCA) include monoparesis/plegia, hemiparesis/plegia, extraocular motor deficit, apraxia, and aphasia. Likewise, anterior cerebral artery (ACA) vasospasm may result in confusion, sluggishness, abulia, urinary incontinence, and the frontal release reflexes of grasp, suck, and palmar mentalis.

The commencement of cerebral vasospasm is delayed in relevance to the onset of aneurysm rupture. Virtually exclusively, cerebral vasospasm does not occur until 3 days after aSAH with the most common period of onset between days 6 and 8, but can also present in delayed fashion. Cerebral vasospasm post-aSAH typically resolves clinically by day 12 and by angiography between days 14 and 28 [152-154]. This 'resolution' of cerebral vasospasm is not necessarily a clinical reversal to baseline but rather a cessation in progression if the ischemia induced by spasm has progressed to infarction.

The severity of clinical consequences from cerebral vasospasm ranges from reversible neurological deficit to stroke and even death. Permanent neurological deficit secondary to ischemic infarction from cerebral vasospasm after aSAH can occur in 7-20% of patients and may be fatal in 7% despite maximal therapy [137, 151, 155]. Of patients who survive the initial rupture of a cerebral aneurysm, vasospasm accounts for nearly 1 out of 2 deaths which can match and even exceed the mortality associated with initial aneurysm rupture and rehemorrhage [156]. As such suspicion for vasospasm must be high. Yet in the comatose patient clinical indicators are often inconspicuous. Thus, practitioners often screen through the peak period of vasospasm onset and if vasospasm has occurred then throughout the period of vasospasm occurrence (approximately days 14 and 21 post-aSAH, respectively).

The most common modality in the screening for and monitoring of cerebral vasospasm is transcranial Doppler (TCD). Absolute increases and increasing trends in blood flow velocity as detected by TCD may precede as well as help explain clinical decline. A stable percentage of cardiac output to the brain in the setting of focal vascular narrowing secondary to vasospasm mandates an increase in blood flow velocity through the affected cerebral artery [157-159]. TCD measures blood flow in centimeters per second. TCD measurements are operator-dependent and require good quality control between examiners at each institution [160-162]. Hence, the natural variability in clinical presentation of cerebral vasospasm in combination with intra- and inter-examiner variability has yielded differing opinions on the sensitivity and specificity of TCD in detecting cerebral vasospasm. In addition, TCD measurement can be affected by alterations in blood pressure, central vascular volume, and in the setting of vasospasm treatment. In this light, the Lindegaard ratio (ratio of the velocity of the cerebral vessel of study to the velocity in the ipsilateral extracranial internal carotid artery) helps distinguish generalized hypertension and hyperemia from cerebral vasospasm [157, 163]. A ratio of 3 is considered normal, while 6 is indicative of severe cerebral vasospasm. A ratio between 3 and 6 may indicate mild vasospasm but with low sensitivity.

The non-invasiveness, relative rapidity, and good correlation at extreme blood flow velocities make TCD an attractive modality. However, the above limitations of TCD have encouraged practitioners to utilize additional modalities in the diagnosis and management of cerebral vasospasm after aSAH. These methods include perfusion- and diffusion-weighted imaging (PWI and DWI) on MRI. DWI demonstrates areas of acute brain ischemia and PWI provides information on the relative perfusion status of the microcirculation. As in stroke, areas of perfusion that exceed the boundaries of diffusion ('perfusion-diffusion mismatch') may indicate zones of brain susceptible to but yet salvageable from infarction. Likewise, xenon CT perfusion can detect global or regional changes in cerebral blood flow but is generally too insensitive to detect a focal perfusion deficit [164]. Recently, continuous quantitative monitoring by EEG has gained some momentum. Vespa et al demonstrated that a decline in the percent of alpha wave (6-14 Hertz) activity was a sooner predictor of cerebral vasospasm than either TCD or angiography [165]. Similarly, a decline in total EEG amplitude was very sensitive for predicting the onset of cerebral vasospasm in aSAH [166]. Many centers utilize the above methods as adjuncts to TCD and time the post-treatment cerebral angiogram with the peak incidence of vasospasm in high-risk patients, thus implementing angiography as both a diagnostic and potentially therapeutic (see below) modality.

As mentioned before, the early treatment of ruptured cerebral aneurysms allows for more aggressive and lower risk management of cerebral vasospasm. The goal of the myriad of potential therapies for cerebral vasospasm is to minimize the effects of cerebral ischemia on neurons, improve cerebral blood flow, and reverse vascular narrowing, thus improving clinical outcome. The early observations that intravascular volume contraction and hypotension are risk factors for the development of delayed cerebral ischemia from vasospasm, led many to imply that the reverse could improve outcomes from cerebral vasospasm [167, 168]. As such, hypertensive hypervolemic hemodilution ('triple-H') therapy was investigated but largely via uncontrolled studies. These investigations described the resolution of neurological deficits and improved outcomes from cerebral vasospasm after aSAH compared with historical controls [169-173]. These and similar studies led to triple-H therapy becoming a mainstay in the treatment of cerebral vasospasm after aSAH **(IIa/B)**. However, in a randomized controlled trial by Lennihan and colleagues, there was no significant difference in cerebral blood flow or volume between groups of patients receiving hypervolemic or normovolemic therapy after aSAH [174]. This was despite increases in central venous and pulmonary artery diastolic pressure in the hypervolemic group versus normovolemic controls. In an analogous prospective randomized control study by Egge *et al*, prophylactic hyperdynamic postoperative fluid therapy was evaluated in the setting of aSAH prior to the onset of cerebral vasospasm [175]. There was no significant difference between the triple-H and normovolemic groups with respect to clinical or sonographic cerebral vasospasm, cerebral blood flow, and 1-year clinical outcome as measured by neuropsychological testing and Glasgow Coma Scale. Additionally, there was greater cost and complications in the triple-H group. These prospective randomized trials were small single-institution investigations with limited power. Furthermore, all patients in the treated and control groups in both studies received nimodipine (see below), possibly masking the potential beneficial effects of hyperdynamic therapy. Importantly one must not extrapolate the above apparent lack of efficacy of prophylactic to therapeutic triple-H therapy, for which there is much practitioner and anecdotal data. Nevertheless and independent of the efficacy of triple-H therapy, the avoidance of hypovolemia and hypotension is advocated after aSAH **(IIa/B)**. Hyperdynamic therapy needs to be taken in balance with its potential and serious complications which include cerebral edema and resultant elevated intracranial pressure, cardiac failure, pulmonary edema, hyponatremia, and bleeding diathesis secondary to dilution of serum clotting factors.

As vasospasm is by definition abnormal narrowing of cerebral vasculature and this is mediated by smooth muscle contraction, intuitively, the inhibition of such contraction should attenuate cerebral vasospasm. Calcium channel blockers disrupt calcium influx through the 'slow-channel' which are localized to smooth and cardiac but not skeletal muscle. As such, it had been theorized that the augmented contraction of smooth muscle during vasospasm may be mitigated by cerebral vasculature calcium channel blockade.

The most widely used calcium channel blocker in the setting of aSAH is nimodipine largely based on its greater selectivity for cerebral vasculature. Interestingly, though nimodipine does not increase vascular caliber or incidence of angiographic vasospasm, it has been demonstrated to improve clinical outcomes in multiple studies **(Ia/A)**. The British Aneurysm Nimodipine Trial demonstrated a significant reduction in cerebral infarctions from 33% to 22% as well as a 40% reduction in poor outcomes with the use of nimodipine in patients with aSAH [176]. In a meta-analysis review, Barker and Ogilvy demonstrated that the prophylactic use of nimodipine after aSAH increased the likelihood of good outcome after aSAH [177] **(Ia/A)**. These benefits have been associated with minimal adverse effects and have been cost-effective [178]. The improved outcome despite no statistically significant improvement in angiographic vasospasm with the use of nimodipine in aSAH patients may be attributable to the other potential physiological effects of this calcium channel blocker including: inhibition of calcium entry into neurons thus diminishing the injury from cerebral ischemia, increased red blood cell deformability and thus blood rheology and flow, an antiplatelet effect with respect to aggregation, and dilation of leptomeningeal arteries thus collateral flow [177, 179-182]. Nicardipine is another L-type calcium channel blocker with regional selectivity on vascular smooth muscle. Nicardipine is administered intravenously and is largely utilized as an antihypertensive agent. Nicardipine has been demonstrated to reduce cerebral vasospasm by 30% [183]. However, there has been no associated improvement in outcome with the use of nicardipine in aSAH patients [184, 185]. In collective, most institutions start aSAH patients on nimodipine shortly after aneurysmal rupture and control the often elevated blood pressure with nicardipine. As such, there may be a serendipitous effect of neuroprotection by nimodipine and decreased cerebral vasospasm and controlled blood pressure by nicardipine. Interestingly, there have been recent trials on the use of prolonged-release nicardipine implants (NPRIs) in basal cisterns during the time of microsurgery for ruptured aneurysms. In a small prospective randomized double-blind investigation, Barth et al demonstrated a significant reduction in angiographic vasospasm (73% vs. 7%), lower incidence of delayed ischemic insults (47% vs. 14%), improved functional outcome, and lower incidence of deaths (38% vs. 6%) comparing controls and patients receiving NPRIs, respectively [186].

There have been many recent investigations in the prevention and treatment of cerebral vasospasm after aSAH, given the as-of-yet limited understanding of the pathophysiological mechanisms driving its onset and progression as well as the associated relative high morbidity and mortality.

Magnesium is one such agent given its inhibitory effect on calcium influx and the necessity of calcium entry for smooth muscle contraction. Hypomagnesemia occurs in over half of patients with aSAH and has been related to the development of delayed cerebral ischemia and poor outcome [187]. In multiple experimental models in rats, magnesium has been shown to be a neuroprotectant, reverse cerebral vasospasm, and reduce the extent of acute ischemic cerebral insult after aSAH [188-191]. These findings are believed to be via the effects of magnesium in non-competitive inhibition of voltage-dependent calcium channels, inhibiting the release of excitatory amino acids, and blocking of the N-methyl-D-aspartate (NMDA) glutamate receptor [192, 193]. In a randomized multicenter control trial by van den Bergh, there was a risk reduction of 34% for the development of delayed cerebral ischemia (defined as hypodense lesions on CT in patients with clinical features of cerebral vasospasm) and at 3 months post-aSAH a 23% reduction in poor outcome (Rankin scale 3) in the magnesium treatment group versus controls. However, in a 2010 randomized double-blinded placebo-controlled phase III trial of aSAH patients, there was no demonstrable benefit of intravenous magnesium over placebo in terms of clinical vasospasm or favorable outcome [194]. Likewise, these investigators found an association between high plasma magnesium concentration and worse clinical outcome after aSAH [195].

Recent investigations have also implicated the role of inflammatory mediators in the development of cerebral vasospasm after aSAH. Integral to this potential pathophysiological mechanism is the leukocyte-endothelial interaction which is mediated by cellular adhesion molecules (CAMs). Upregulation of CAMs on endothelial cell membranes after aSAH promotes the diapedesis of neutrophils into the subarachnoid and depletion of nitric oxide (NO) [196-200].

Endothelin (ET) is a potent endogenous vasoconstrictor and has been implicated in the pathogenesis of cerebral vasospasm after aSAH [201-203]. The impetus for these investigations is driven by several associated observations. Concentrations of ET in serum and CSF are increased in aSAH and especially after the development of cerebral vasospasm [204]. After aSAH, oxyhemoglobin and thrombin are present in high concentrations in CSF and result in elevated levels of ET [205]. Experimentally, cerebral vasospasm can be induced with the cisternal administration of ET [206]. Conversely, administration of ET antagonists attenuates cerebral vasospasm in aSAH experimental models [207]. The production of ET appears to be present in multitude as it has been attributed to endothelial and smooth muscle cells, neurons, astrocytes, and leukocytes. The vasoconstrictive effect of ET on vasculature is primarily mediated through the endothelin-A (ET-A) receptor located on vascular smooth muscle cells. Clazosentan is a selective antagonist of the ET-A receptor. In a small randomized double-blinded placebo-controlled phase IIa study, Vajkoczy and colleagues demonstrated a reduced incidence of angiographic vasospasm with the use of clazosentan in Hunt and Hess grade III and IV and Fisher grade 3 aSAH patients [208]. The incidence and severity of adverse events were comparable between the treated and placebo groups. This early study led to the larger randomized double-blinded placebo-controlled phase II investigation by Macdonald et al [209]. In this study, clazosentan resulted in a significant decrease in moderate and severe vasospasm from 66% in the placebo group to 23% in the clazosentan group and this was in a dose-dependent manner. There was also a trend towards reduced vasospasm-related morbidity and mortality. The adverse effects of clazosentan (anemia, hypotension, and pulmonary complications) were reported by the authors as manageable and not considered serious. In a recent meta-analysis by Kramer and Fletcher of two ET-A receptor antagonist trials and one ET-A/B receptor antagonist (TAK-044) trial, there was no demonstrable evidence that ET receptor antagonists have an impact on mortality or poor neurological outcome despite reductions in radiographic vasospasm and DIND [210, 211]. Endothelin receptor antagonists show promise in the setting of cerebral vasospasm after aSAH; whether this translates into improved outcome remains to be elucidated.

Inherent in the sequence of events leading to cerebral vasospasm is the extraluminal release of oxyhemoglobin after aSAH [212, 213]. Extraluminal oxyhemoglobin is converted to methemoglobin with the release of superoxide (O_2^-) and is also known to elicit the generation of hydroxyl radicals ($OH^\bullet$) [214-217]. Free radicals are known to induce lipid peroxidation and this has been implicated in cerebral vasospasm [218, 219]. In this light, there have been several investigations on the effects of hydroxyl radical scavengers and inhibitors of lipid peroxidation as cytoprotective agents in aSAH. In a placebo-controlled double-blind trial of aSAH patients by Asano et al, a synthetic $OH^\bullet$ specific scavenger provided a significant reduction in DIND in the treated versus control groups, 54.2% versus 35.5%, respectively [220]. Also, there was improvement in functional outcome at 1 month post-aSAH. Though this improvement in functional outcome became marginal at 3 months, there was a significant reduction in incidence of death at 3 months in the treated group. In a study to investigate the safety and efficacy of the lipid peroxidation inhibitor, tirilazad mesylate, Kassell and colleagues demonstrated increased frequency of good recovery and reduced mortality in the treated group at 3 months post-aSAH [221]. However, in a follow-up study in North America there was no demonstrable difference between tirilazad mesylate administered and control groups after aSAH [222]. This difference in efficacy of tirilazad mesylate was attributable, by the latter investigators, to differences in admission characteristics, management protocols, and use of anticonvulsants. Other studies have concurred that inhibitors of lipid peroxidation may reduce the incidence of symptomatic vasospasm but not mortality or functional outcome [223]. These and other agents under study in acute ischemic stroke models, which mediate their effects through free radicals, are areas of investigation with potential promise. However, currently there is no strong evidence supporting their use in cerebral vasospasm after aSAH.

As ET has been implicated in initiating vasoconstrictor tone, NO has for vasodilation. The imbalance between the vasoconstrictive and vasodilatory effects of ET and NO, respectively, are thought to be one potential mechanism involved in the pathogenesis of cerebral vasospasm after aSAH. NO is released from vascular endothelium and is partially responsible for matching the supply of vascular tone to the demand from recipient tissue. This equilibrium if not in balance due to reduced levels of local NO has been offered as a potential mechanism involved in the genesis of cerebral vasospasm post-aSAH [224, 225]. Reduced local levels of NO after aSAH may be the result of several processes including sequestration of NO by oxyhemoglobin and reduced endogenous levels of NO synthase (NOS) [226-228]. In experimental and early models, there has been an association between reduced levels of NO or NOS and cerebral vasospasm after aSAH as well as an amelioration of cerebral vasospasm after administration of NO or NOS substrates [229-233]. The short half-life and potentially wide side-effect profile, has limited the peripheral administration of NO in the setting of cerebral vasospasm. To assist in addressing these limitations, investigators have studied the intrathecal, intravascular, and local administration of NO or NOS substrates [234-236]. These investigations demonstrated angiographic improvement in cerebral vasospasm but their clinical translation may be limited by the hypotension, increased intracranial pressure, and cerebral blood flow shunting away (a 'steal' phenomenon) from the desired region with NO or NOS substrate administration [237, 238]. There have been mixed results in the use of intrathecal NO or NOS substrates in cerebral vasospasm [235, 237, 239, 240]. Also, the inherent shortcomings of variable and non-specific drug distribution and preferential effect on vasculature not encased in aSAH/clot may hinder use of this delivery method. A method to overcome these limitations is direct delivery of vasodilatory agents near spastic vasculature. Gabikian *et al* report on the beneficial effects of NO delivery via the placement of a controlled release polymer embedded with NO at the time of surgery [225]. But what of the patients who do not undergo open surgery or are treated by endovascular means. Recent investigations have concentrated on nitrite as a storage molecule and an 'on-demand' donor of NO. Nitrite can be reduced to NO by both enzymatic and non-enzymatic means [241, 242]. Importantly in SAH, deoxyhemoglobin can reduce nitrite to form NO [243]. In this light, Pluta *et al* investigated the efficacy of intravenous nitrite infusion in a primate model of SAH [227]. Nearly half of the control monkeys developed cerebral vasospasm by arteriography compared to none of the nitrite-treated monkeys and there were no significant deleterious effects with such therapy. Interestingly, there was also an indirect correlation between CSF nitrite concentration and development of cerebral vasospasm. These investigations are promising and may yield the potential clinical use of NO, NOS substrates, or similar compounds. Currently, such a recommendation cannot be made.

In addition to their cholesterol-lowering effect, 3-hydroxy-3-methylgluteryl coenzyme A (HMG-CoA) reductase inhibitors ('statins') may have a neuroprotectant role. In the setting of cerebral ischemia, statins improve vasomotor reactivity, fibrinolytic activity, and reduce platelet activation, the genesis of thrombosis, and cytokine production [244, 245]. Statins also have direct effects on endothelial NOS (eNOS). Statins upregulate eNOS resulting in improved vasomotor activity leading to increased cerebral blood flow [246]. Thus, the potential neuroprotectant effects of statins may be mediated through several avenues. In a 2005 randomized placebo-controlled trial of aSAH patients, Tseng and colleagues demonstrated a significant reduction in cerebral vasospasm, DIND, and mortality in the pravastatin treated group compared to controls [247]. Similarly, in a pilot study, the administration of simvastatin within 48 hours of aSAH was associated with decreased serum markers of brain injury, angiographic vasospasm, and DIND [248]. In a meta-analysis by Sillberg et al, the potential beneficial effects of statins were expanded into 'recommendations' but this was justifiably received with criticism [249, 250]. In a 2009 double-blind placebo-controlled randomized trial, there was no statistical benefit of simvastatin in aSAH patients in terms of incidence of cerebral vasospasm by TCD, DIND, and poor outcome [251]. Likewise in a 2010 meta-analysis, Vergouwen and colleagues confirmed the lack of evidence that statins reduce cerebral vasospasm, DIND, poor outcome, or mortality associated with aSAH [252]. Currently, there is no evidence to support the routine use of statins in the prevention or treatment of cerebral vasospasm associated with aSAH.

With failed medical therapy of cerebral vasospasm of secured ruptured aneurysm, more direct measures are often sought to halt the effects of spastic cerebral vasculature in aSAH. Invasive measures to treat cerebral vasospasm after aSAH include intra-arterial administration of vasodilators and balloon angioplasty. Balloon angioplasty is effective in reversing cerebral vasospasm in large proximal intracranial vessels – basilar artery and the proximal portions of the anterior, middle, and posterior cerebral arteries – and is not safe in distal perforating branches beyond the second-order segments [253-255] (IIb/B). The ultimate goal of balloon angioplasty is to increase the caliber of the treated vessel thereby improving cerebral blood flow and to do this in a manner with persistent effect but minimal risk. Multiple investigations have demonstrated the efficacy of balloon angioplasty in reducing angiographic vasospasm and ischemic deficit while increasing cerebral blood flow [256-258] (IIb/B). However, this has not been demonstrated in a prospective randomized fashion. In a large case series of 109 aSAH patients treated with balloon angioplasty after the onset of DIND, clinical improvement was noted in only 44% of patients with 28% of patients demonstrating further clinical decline after treatment [259]. Prophylactic balloon angioplasty has not been demonstrated to improve clinical outcome in high Fisher grade patients despite the decreased incidence of cerebral vasospasm and the need for therapeutic angioplasty [260]. However, early treatment with balloon angioplasty may translate into persistent clinical improvement [261, 262].

The technical limitation of balloon angioplasty in terms of vessel diameter is overcome by microcatheterization of third and fourth order cerebral vessels in order to administer intra-arterial vasodilators. There have been several reports on the effective use of intra-arterial papaverine in reversing the cerebral vasospasm associated with aSAH; however, these vasodilatory and cerebral blood flow effects have been short-lived given its half-life of 2 hours [263-266]. Verapamil and other calcium channel blockers are also intra-arterial agents used in the treatment of cerebral vasospasm post-aSAH. These agents are attractive given their longer half-lives (verapamil ~7 hours; nimodipine ~9 hours and nicardipine ~16 hours) and apparent lower side-effect profiles and improved clinical outcome with treatment of aSAH patients with cerebral vasospasm [267-271].

Thus, to date, the only demonstrable agent that reduces the incidence of cerebral vasospasm, DIND, and poor outcome is the calcium channel antagonist, nimodipine (Ia/A). As with many promising therapeutic interventions, optimistic experimental, animal, and initial human trials of prophylactic and attenuating agents of cerebral vasospasm do not often translate into the clinical arena. Procedural interventions such as balloon angioplasty and intra-arterial administration of vasodilatory compounds hold promise but must provide longer efficacy and translate into improved clinical outcome in aSAH patients with cerebral vasospasm. The above investigations have laid the groundwork for future studies and trials that may yield measures to ameliorate upon the current limited options in the prevention and treatment of cerebral vasospasm after aSAH.

Conclusions

Ruptured cerebral aneurysms are common causes of neurological deterioration and death. The morbidity and mortality of ruptured cerebral aneurysms is not only at the time of hemorrhage but also in the subsequent days that follow. Though certain conditions have been associated in the development of cerebral aneurysms, most are believed to be sporadic with possible associated risk factors. The natural history of unruptured cerebral aneurysms is a controversial topic that needs to take into account patient age and aneurysm size, location, morphology, and rate of growth. The diagnosis of aSAH is based on clinical presentation as well as diagnostic imaging modalities and lumbar puncture, which are not always in concordance. Several clinical and radiographic grading systems have developed over the years to minimize intra- and inter-observer variability thus facilitating care. Recurrent hemorrhage and cerebral vasospasm are the leading causes of morbidity and mortality in patients who survive the initial rupture. Though common practices of bed rest and blood pressure control are widely implemented, microneurosurgical clipping or endovascular coiling are the only current definitive treatments of ruptured cerebral aneurysms. Given the high mortality associated with re-rupture, early definitive therapy is recommended. The decision between microneurosurgical or endovascular treatment should not be an argument of 'versus' but rather a consultation between surgical and endovascular experts towards individualized efficacy. Though a myriad of agents have been studied in the prophylaxis and treatment of cerebral vasospasm following aSAH, to date only nimodipine has been demonstrated to reduce the incidence of cerebral vasospasm, DIND, and poor outcome. Endovascular options offer good angiographic reversal of cerebral vasospasm post-aSAH, but their long-term efficacy and translation into improved clinical outcome needs to be further investigated.

The management of ruptured cerebral aneurysms and aSAH is one in evolution which will be frequently modified as historical, current, and future trends are tested against emerging evidence-based treatment paradigms (see key points).

Key points	Evidence level
Risk factors for cerebral aneurysms and aSAH	
◆ The association between hypertension and aSAH is not certain. However, the treatment of hypertension with antihypertensives is recommended to prevent ischemic stroke, intracerebral hemorrhage, and end organ injury.	I/A
◆ Cessation of cigarette smoking is reasonable to reduce the risk of aneurysm rupture but this relationship is not direct.	IIa/B
◆ Screening of high-risk patients for unruptured cerebral aneurysms is uncertain in its value. This may change with the use of non-invasive screening modalities.	IIb/B
Natural history and outcome of aSAH	
◆ Ruptured untreated cerebral aneurysms have a significant risk of rehemorrhage – greatest in the first 24 hours but remains elevated for months post-initial aSAH.	Ib/A
◆ The natural history or risk of hemorrhage of unruptured cerebral aneurysms remains a controversial topic. There was a discrepancy between historical norms and expert opinion and the largest investigation to date, ISUIA, in terms of risk of rupture of unruptured cerebral aneurysms.	Ib/A
Diagnosis of aSAH	
◆ The sudden onset of severe headache should prompt clinical suspicion of aSAH.	Ib/A
◆ In suspected aSAH patients, a non-contrast head CT should be promptly performed.	Ib/A
◆ If clinical suspicion remains for aSAH after a negative non-contrast head CT, a lumbar puncture is recommended.	Ib/A
◆ Cerebral angiography is the study of choice in the diagnosis and anatomic characterization of cerebral aneurysms.	Ib/A
◆ CTA and MRA are non-invasive alternatives to catheter angiography in the detection of cerebral aneurysms, especially those ≥5mm.	IIb/B
Continued	

Key points *continued*	Evidence level

Grading of aSAH
- The clinical and radiographic grading of aSAH is useful in prognosis and triage. — IIa/B

Medical measures to prevent rehemorrhage after aSAH
- Bed rest is not suffice in preventing rehemorrhage after initial aneurysm rupture. — IIb/B
- Blood pressure should be monitored and controlled in an attempt to balance the risk of rehemorrhage associated with hypertension and maintenance of adequate cerebral perfusion pressure. — Ib/A
- The beneficial effects of antifibrinolytics in reducing rehemorrhage after initial aneurysm rupture may need to be balanced by the potential increased likelihood of cerebral ischemia with their use, but recent evidence suggests that an early and short course use of antifibrinolytic therapy combined with nimodipine may offer overall benefit but further investigation is needed. — IIb/B

Timing of definitive treatment
- Although previous investigations have shown that outcome between early and delayed surgery was similar, early definitive treatment may offer overall benefit and is probably indicated in the majority of cases. — IIb/B

Type of definitive treatment
- Microneurosurgical clipping or endovascular coiling should be performed to reduce the rate of re-rupture and its high associated mortality rate after initial aSAH. — Ib/A
- In ruptured cerebral aneurysms in which either microneurosurgical clipping or endovascular coiling are amenable as judged by respective experts in each field, endovascular coiling can be beneficial. — Ib/A
- However, individual patient and aneurysm characteristics need to be considered in deciding the most appropriate intervention. — IIa/B

Cerebral vasospasm
- Management of cerebral vasospasm after aSAH should begin with early definitive treatment in conjunction with maintenance of normal circulating blood volume and avoidance of hypovolemia and hypotension. — IIa/B

Continued

Key points *continued*	Evidence level
♦ Oral nimodipine is indicated to reduce the incidence of cerebral vasospasm, DIND, and poor outcome after aSAH.	I/A
♦ In the management of symptomatic cerebral vasospasm, the induction of intravascular volume expansion, hypertension, and hemodilution may be a reasonable approach.	IIa/B
♦ Cerebral balloon angioplasty or intra-arterial vasodilator administration may be reasonable in symptomatic cerebral vasospasm despite maximal medical therapy, but further investigation is needed to determine the long-term effects of these interventions in outcome.	IIb/B

References

1. Bederson JB, Connolly ES, Jr., Batjer HH, Dacey RG, Dion JE, Diringer MN, *et al*. Guidelines for the management of aneurysmal subarachnoid hemorrhage: a statement for healthcare professionals from a special writing group of the Stroke Council, American Heart Association. *Stroke* 2009; 40(3): 994-1025.
2. King JT, Jr. Epidemiology of aneurysmal subarachnoid hemorrhage. *Neuroimaging Clin N Am* 1997; 7(4): 659-68.
3. Ingall T, Asplund K, Mahonen M, Bonita R. A multinational comparison of subarachnoid hemorrhage epidemiology in the WHO MONICA stroke study. *Stroke* 2000; 31(5): 1054-61.
4. Linn FH, Rinkel GJ, Algra A, van Gijn J. Incidence of subarachnoid hemorrhage: role of region, year, and rate of computed tomography: a meta-analysis. *Stroke* 1996; 27(4): 625-9.
5. Broderick JP, Brott T, Tomsick T, Miller R, Huster G. Intracerebral hemorrhage more than twice as common as subarachnoid hemorrhage. *J Neurosurg* 1993; 78(2): 188-91.
6. Kassell NF, Torner JC, Haley EC, Jr., Jane JA, Adams HP, Kongable GL. The International Cooperative Study on the Timing of Aneurysm Surgery. Part 1: Overall management results. *J Neurosurg* 1990; 73(1): 18-36.
7. van Gijn J, Rinkel GJ. Subarachnoid haemorrhage: diagnosis, causes and management. *Brain* 2001; 124(Pt 2): 249-78.
8. Rinkel GJ, Djibuti M, Algra A, van Gijn J. Prevalence and risk of rupture of intracranial aneurysms: a systematic review. *Stroke* 1998; 29(1): 251-6.
9. Longstreth WT, Nelson LM, Koepsell TD, van Belle G. Subarachnoid hemorrhage and hormonal factors in women. A population-based case-control study. *Ann Intern Med* 1994; 121(3): 168-73.
10. Okamoto K, Horisawa R, Kawamura T, Asai A, Ogino M, Takagi T, *et al*. Menstrual and reproductive factors for subarachnoid hemorrhage risk in women: a case-control study in Nagoya, Japan. *Stroke* 2001; 32(12): 2841-4.
11. Wiebers DO, Whisnant JP, Sundt TM, Jr., O'Fallon WM. The significance of unruptured intracranial saccular aneurysms. *J Neurosurg* 1987; 66(1): 23-9.
12. Mohr JP, Caplan LR, Melski JW, Goldstein RJ, Duncan GW, Kistler JP, *et al*. The Harvard Cooperative Stroke Registry: a prospective registry. *Neurology* 1978; 28(8): 754-62.
13. Greene KA, Marciano FF, Johnson BA, Jacobowitz R, Spetzler RF, Harrington TR. Impact of traumatic subarachnoid hemorrhage on outcome in nonpenetrating head injury. Part I: A proposed computerized tomography grading scale. *J Neurosurg* 1995; 83(3): 445-52.
14. Taneda M, Kataoka K, Akai F, Asai T, Sakata I. Traumatic subarachnoid hemorrhage as a predictable indicator of delayed ischemic symptoms. *J Neurosurg* 1996; 84(5): 762-8.
15. Wirth FP. Surgical treatment of incidental intracranial aneurysms. *Clin Neurosurg* 1986; 33: 125-35.
16. Greenberg MS. *Handbook of Neurosurgery*, 6th ed. New York, USA: Thieme Medical Publisher, 2006.

17. Cioffi F, Pasqualin A, Cavazzani P, Da Pian R. Subarachnoid haemorrhage of unknown origin: clinical and tomographical aspects. *Acta Neurochir* (Wien) 1989; 97(1-2): 31-9.

18. Iwanaga H, Wakai S, Ochiai C, Narita J, Inoh S, Nagai M. Ruptured cerebral aneurysms missed by initial angiographic study. *Neurosurgery* 1990; 27(1): 45-51.

19. Farres MT, Ferraz-Leite H, Schindler E, Muhlbauer M. Spontaneous subarachnoid hemorrhage with negative angiography: CT findings. *J Comput Assist Tomogr* 1992; 16(4): 534-7.

20. Tatter SB, Crowell RM, Ogilvy CS. Aneurysmal and microaneurysmal 'angiogram-negative' subarachnoid hemorrhage. *Neurosurgery* 1995; 37(1): 48-55.

21. Fang H. A comparison of blood vessels of the brain and peripheral blood vessels. In: *Cerebral Vascular Diseases*. Wright IS, Millikan CH, Eds. New York, USA: Grune and Stratton, 1958: 17-22.

22. Wilkinson IM. The vertebral artery. Extracranial and intracranial structure. *Arch Neurol* 1972; 27(5): 392-6.

23. *Youmans' Neurological Surgery*, 3rd ed. Youmans JR, Ed. Philadelphia, USA: W.B. Saunders, 1989.

24. Nixon AM, Gunel M, Sumpio BE. The critical role of hemodynamics in the development of cerebral vascular disease. *J Neurosurg* 2010; 112(6): 1240-53.

25. Rhoton AL, Jr., Merz W. Suction tubes for conventional and microscopic neurosurgery. *Surg Neurol* 1981; 15(2): 120-4.

26. Ferguson GG. Physical factors in the initiation, growth, and rupture of human intracranial saccular aneurysms. *J Neurosurg* 1972; 37(6): 666-77.

27. Hoi Y, Meng H, Woodward SH, Bendok BR, Hanel RA, Guterman LR, *et al.* Effects of arterial geometry on aneurysm growth: three-dimensional computational fluid dynamics study. *J Neurosurg* 2004; 101(4): 676-81.

28. Qureshi AI, Suri MF, Yahia AM, Suarez JI, Guterman LR, Hopkins LN, *et al.* Risk factors for subarachnoid hemorrhage. *Neurosurgery* 2001; 49(3): 607-12; discussion 12-3.

29. Taylor CL, Yuan Z, Selman WR, Ratcheson RA, Rimm AA. Cerebral arterial aneurysm formation and rupture in 20,767 elderly patients: hypertension and other risk factors. *J Neurosurg* 1995; 83(5): 812-9.

30. Kubota M, Yamaura A, Ono J. Prevalence of risk factors for aneurysmal subarachnoid haemorrhage: results of a Japanese multicentre case control study for stroke. *Br J Neurosurg* 2001; 15(6): 474-8.

31. Knekt P, Reunanen A, Aho K, Heliovaara M, Rissanen A, Aromaa A, *et al.* Risk factors for subarachnoid hemorrhage in a longitudinal population study. *J Clin Epidemiol* 1991; 44(9): 933-9.

32. Juvela S, Hillbom M, Numminen H, Koskinen P. Cigarette smoking and alcohol consumption as risk factors for aneurysmal subarachnoid hemorrhage. *Stroke* 1993; 24(5): 639-46.

33. Oyesiku NM, Colohan AR, Barrow DL, Reisner A. Cocaine-induced aneurysmal rupture: an emergent negative factor in the natural history of intracranial aneurysms? *Neurosurgery* 1993; 32(4): 518-25; discussion 25-6.

34. Kernan WN, Viscoli CM, Brass LM, Broderick JP, Brott T, Feldmann E, *et al.* Phenylpropanolamine and the risk of hemorrhagic stroke. *N Engl J Med* 2000; 343(25): 1826-32.

35. Tsementzis SA, Gill JS, Hitchcock ER, Gill SK, Beevers DG. Diurnal variation of and activity during the onset of stroke. *Neurosurgery* 1985; 17(6): 901-4.

36. Dias MS, Sekhar LN. Intracranial hemorrhage from aneurysms and arteriovenous malformations during pregnancy and the puerperium. *Neurosurgery* 1990; 27(6): 855-65; discussion 65-6.

37. Fountas KN, Kapsalaki EZ, Machinis T, Karampelas I, Smisson HF, Robinson JS. Review of the literature regarding the relationship of rebleeding and external ventricular drainage in patients with subarachnoid hemorrhage of aneurysmal origin. *Neurosurg Rev* 2006; 29(1): 14-8; discussion 9-20.

38. Qureshi AI, Suarez JI, Parekh PD, Sung G, Geocadin R, Bhardwaj A, *et al.* Risk factors for multiple intracranial aneurysms. *Neurosurgery* 1998; 43(1): 22-6; discussion 6-7.

39. Juvela S. Risk factors for multiple intracranial aneurysms. *Stroke* 2000; 31(2): 392-7.

40. Ellamushi HE, Grieve JP, Jager HR, Kitchen ND. Risk factors for the formation of multiple intracranial aneurysms. *J Neurosurg* 2001; 94(5): 728-32.

41. Butler WE, Barker FG, 2nd, Crowell RM. Patients with polycystic kidney disease would benefit from routine magnetic resonance angiographic screening for intracerebral aneurysms: a decision analysis. *Neurosurgery* 1996; 38(3): 506-15; discussion 15-6.

42. Levey AS, Pauker SG, Kassirer JP. Occult intracranial aneurysms in polycystic kidney disease. When is cerebral arteriography indicated? *N Engl J Med* 1983; 308(17): 986-94.

43. Schievink WI, Prendergast V, Zabramski JM. Rupture of a previously documented small asymptomatic intracranial aneurysm in a patient with autosomal dominant polycystic kidney disease. Case report. *J Neurosurg* 1998; 89(3): 479-82.

44. Schievink WI, Torres VE, Piepgras DG, Wiebers DO. Saccular intracranial aneurysms in autosomal dominant polycystic kidney disease. *J Am Soc Nephrol* 1992; 3(1): 88-95.

45. Batjer H, Suss RA, Samson D. Intracranial arteriovenous malformations associated with aneurysms. *Neurosurgery* 1986; 18(1): 29-35.

46. Fisher W. Concomitant intracranial aneurysms and arteriovenous malformations. In: *Neurosurgery*. Wilkins RH RS, Ed. New York, USA: McGraw Hill, 1996.

47. Redekop G, TerBrugge K, Montanera W, Willinsky R. Arterial aneurysms associated with cerebral arteriovenous malformations: classification, incidence, and risk of hemorrhage. *J Neurosurg* 1998; 89(4): 539-46.

48. Cloft HJ, Kallmes DF, Kallmes MH, Goldstein JH, Jensen ME, Dion JE. Prevalence of cerebral aneurysms in patients with fibromuscular dysplasia: a reassessment. *J Neurosurg* 1998; 88(3): 436-40.

49. Kissela BM, Sauerbeck L, Woo D, Khoury J, Carrozzella J, Pancioli A, *et al*. Subarachnoid hemorrhage: a preventable disease with a heritable component. *Stroke* 2002; 33(5): 1321-6.

50. Alberts MJ, Quinones A, Graffagnino C, Friedman A, Roses AD. Risk of intracranial aneurysms in families with subarachnoid hemorrhage. *Can J Neurol Sci* 1995; 22(2): 121-5.

51. Raaymakers TW, Rinkel GJ, Ramos LM. Initial and follow-up screening for aneurysms in families with familial subarachnoid hemorrhage. *Neurology* 1998; 51(4): 1125-30.

52. Sarti C, Tuomilehto J, Salomaa V, Sivenius J, Kaarsalo E, Narva EV, *et al*. Epidemiology of subarachnoid hemorrhage in Finland from 1983 to 1985. *Stroke* 1991; 22(7): 848-53.

53. Wills S, Ronkainen A, van der Voet M, Kuivaniemi H, Helin K, Leinonen E, *et al*. Familial intracranial aneurysms: an analysis of 346 multiplex Finnish families. *Stroke* 2003; 34(6): 1370-4.

54. Rinne JK, Hernesniemi JA. De novo aneurysms: special multiple intracranial aneurysms. *Neurosurgery* 1993; 33(6): 981-5.

55. David CA, Vishteh AG, Spetzler RF, Lemole M, Lawton MT, Partovi S. Late angiographic follow-up review of surgically treated aneurysms. *J Neurosurg* 1999; 91(3): 396-401.

56. Juvela S, Porras M, Poussa K. Natural history of unruptured intracranial aneurysms: probability of and risk factors for aneurysm rupture. *J Neurosurg* 2000; 93(3): 379-87.

57. Yasui N, Suzuki A, Nishimura H, Suzuki K, Abe T. Long-term follow-up study of unruptured intracranial aneurysms. *Neurosurgery* 1997; 40(6): 1155-9; discussion 9-60.

58. Unruptured intracranial aneurysms - risk of rupture and risks of surgical intervention. International Study of Unruptured Intracranial Aneurysms Investigators. *N Engl J Med* 1998; 339(24): 1725-33.

59. Bederson JB, Awad IA, Wiebers DO, Piepgras D, Haley EC, Jr., Brott T, *et al*. Recommendations for the management of patients with unruptured intracranial aneurysms: a statement for healthcare professionals from the Stroke Council of the American Heart Association. *Stroke* 2000; 31(11): 2742-50.

60. Wiebers DO, Whisnant JP, Huston J, 3rd, Meissner I, Brown RD, Jr., Piepgras DG, *et al*. Unruptured intracranial aneurysms: natural history, clinical outcome, and risks of surgical and endovascular treatment. *Lancet* 2003; 362(9378): 103-10.

61. Broderick JP, Brott TG, Duldner JE, Tomsick T, Leach A. Initial and recurrent bleeding are the major causes of death following subarachnoid hemorrhage. *Stroke* 1994; 25(7): 1342-7.

62. Schievink WI. Intracranial aneurysms. *N Engl J Med* 1997; 336(1): 28-40.

63. Mount LA. *Practical Applications*. Philadelphia, USA: Lippincott, 1969.

64. Johnston SC, Selvin S, Gress DR. The burden, trends, and demographics of mortality from subarachnoid hemorrhage. *Neurology* 1998; 50(5): 1413-8.

65. Hop JW, Rinkel GJ, Algra A, van Gijn J. Case-fatality rates and functional outcome after subarachnoid hemorrhage: a systematic review. *Stroke* 1997; 28(3): 660-4.

66. Drake CG. Progress in cerebrovascular disease. Management of cerebral aneurysm. *Stroke* 1981; 12(3): 273-83.

67. Kassell NF, Drake CG. Review of the management of saccular aneurysms. *Neurol Clin* 1983; 1(1): 73-86.

68. Mayberg MR, Batjer HH, Dacey R, Diringer M, Haley EC, Heros RC, *et al*. Guidelines for the management of aneurysmal subarachnoid hemorrhage. A statement for healthcare professionals from a special writing group of the Stroke Council, American Heart Association. *Circulation* 1994; 90(5): 2592-605.

69. Winn HR, Richardson AE, Jane JA. The long-term prognosis in untreated cerebral aneurysms: I. The incidence of late hemorrhage in cerebral aneurysm: a 10-year evaluation of 364 patients. *Ann Neurol* 1977; 1(4): 358-70.

70. Richardson AE, Jane JA, Payne PM. Assessment of the Natural History of Anterior Communicating Aneurysms. *J Neurosurg* 1964; 21: 266-74.

71. Henderson WG, Torner JC, Nibbelink DW. Intracranial aneurysms and subarachnoid hemorrhage - report on a randomized treatment study. IV-B. Regulated bed rest - statistical evaluation. *Stroke* 1977; 8(5): 579-89.

72. Bassi P, Bandera R, Loiero M, Tognoni G, Mangoni A. Warning signs in subarachnoid hemorrhage: a cooperative study. *Acta Neurol Scand* 1991; 84(4): 277-81.

73. Leblanc R. The minor leak preceding subarachnoid hemorrhage. *J Neurosurg* 1987; 66(1): 35-9.

74. Hauerberg J, Andersen BB, Eskesen V, Rosenorn J, Schmidt K. Importance of the recognition of a warning leak as a sign of a ruptured intracranial aneurysm. *Acta Neurol Scand* 1991; 83(1): 61-4.

75. Juvela S. Minor leak before rupture of an intracranial aneurysm and subarachnoid hemorrhage of unknown etiology. *Neurosurgery* 1992; 30(1): 7-11.

76. Verweij RD, Wijdicks EF, van Gijn J. Warning headache in aneurysmal subarachnoid hemorrhage. A case-control study. *Arch Neurol* 1988; 45(9): 1019-20.

77. Fisher CM. Honored guest presentation: painful states: a neurological commentary. *Clin Neurosurg* 1983; 31: 32-53.

78. Linn FH, Rinkel GJ, Algra A, van Gijn J. Headache characteristics in subarachnoid haemorrhage and benign thunderclap headache. *J Neurol Neurosurg Psychiatry* 1998; 65(5): 791-3.

79. Edlow JA. Diagnosis of subarachnoid hemorrhage in the emergency department. *Emerg Med Clin North Am* 2003; 21(1): 73-87.

80. Kowalski RG, Claassen J, Kreiter KT, Bates JE, Ostapkovich ND, Connolly ES, *et al.* Initial misdiagnosis and outcome after subarachnoid hemorrhage. *JAMA* 2004; 291(7): 866-9.

81. Edlow JA. Diagnosis of subarachnoid hemorrhage. *Neurocrit Care* 2005; 2(2): 99-109.

82. Fontanarosa PB. Recognition of subarachnoid hemorrhage. *Ann Emerg Med* 1989; 18(11): 1199-205.

83. Ogilvy CS, Rordorf G. Mechanisms and treatment of coma after subarachnoid hemorrhage In: *Subarachnoid Hemorrhage: Pathophysiology and Management.* Bederson JB, Ed. Park Ridge, IL, USA: Neurosurgical topics. Committee AP. American Association of Neurological Surgeons, 1997: 157-71.

84. Sundaram MB, Chow F. Seizures associated with spontaneous subarachnoid hemorrhage. *Can J Neurol Sci* 1986; 13(3): 229-31.

85. Ohman J. Hypertension as a risk factor for epilepsy after aneurysmal subarachnoid hemorrhage and surgery. *Neurosurgery* 1990; 27(4): 578-81.

86. Manschot WA. Subarachnoid hemorrhage; intraocular symptoms and their pathogenesis. *Am J Ophthalmol* 1954; 38(4): 501-5.

87. Garfinkle AM, Danys IR, Nicolle DA, Colohan AR, Brem S. Terson's syndrome: a reversible cause of blindness following subarachnoid hemorrhage. *J Neurosurg* 1992; 76(5): 766-71.

88. Pfausler B, Belcl R, Metzler R, Mohsenipour I, Schmutzhard E. Terson's syndrome in spontaneous subarachnoid hemorrhage: a prospective study in 60 consecutive patients. *J Neurosurg* 1996; 85(3): 392-4.

89. Vanderlinden RG, Chisholm LD. Vitreous hemorrhages and sudden increased intracranial pressure. *J Neurosurg* 1974; 41(2): 167-76.

90. Keithahn MA, Bennett SR, Cameron D, Mieler WF. Retinal folds in Terson syndrome. *Ophthalmology* 1993; 100(8): 1187-90.

91. Schultz PN, Sobol WM, Weingeist TA. Long-term visual outcome in Terson syndrome. *Ophthalmology* 1991; 98(12): 1814-9.

92. Morgenstern LB, Luna-Gonzales H, Huber JC, Jr., Wong SS, Uthman MO, Gurian JH, *et al.* Worst headache and subarachnoid hemorrhage: prospective, modern computed tomography and spinal fluid analysis. *Ann Emerg Med* 1998; 32(3 Pt 1): 297-304.

93. van der Wee N, Rinkel GJ, Hasan D, van Gijn J. Detection of subarachnoid haemorrhage on early CT: is lumbar puncture still needed after a negative scan? *J Neurol Neurosurg Psychiatry* 1995; 58(3): 357-9.

94. Sames TA, Storrow AB, Finkelstein JA, Magoon MR. Sensitivity of new-generation computed tomography in subarachnoid hemorrhage. *Acad Emerg Med* 1996; 3(1): 16-20.

95. van Gijn J, van Dongen KJ. The time course of aneurysmal haemorrhage on computed tomograms. *Neuroradiology* 1982; 23(3): 153-6.

96. Cortnum S, Sorensen P, Jorgensen J. Determining the sensitivity of computed tomography scanning in early detection of subarachnoid hemorrhage. *Neurosurgery* 2010; 66(5): 900-2; discussion 3.

97. Shah KH, Edlow JA. Distinguishing traumatic lumbar puncture from true subarachnoid hemorrhage. *J Emerg Med* 2002; 23(1): 67-74.

98. Mitchell P, Wilkinson ID, Hoggard N, Paley MN, Jellinek DA, Powell T, *et al.* Detection of subarachnoid haemorrhage with magnetic resonance imaging. *J Neurol Neurosurg Psychiatry* 2001; 70(2): 205-11.

99. da Rocha AJ, da Silva CJ, Gama HP, Baccin CE, Braga FT, Cesare Fde A, *et al.* Comparison of magnetic resonance imaging sequences with computed tomography to detect low-grade subarachnoid hemorrhage: role of fluid-attenuated inversion recovery sequence. *J Comput Assist Tomogr* 2006; 30(2): 295-303.

100. Vieco PT, Shuman WP, Alsofrom GF, Gross CE. Detection of circle of Willis aneurysms in patients with acute subarachnoid hemorrhage: a comparison of CT angiography and digital subtraction angiography. *AJR Am J Roentgenol* 1995; 165(2): 425-30.

101. Hope JK, Wilson JL, Thomson FJ. Three-dimensional CT angiography in the detection and characterization of intracranial berry aneurysms. *AJNR Am J Neuroradiol* 1996; 17(3): 439-45.

102. Uysal E, Yanbuloglu B, Erturk M, Kilinc BM, Basak M. Spiral CT angiography in diagnosis of cerebral aneurysms of cases with acute subarachnoid hemorrhage. *Diagn Interv Radiol* 2005; 11(2): 77-82.

103. Wilms G, Guffens M, Gryspeerdt S, Bosmans H, Maaly M, Boulanger T, *et al.* Spiral CT of intracranial aneurysms: correlation with digital subtraction and magnetic resonance angiography. *Neuroradiology* 1996; 38 Suppl 1: S20-5.

104. Ogawa T, Okudera T, Noguchi K, Sasaki N, Inugami A, Uemura K, *et al.* Cerebral aneurysms: evaluation with three-dimensional CT angiography. *AJNR Am J Neuroradiol* 1996; 17(3): 447-54.

105. Villablanca JP, Jahan R, Hooshi P, Lim S, Duckwiler G, Patel A, *et al.* Detection and characterization of very small cerebral aneurysms by using 2D and 3D helical CT angiography. *AJNR Am J Neuroradiol* 2002; 23(7): 1187-98.

106. Velthuis BK, Rinkel GJ, Ramos LM, Witkamp TD, Berkelbach van der Sprenkel JW, Vandertop WP, *et al.* Subarachnoid hemorrhage: aneurysm detection and preoperative evaluation with CT angiography. *Radiology* 1998; 208(2): 423-30.

107. Korogi Y, Takahashi M, Katada K, Ogura Y, Hasuo K, Ochi M, *et al.* Intracranial aneurysms: detection with three-dimensional CT angiography with volume rendering - comparison with conventional angiographic and surgical findings. *Radiology* 1999; 211(2): 497-506.

108. Huston J, 3rd, Nichols DA, Luetmer PH, Goodwin JT, Meyer FB, Wiebers DO, *et al.* Blinded prospective evaluation of sensitivity of MR angiography to known intracranial aneurysms: importance of aneurysm size. *AJNR Am J Neuroradiol* 1994; 15(9): 1607-14.

109. Schuierer G, Huk WJ, Laub G. Magnetic resonance angiography of intracranial aneurysms: comparison with intra-arterial digital subtraction angiography. *Neuroradiology* 1992; 35(1): 50-4.

110. Anzalone N, Triulzi F, Scotti G. Acute subarachnoid haemorrhage: 3D time-of-flight MR angiography versus intra-arterial digital angiography. *Neuroradiology* 1995; 37(4): 257-61.

111. Horikoshi T, Fukamachi A, Nishi H, Fukasawa I. Detection of intracranial aneurysms by three-dimensional time-of-flight magnetic resonance angiography. *Neuroradiology* 1994; 36(3): 203-7.

112. Atlas SW. Magnetic resonance imaging of intracranial aneurysms. *Neuroimaging Clin N Am* 1997; 7(4): 709-20.

113. Wilcock D, Jaspan T, Holland I, Cherryman G, Worthington B. Comparison of magnetic resonance angiography with conventional angiography in the detection of intracranial aneurysms in patients presenting with subarachnoid haemorrhage. *Clin Radiol* 1996; 51(5): 330-4.

114. Hunt WE, Hess RM. Surgical risk as related to time of intervention in the repair of intracranial aneurysms. *J Neurosurg* 1968; 28(1): 14-20.

115. Hunt WE, Kosnik EJ. Timing and perioperative care in intracranial aneurysm surgery. *Clin Neurosurg* 1974; 21: 79-89.

116. Report of World Federation of Neurological Surgeons Committee on a Universal Subarachnoid Hemorrhage Grading Scale. *J Neurosurg* 1988; 68(6): 985-6.

117. Teasdale G, Jennett B. Assessment of coma and impaired consciousness. A practical scale. *Lancet* 1974; 2(7872): 81-4.

118. Fisher CM, Kistler JP, Davis JM. Relation of cerebral vasospasm to subarachnoid hemorrhage visualized by computerized tomographic scanning. *Neurosurgery* 1980; 6(1): 1-9.

119. Ogilvy CS, Carter BS. A proposed comprehensive grading system to predict outcome for surgical management of intracranial aneurysms. *Neurosurgery* 1998; 42(5): 959-68; discussion 68-70.

120. Inagawa T, Kamiya K, Ogasawara H, Yano T. Rebleeding of ruptured intracranial aneurysms in the acute stage. *Surg Neurol* 1987; 28(2): 93-9.

121. Wijdicks EF, Vermeulen M, Murray GD, Hijdra A, van Gijn J. The effects of treating hypertension following aneurysmal subarachnoid hemorrhage. *Clin Neurol Neurosurg* 1990; 92(2): 111-7.

122. Fujii Y, Takeuchi S, Sasaki O, Minakawa T, Koike T, Tanaka R. Ultra-early rebleeding in spontaneous subarachnoid hemorrhage. *J Neurosurg* 1996; 84(1): 35-42.

123. Naidech AM, Janjua N, Kreiter KT, Ostapkovich ND, Fitzsimmons BF, Parra A, et al. Predictors and impact of aneurysm rebleeding after subarachnoid hemorrhage. *Arch Neurol* 2005; 62(3): 410-6.

124. Stornelli SA, French JD. Subarachnoid hemorrhage - factors in prognosis and management. *J Neurosurg* 1964; 21: 769-80.

125. Gibbs JR, O'Gorman P. Fibrinolysis in subarachnoid haemorrhage. *Postgrad Med J* 1967; 43(506): 779-84.

126. Torner JC, Kassell NF, Wallace RB, Adams HP, Jr. Preoperative prognostic factors for rebleeding and survival in aneurysm patients receiving antifibrinolytic therapy: report of the Cooperative Aneurysm Study. *Neurosurgery* 1981; 9(5): 506-13.

127. Kassell NF, Torner JC, Adams HP, Jr. Antifibrinolytic therapy in the acute period following aneurysmal subarachnoid hemorrhage. Preliminary observations from the Cooperative Aneurysm Study. *J Neurosurg* 1984; 61(2): 225-30.

128. Hillman J, Fridriksson S, Nilsson O, Yu Z, Saveland H, Jakobsson KE. Immediate administration of tranexamic acid and reduced incidence of early rebleeding after aneurysmal subarachnoid hemorrhage: a prospective randomized study. *J Neurosurg* 2002; 97(4): 771-8.

129. Roos Y, Rinkel G, Vermeulen M, Algra A, van Gijn J. Antifibrinolytic therapy for aneurysmal subarachnoid hemorrhage: a major update of a Cochrane review. *Stroke* 2003; 34(9): 2308-9.

130. Roos Y. Antifibrinolytic treatment in subarachnoid hemorrhage: a randomized placebo-controlled trial. STAR Study Group. *Neurology* 2000; 54(1): 77-82.

131. Drake CG. Cerebral aneurysm surgery: an update. In: *Cerebrovascular Diseases*, Tenth Princeton Conference. Scheinberg P, Ed. New York, USA: Raven Press, 1976: 289-310.

132. Sundt TM, Jr., Whisnant JP. Subarachnoid hemorrhage from intracranial aneurysms. Surgical management and natural history of disease. *N Engl J Med* 1978; 299(3): 116-22.

133. Kassell NF, Drake CG. Timing of aneurysm surgery. *Neurosurgery* 1982; 10(4): 514-9.

134. Suzuki J, Yoshimoto T, Onuma T. Early operations for ruptured intracranial aneurysms - study of 31 cases operated on within the first four days after ruptured aneurysm. *Neurol Med Chir* (Tokyo) 1978; 18(1 Pt 1): 82-9.

135. Mizukami M, Kawase T, Usami T, Tazawa T. Prevention of vasospasm by early operation with removal of subarachnoid blood. *Neurosurgery* 1982; 10(3): 301-7.

136. Kassell NF, Torner JC, Jane JA, Haley EC, Jr., Adams HP. The International Cooperative Study on the Timing of Aneurysm Surgery. Part 2: Surgical results. *J Neurosurg* 1990; 73(1): 37-47.

137. Haley EC, Jr., Kassell NF, Torner JC. The International Cooperative Study on the Timing of Aneurysm Surgery. The North American experience. *Stroke* 1992; 23(2): 205-14.

138. Fogelholm R, Hernesniemi J, Vapalahti M. Impact of early surgery on outcome after aneurysmal subarachnoid hemorrhage. A population-based study. *Stroke* 1993; 24(11): 1649-54.

139. Ohman J, Heiskanen O. Timing of operation for ruptured supratentorial aneurysms: a prospective randomized study. *J Neurosurg* 1989; 70(1): 55-60.

140. Disney L, Weir B, Grace M. Factors influencing the outcome of aneurysm rupture in poor grade patients: a prospective series. *Neurosurgery* 1988; 23(1): 1-9.

141. Le Roux PD, Elliott JP, Newell DW, Grady MS, Winn HR. Predicting outcome in poor-grade patients with subarachnoid hemorrhage: a retrospective review of 159 aggressively managed cases. *J Neurosurg* 1996; 85(1): 39-49.

142. Le Roux PD, Elliot JP, Newell DW, Grady MS, Winn HR. The incidence of surgical complications is similar in good and poor grade patients undergoing repair of ruptured anterior circulation aneurysms: a retrospective review of 355 patients. *Neurosurgery* 1996; 38(5): 887-93; discussion 93-5.

143. Lawson MF, Chi YY, Velat GJ, Mocco J, Hoh BL. Timing of aneurysm surgery: the International Cooperative Study revisited in the era of endovascular coiling. *Journal of NeuroInterventional Surgery* 2010; 2(2): 131-4.

144. Raymond J, Roy D. Safety and efficacy of endovascular treatment of acutely ruptured aneurysms. *Neurosurgery* 1997; 41(6): 1235-45; discussion 45-6.

145. Debrun GM, Aletich VA, Kehrli P, Misra M, Ausman JI, Charbel F. Selection of cerebral aneurysms for treatment using Guglielmi detachable coils: the preliminary University of Illinois at Chicago experience. *Neurosurgery* 1998; 43(6): 1281-95; discussion 96-7.

146. Vanninen R, Koivisto T, Saari T, Hernesniemi J, Vapalahti M. Ruptured intracranial aneurysms: acute endovascular treatment with electrolytically detachable coils - a prospective randomized study. *Radiology* 1999; 211(2): 325-36.

147. Koivisto T, Vanninen R, Hurskainen H, Saari T, Hernesniemi J, Vapalahti M. Outcomes of early endovascular versus surgical treatment of ruptured cerebral aneurysms. A prospective randomized study. *Stroke* 2000; 31(10): 2369-77.

148. Molyneux A, Kerr R, Stratton I, Sandercock P, Clarke M, Shrimpton J, *et al.* International Subarachnoid Aneurysm Trial (ISAT) of neurosurgical clipping versus endovascular coiling in 2143 patients with ruptured intracranial aneurysms: a randomised trial. *Lancet* 2002; 360(9342): 1267-74.

149. Molyneux AJ, Kerr RS, Yu LM, Clarke M, Sneade M, Yarnold JA, *et al.* International subarachnoid aneurysm trial (ISAT) of neurosurgical clipping versus endovascular coiling in 2143 patients with ruptured intracranial aneurysms: a randomised comparison of effects on survival, dependency, seizures, rebleeding, subgroups, and aneurysm occlusion. *Lancet* 2005; 366(9488): 809-17.

150. Molyneux AJ, Kerr RS, Birks J, Ramzi N, Yarnold J, Sneade M, *et al.* Risk of recurrent subarachnoid haemorrhage, death, or dependence and standardised mortality ratios after clipping or coiling of an intracranial aneurysm in the International Subarachnoid Aneurysm Trial (ISAT): long-term follow-up. *Lancet Neurol* 2009; 8(5): 427-33.

151. Kassell NF, Sasaki T, Colohan AR, Nazar G. Cerebral vasospasm following aneurysmal subarachnoid hemorrhage. *Stroke* 1985; 16(4): 562-72.

152. Weir B, Grace M, Hansen J, Rothberg C. Time course of vasospasm in man. *J Neurosurg* 1978; 48(2): 173-8.

153. Heros RC, Zervas NT, Varsos V. Cerebral vasospasm after subarachnoid hemorrhage: an update. *Ann Neurol* 1983; 14(6): 599-608.

154. Fisher CM, Roberson GH, Ojemann RG. Cerebral vasospasm with ruptured saccular aneurysm - the clinical manifestations. *Neurosurgery* 1977; 1(3): 245-8.

155. Longstreth WT, Jr., Nelson LM, Koepsell TD, van Belle G. Clinical course of spontaneous subarachnoid hemorrhage: a population-based study in King County, Washington. *Neurology* 1993; 43(4): 712-8.

156. Kassell NF, Boarini DJ, Adams HP, Jr., Sahs AL, Graf CJ, Torner JC, *et al.* Overall management of ruptured aneurysm: comparison of early and late operation. *Neurosurgery* 1981; 9(2): 120-8.

157. Lindegaard KF, Nornes H, Bakke SJ, Sorteberg W, Nakstad P. Cerebral vasospasm after subarachnoid haemorrhage investigated by means of transcranial Doppler ultrasound. *Acta Neurochir Suppl* (Wien) 1988; 42: 81-4.

158. Seiler RW, Grolimund P, Aaslid R, Huber P, Nornes H. Cerebral vasospasm evaluated by transcranial ultrasound correlated with clinical grade and CT-visualized subarachnoid hemorrhage. *J Neurosurg* 1986; 64(4): 594-600.

159. Sekhar LN, Wechsler LR, Yonas H, Luyckx K, Obrist W. Value of transcranial Doppler examination in the diagnosis of cerebral vasospasm after subarachnoid hemorrhage. *Neurosurgery* 1988; 22(5): 813-21.

160. Aaslid R, Markwalder TM, Nornes H. Noninvasive transcranial Doppler ultrasound recording of flow velocity in basal cerebral arteries. *J Neurosurg* 1982; 57(6): 769-74.

161. Aaslid R, Huber P, Nornes H. Evaluation of cerebrovascular spasm with transcranial Doppler ultrasound. *J Neurosurg* 1984; 60(1): 37-41.

162. Aaslid R, Huber P, Nornes H. A transcranial Doppler method in the evaluation of cerebrovascular spasm. *Neuroradiology* 1986; 28(1): 11-6.

163. Lindegaard KF, Nornes H, Bakke SJ, Sorteberg W, Nakstad P. Cerebral vasospasm diagnosis by means of angiography and blood velocity measurements. *Acta Neurochir* (Wien) 1989; 100(1-2): 12-24.

164. Weir B, Menon D, Overton T. Regional cerebral blood flow in patients with aneurysms: estimation by Xenon 133 inhalation. *Can J Neurol Sci* 1978; 5(3): 301-5.

165. Vespa PM, Nuwer MR, Juhasz C, Alexander M, Nenov V, Martin N, *et al.* Early detection of vasospasm after acute subarachnoid hemorrhage using continuous EEG ICU monitoring. *Electroencephalogr Clin Neurophysiol* 1997; 103(6): 607-15.

166. Labar DR, Fisch BJ, Pedley TA, Fink ME, Solomon RA. Quantitative EEG monitoring for patients with subarachnoid hemorrhage. *Electroencephalogr Clin Neurophysiol* 1991; 78(5): 325-32.

167. Maroon JC, Nelson PB. Hypovolemia in patients with subarachnoid hemorrhage: therapeutic implications. *Neurosurgery* 1979; 4(3): 223-6.

168. Kosnik EJ, Hunt WE. Postoperative hypertension in the management of patients with intracranial arterial aneurysms. *J Neurosurg* 1976; 45(2): 148-54.

169. Kindt GW, McGillicuddy JE, Giannotta SL, Pritz MD. The reversal of neurologic deficit in patients with acute cerebral ischemia by profound increases in intravascular volume. *Acta Neurologica Scandinavica* 1979; 60(Suppl 72): 468-9.

170. Kassell NF, Peerless SJ, Durward QJ, Beck DW, Drake CG, Adams HP. Treatment of ischemic deficits from vasospasm with intravascular volume expansion and induced arterial hypertension. *Neurosurgery* 1982; 11(3): 337-43.

171. Awad IA, Carter LP, Spetzler RF, Medina M, Williams FC, Jr. Clinical vasospasm after subarachnoid hemorrhage: response to hypervolemic hemodilution and arterial hypertension. *Stroke* 1987; 18(2): 365-72.

172. Solomon RA, Post KD, McMurtry JG, 3rd. Depression of circulating blood volume in patients after subarachnoid hemorrhage: implications for the management of symptomatic vasospasm. *Neurosurgery* 1984; 15(3): 354-61.

173. Muizelaar JP, Becker DP. Induced hypertension for the treatment of cerebral ischemia after subarachnoid hemorrhage. Direct effect on cerebral blood flow. *Surg Neurol* 1986; 25(4): 317-25.

174. Lennihan L, Mayer SA, Fink ME, Beckford A, Paik MC, Zhang H, et al. Effect of hypervolemic therapy on cerebral blood flow after subarachnoid hemorrhage: a randomized controlled trial. *Stroke* 2000; 31(2): 383-91.

175. Egge A, Waterloo K, Sjoholm H, Solberg T, Ingebrigtsen T, Romner B. Prophylactic hyperdynamic postoperative fluid therapy after aneurysmal subarachnoid hemorrhage: a clinical, prospective, randomized, controlled study. *Neurosurgery* 2001; 49(3): 593-605; discussion -6.

176. Pickard JD, Murray GD, Illingworth R, Shaw MD, Teasdale GM, Foy PM, et al. Effect of oral nimodipine on cerebral infarction and outcome after subarachnoid haemorrhage: British Aneurysm Nimodipine Trial. *BMJ* 1989; 298(6674): 636-42.

177. Barker FG, 2nd, Ogilvy CS. Efficacy of prophylactic nimodipine for delayed ischemic deficit after subarachnoid hemorrhage: a meta-analysis. *J Neurosurg* 1996; 84(3): 405-14.

178. Karinen P, Koivukangas P, Ohinmaa A, Koivukangas J, Ohman J. Cost-effectiveness analysis of nimodipine treatment after aneurysmal subarachnoid hemorrhage and surgery. *Neurosurgery* 1999; 45(4): 780-4; discussion 4-5.

179. Allen GS, Ahn HS, Preziosi TJ, Battye R, Boone SC, Chou SN, et al. Cerebral arterial spasm - a controlled trial of nimodipine in patients with subarachnoid hemorrhage. *N Engl J Med* 1983; 308(11): 619-24.

180. Schanne FA, Kane AB, Young EE, Farber JL. Calcium dependence of toxic cell death: a final common pathway. *Science* 1979; 206(4419): 700-2.

181. Dale J, Landmark KH, Myhre E. The effects of nifedipine, a calcium antagonist, on platelet function. *Am Heart J* 1983; 105(1): 103-5.

182. Auer LM. Pial arterial vasodilation by intravenous nimodipine in cats. *Arzneimittelforschung* 1981; 31(9): 1423-5.

183. Flamm ES, Adams HP, Jr., Beck DW, Pinto RS, Marler JR, Walker MD, et al. Dose-escalation study of intravenous nicardipine in patients with aneurysmal subarachnoid hemorrhage. *J Neurosurg* 1988; 68(3): 393-400.

184. Haley EC, Jr., Kassell NF, Torner JC. A randomized controlled trial of high-dose intravenous nicardipine in aneurysmal subarachnoid hemorrhage. A report of the Cooperative Aneurysm Study. *J Neurosurg* 1993; 78(4): 537-47.

185. Haley EC, Jr., Kassell NF, Torner JC. A randomized trial of nicardipine in subarachnoid hemorrhage: angiographic and transcranial Doppler ultrasound results. A report of the Cooperative Aneurysm Study. *J Neurosurg* 1993; 78(4): 548-53.

186. Barth M, Capelle HH, Weidauer S, Weiss C, Munch E, Thome C, et al. Effect of nicardipine prolonged-release implants on cerebral vasospasm and clinical outcome after severe aneurysmal subarachnoid hemorrhage: a prospective, randomized, double-blind phase IIa study. *Stroke* 2007; 38(2): 330-6.

187. van den Bergh WM, Algra A, van der Sprenkel JW, Tulleken CA, Rinkel GJ. Hypomagnesemia after aneurysmal subarachnoid hemorrhage. *Neurosurgery* 2003; 52(2): 276-81; discussion 81-2.

188. Marinov MB, Harbaugh KS, Hoopes PJ, Pikus HJ, Harbaugh RE. Neuroprotective effects of preischemia intra-arterial magnesium sulfate in reversible focal cerebral ischemia. *J Neurosurg* 1996; 85(1): 117-24.

189. Ram Z, Sadeh M, Shacked I, Sahar A, Hadani M. Magnesium sulfate reverses experimental delayed cerebral vasospasm after subarachnoid hemorrhage in rats. *Stroke* 1991; 22(7): 922-7.

190. van den Bergh WM, Dijkhuizen RM, Rinkel GJ. Potentials of magnesium treatment in subarachnoid haemorrhage. *Magnes Res* 2004; 17(4): 301-13.

191. van den Bergh WM, Zuur JK, Kamerling NA, van Asseldonk JT, Rinkel GJ, Tulleken CA, et al. Role of magnesium in the reduction of ischemic depolarization and lesion volume after experimental subarachnoid hemorrhage. *J Neurosurg* 2002; 97(2): 416-22.

192. Johnson JW, Ascher P. Voltage-dependent block by intracellular Mg2+ of N-methyl-D-aspartate-activated channels. *Biophys J* 1990; 57(5): 1085-90.

193. Rothman S. Synaptic release of excitatory amino acid neurotransmitter mediates anoxic neuronal death. *J Neurosci* 1984; 4(7): 1884-91.

194. Wong GK, Poon WS, Chan MT, Boet R, Gin T, Ng SC, et al. Intravenous magnesium sulphate for aneurysmal subarachnoid hemorrhage (IMASH): a randomized, double-blinded, placebo-controlled, multicenter phase III trial. *Stroke* 2010; 41(5): 921-6.

195. Wong GK, Poon WS, Chan MT, Boet R, Gin T, Ng SC, et al. Plasma magnesium concentrations and clinical outcomes in aneurysmal subarachnoid hemorrhage patients: post hoc analysis of intravenous magnesium sulphate for aneurysmal subarachnoid hemorrhage trial. *Stroke* 2010; 41(8): 1841-4.

196. Dietrich HH, Dacey RG, Jr. Molecular keys to the problems of cerebral vasospasm. *Neurosurgery* 2000; 46(3): 517-30.

197. Sercombe R, Dinh YR, Gomis P. Cerebrovascular inflammation following subarachnoid hemorrhage. *Jpn J Pharmacol* 2002; 88(3): 227-49.

198. Provencio JJ, Vora N. Subarachnoid hemorrhage and inflammation: bench to bedside and back. *Semin Neurol* 2005; 25(4): 435-44.

199. Kaynar MY, Tanriverdi T, Kafadar AM, Kacira T, Uzun H, Aydin S, et al. Detection of soluble intercellular adhesion molecule-1 and vascular cell adhesion molecule-1 in both cerebrospinal fluid and serum of patients after aneurysmal subarachnoid hemorrhage. *J Neurosurg* 2004; 101(6): 1030-6.

200. Mocco J, Mack WJ, Kim GH, Lozier AP, Laufer I, Kreiter KT, et al. Rise in serum soluble intercellular adhesion molecule-1 levels with vasospasm following aneurysmal subarachnoid hemorrhage. *J Neurosurg* 2002; 97(3): 537-41.

201. Hansen-Schwartz J, Nordstrom CH, Edvinsson L. Human endothelin subtype A receptor enhancement during tissue culture via de novo transcription. *Neurosurgery* 2002; 50(1): 127-33; discussion 33-5.

202. Juvela S. Plasma endothelin concentrations after aneurysmal subarachnoid hemorrhage. *J Neurosurg* 2000; 92(3): 390-400.

203. Suzuki K, Meguro K, Sakurai T, Saitoh Y, Takeuchi S, Nose T. Endothelin-1 concentration increases in the cerebrospinal fluid in cerebral vasospasm caused by subarachnoid hemorrhage. *Surg Neurol* 2000; 53(2): 131-5.

204. Mascia L, Fedorko L, Stewart DJ, Mohamed F, terBrugge K, Ranieri VM, et al. Temporal relationship between endothelin-1 concentrations and cerebral vasospasm in patients with aneurysmal subarachnoid hemorrhage. *Stroke* 2001; 32(5): 1185-90.

205. Kasuya H, Weir BK, White DM, Stefansson K. Mechanism of oxyhemoglobin-induced release of endothelin-1 from cultured vascular endothelial cells and smooth-muscle cells. *J Neurosurg* 1993; 79(6): 892-8.

206. Zubkov AY, Rollins KS, Parent AD, Zhang J, Bryan RM, Jr. Mechanism of endothelin-1-induced contraction in rabbit basilar artery. *Stroke* 2000; 31(2): 526-33.

207. Zuccarello M, Soattin GB, Lewis AI, Breu V, Hallak H, Rapoport RM. Prevention of subarachnoid hemorrhage-induced cerebral vasospasm by oral administration of endothelin receptor antagonists. *J Neurosurg* 1996; 84(3): 503-7.

208. Vajkoczy P, Meyer B, Weidauer S, Raabe A, Thome C, Ringel F, et al. Clazosentan (AXV-034343), a selective endothelin A receptor antagonist, in the prevention of cerebral vasospasm following severe aneurysmal subarachnoid hemorrhage: results of a randomized, double-blind, placebo-controlled, multicenter phase IIa study. *J Neurosurg* 2005; 103(1): 9-17.

209. Macdonald RL, Kassell NF, Mayer S, Ruefenacht D, Schmiedek P, Weidauer S, et al. Clazosentan to overcome neurological ischemia and infarction occurring after subarachnoid hemorrhage (CONSCIOUS-1): randomized, double-blind, placebo-controlled phase 2 dose-finding trial. *Stroke* 2008; 39(11): 3015-21.

210. Kramer A, Fletcher J. Do endothelin-receptor antagonists prevent delayed neurological deficits and poor outcomes after aneurysmal subarachnoid hemorrhage?: a meta-analysis. *Stroke* 2009; 40(10): 3403-6.

211. Shaw MD, Vermeulen M, Murray GD, Pickard JD, Bell BA, Teasdale GM. Efficacy and safety of the endothelin, receptor antagonist TAK-044 in treating subarachnoid hemorrhage: a report by the Steering Committee on behalf of the UK/Netherlands/Eire TAK-044 Subarachnoid Haemorrhage Study Group. *J Neurosurg* 2000; 93(6): 992-7.

212. Macdonald RL, Weir BK. A review of hemoglobin and the pathogenesis of cerebral vasospasm. *Stroke* 1991; 22(8): 971-82.

213. Macdonald RL, Weir BK, Runzer TD, Grace MG, Findlay JM, Saito K, et al. Etiology of cerebral vasospasm in primates. *J Neurosurg* 1991; 75(3): 415-24.

214. Misra HP, Fridovich I. The generation of superoxide radical during the autoxidation of hemoglobin. *J Biol Chem* 1972; 247(21): 6960-2.

215. Winterbourn CC, McGrath BM, Carrell RW. Reactions involving superoxide and normal and unstable haemoglobins. *Biochem J* 1976; 155(3): 493-502.

216. Halliwell B, Gutteridge JMC. *Free Radicals in Biology and Medicine*. New York, USA: Oxford University Press, 1985.

217. Gutteridge JM. Iron promoters of the Fenton reaction and lipid peroxidation can be released from haemoglobin by peroxides. *FEBS Lett* 1986; 201(2): 291-5.

218. Schmidley JW. Free radicals in central nervous system ischemia. *Stroke* 1990; 21(7): 1086-90.

219. Kamezaki T, Yanaka K, Nagase S, Fujita K, Kato N, Nose T. Increased levels of lipid peroxides as predictive of symptomatic vasospasm and poor outcome after aneurysmal subarachnoid hemorrhage. *J Neurosurg* 2002; 97(6): 1302-5.

220. Asano T, Takakura K, Sano K, Kikuchi H, Nagai H, Saito I, et al. Effects of a hydroxyl radical scavenger on delayed ischemic neurological deficits following aneurysmal subarachnoid hemorrhage: results of a multicenter, placebo-controlled double-blind trial. *J Neurosurg* 1996; 84(5): 792-803.

221. Kassell NF, Haley EC, Jr., Apperson-Hansen C, Alves WM. Randomized, double-blind, vehicle-controlled trial of tirilazad mesylate in patients with aneurysmal subarachnoid hemorrhage: a cooperative study in Europe, Australia, and New Zealand. *J Neurosurg* 1996; 84(2): 221-8.

222. Haley EC, Jr., Kassell NF, Apperson-Hansen C, Maile MH, Alves WM. A randomized, double-blind, vehicle-controlled trial of tirilazad mesylate in patients with aneurysmal subarachnoid hemorrhage: a cooperative study in North America. *J Neurosurg* 1997; 86(3): 467-74.

223. Lanzino G, Kassell NF, Dorsch NW, Pasqualin A, Brandt L, Schmiedek P, et al. Double-blind, randomized, vehicle-controlled study of high-dose tirilazad mesylate in women with aneurysmal subarachnoid hemorrhage. Part I. A cooperative study in Europe, Australia, New Zealand, and South Africa. *J Neurosurg* 1999; 90(6): 1011-7.

224. Faraci FM. Role of nitric oxide in regulation of basilar artery tone *in vivo*. *Am J Physiol* 1990; 259(4 Pt 2): H1216-21.

225. Gabikian P, Clatterbuck RE, Eberhart CG, Tyler BM, Tierney TS, Tamargo RJ. Prevention of experimental cerebral vasospasm by intracranial delivery of a nitric oxide donor from a controlled-release polymer: toxicity and efficacy studies in rabbits and rats. *Stroke* 2002; 33(11): 2681-6.

226. Ignarro LJ. Biosynthesis and metabolism of endothelium-derived nitric oxide. *Annu Rev Pharmacol Toxicol* 1990; 30: 535-60.

227. Pluta RM, Dejam A, Grimes G, Gladwin MT, Oldfield EH. Nitrite infusions to prevent delayed cerebral vasospasm in a primate model of subarachnoid hemorrhage. *JAMA* 2005; 293(12): 1477-84.

228. Jung CS, Iuliano BA, Harvey-White J, Espey MG, Oldfield EH, Pluta RM. Association between cerebrospinal fluid levels of asymmetric dimethyl-L-arginine, an endogenous inhibitor of endothelial nitric oxide synthase, and cerebral vasospasm in a primate model of subarachnoid hemorrhage. *J Neurosurg* 2004; 101(5): 836-42.

229. Heros RC, Zervas NT, Lavyne MH, Pickren KS. Reversal of experimental cerebral vasospasm by intravenous nitroprusside therapy. *Surg Neurol* 1976; 6(4): 227-9.

230. Pluta RM, Oldfield EH, Boock RJ. Reversal and prevention of cerebral vasospasm by intracarotid infusions of nitric oxide donors in a primate model of subarachnoid hemorrhage. *J Neurosurg* 1997; 87(5): 746-51.

231. Pluta RM, Thompson BG, Dawson TM, Snyder SH, Boock RJ, Oldfield EH. Loss of nitric oxide synthase immunoreactivity in cerebral vasospasm. *J Neurosurg* 1996; 84(4): 648-54.

232. Thomas JE, Nemirovsky A, Zelman V, Giannotta SL. Rapid reversal of endothelin-1-induced cerebral vasoconstriction by intrathecal administration of nitric oxide donors. *Neurosurgery* 1997; 40(6): 1245-9.

233. Thomas JE, Rosenwasser RH. Reversal of severe cerebral vasospasm in three patients after aneurysmal subarachnoid hemorrhage: initial observations regarding the use of intraventricular sodium nitroprusside in humans. *Neurosurgery* 1999; 44(1): 48-57; discussion -8.

234. Hirsh LF. Intra-arterial nitroprusside treatment of acute experimental vasospasm. *Stroke* 1980; 11(6): 601-5.

235. Thomas JE, Rosenwasser RH, Armonda RA, Harrop J, Mitchell W, Galaria I. Safety of intrathecal sodium nitroprusside for the treatment and prevention of refractory cerebral vasospasm and ischemia in humans. *Stroke* 1999; 30(7): 1409-16.

236. Tierney TS, Clatterbuck RE, Lawson C, Thai QA, Rhines LD, Tamargo RJ. Prevention and reversal of experimental posthemorrhagic vasospasm by the periadventitial administration of nitric oxide from a controlled-release polymer. *Neurosurgery* 2001; 49(4): 945-51; discussion 51-3.

237. Egemen N, Turker RK, Sanlidilek U, Zorlutuna A, Bilgic S, Baskaya M, et al. The effect of intrathecal sodium nitroprusside on severe chronic vasospasm. *Neurol Res* 1993; 15(5): 310-5.

238. Paulson OB. Regional cerebral blood flow in apoplexy due to occlusion of the middle cerebral artery. *Neurology* 1970; 20(1): 63-77.

239. Wolf EW, Banerjee A, Soble-Smith J, Dohan FC, Jr., White RP, Robertson JT. Reversal of cerebral vasospasm using an intrathecally administered nitric oxide donor. *J Neurosurg* 1998; 89(2): 279-88.

240. Raabe A, Zimmermann M, Setzer M, Vatter H, Berkefeld J, Seifert V. Effect of intraventricular sodium nitroprusside on cerebral hemodynamics and oxygenation in poor-grade aneurysm patients with severe, medically refractory vasospasm. *Neurosurgery* 2002; 50(5): 1006-13; discussion 13-4.

241. Millar TM, Stevens CR, Benjamin N, Eisenthal R, Harrison R, Blake DR. Xanthine oxidoreductase catalyses the reduction of nitrates and nitrite to nitric oxide under hypoxic conditions. *FEBS Lett* 1998; 427(2): 225-8.

242. Zweier JL, Wang P, Samouilov A, Kuppusamy P. Enzyme-independent formation of nitric oxide in biological tissues. *Nat Med* 1995; 1(8): 804-9.

243. Nagababu E, Ramasamy S, Abernethy DR, Rifkind JM. Active nitric oxide produced in the red cell under hypoxic conditions by deoxyhemoglobin-mediated nitrite reduction. *J Biol Chem* 2003; 278(47): 46349-56.

244. Delanty N, Vaughan CJ. Vascular effects of statins in stroke. *Stroke* 1997; 28(11): 2315-20.

245. Sterzer P, Meintzschel F, Rosler A, Lanfermann H, Steinmetz H, Sitzer M. Pravastatin improves cerebral vasomotor reactivity in patients with subcortical small-vessel disease. *Stroke* 2001; 32(12): 2817-20.

246. Endres M, Laufs U, Huang Z, Nakamura T, Huang P, Moskowitz MA, et al. Stroke protection by 3-hydroxy-3-methylglutaryl (HMG)-CoA reductase inhibitors mediated by endothelial nitric oxide synthase. *Proc Natl Acad Sci USA* 1998; 95(15): 8880-5.

247. Tseng MY, Czosnyka M, Richards H, Pickard JD, Kirkpatrick PJ. Effects of acute treatment with pravastatin on cerebral vasospasm, autoregulation, and delayed ischemic deficits after aneurysmal subarachnoid hemorrhage: a phase II randomized placebo-controlled trial. *Stroke* 2005; 36(8): 1627-32.

248. Lynch JR, Wang H, McGirt MJ, Floyd J, Friedman AH, Coon AL, et al. Simvastatin reduces vasospasm after aneurysmal subarachnoid hemorrhage: results of a pilot randomized clinical trial. *Stroke* 2005; 36(9): 2024-6.

249. Sillberg VA, Wells GA, Perry JJ. Do statins improve outcomes and reduce the incidence of vasospasm after aneurysmal subarachnoid hemorrhage: a meta-analysis. *Stroke* 2008; 39(9): 2622-6.

250. Cook AM, Hessel EA, 2nd. Meta-analysis of statins for aneurysmal subarachnoid hemorrhage falls short. *Stroke* 2009; 40(3): e79; author reply e82.

251. Vergouwen MD, Meijers JC, Geskus RB, Coert BA, Horn J, Stroes ES, et al. Biologic effects of simvastatin in patients with aneurysmal subarachnoid hemorrhage: a double-blind, placebo-controlled randomized trial. *J Cereb Blood Flow Metab* 2009; 29(8): 1444-53.

252. Vergouwen MD, de Haan RJ, Vermeulen M, Roos YB. Effect of statin treatment on vasospasm, delayed cerebral ischemia, and functional outcome in patients with aneurysmal subarachnoid hemorrhage: a systematic review and meta-analysis update. *Stroke* 2010; 41(1): e47-52.

253. Bendok BR, Getch CC, Malisch TW, Batjer HH. Treatment of aneurysmal subarachnoid hemorrhage. *Semin Neurol* 1998; 18(4): 521-31.

254. Eskridge JM, Song JK. A practical approach to the treatment of vasospasm. *AJNR Am J Neuroradiol* 1997; 18(9): 1653-60.

255. Eskridge JM, Newell DW, Winn HR. Endovascular treatment of vasospasm. *Neurosurg Clin N Am* 1994; 5(3): 437-47.

256. Newell DW, Eskridge JM, Mayberg MR, Grady MS, Winn HR. Angioplasty for the treatment of symptomatic vasospasm following subarachnoid hemorrhage. *J Neurosurg* 1989; 71(5 Pt 1): 654-60.

257. Polin RS, Coenen VA, Hansen CA, Shin P, Baskaya MK, Nanda A, *et al.* Efficacy of transluminal angioplasty for the management of symptomatic cerebral vasospasm following aneurysmal subarachnoid hemorrhage. *J Neurosurg* 2000; 92(2): 284-90.

258. Firlik AD, Kaufmann AM, Jungreis CA, Yonas H. Effect of transluminal angioplasty on cerebral blood flow in the management of symptomatic vasospasm following aneurysmal subarachnoid hemorrhage. *J Neurosurg* 1997; 86(5): 830-9.

259. Newell DW, Eskridge JM, Aaslid R. Current indications and results of cerebral angioplasty. *Acta Neurochir Suppl* 2001; 77: 181-3.

260. Zwienenberg-Lee M, Hartman J, Rudisill N, Madden LK, Smith K, Eskridge J, *et al.* Effect of prophylactic transluminal balloon angioplasty on cerebral vasospasm and outcome in patients with Fisher grade III subarachnoid hemorrhage: results of a phase II multicenter, randomized, clinical trial. *Stroke* 2008; 39(6): 1759-65.

261. Bejjani GK, Bank WO, Olan WJ, Sekhar LN. The efficacy and safety of angioplasty for cerebral vasospasm after subarachnoid hemorrhage. *Neurosurgery* 1998; 42(5): 979-86; discussion 86-7.

262. Rosenwasser RH, Armonda RA, Thomas JE, Benitez RP, Gannon PM, Harrop J. Therapeutic modalities for the management of cerebral vasospasm: timing of endovascular options. *Neurosurgery* 1999; 44(5): 975-9; discussion 9-80.

263. Kassell NF, Helm G, Simmons N, Phillips CD, Cail WS. Treatment of cerebral vasospasm with intra-arterial papaverine. *J Neurosurg* 1992; 77(6): 848-52.

264. Milburn JM, Moran CJ, Cross DT, 3rd, Diringer MN, Pilgram TK, Dacey RG, Jr. Increase in diameters of vasospastic intracranial arteries by intra-arterial papaverine administration. *J Neurosurg* 1998; 88(1): 38-42.

265. Liu JK, Couldwell WT. Intra-arterial papaverine infusions for the treatment of cerebral vasospasm induced by aneurysmal subarachnoid hemorrhage. *Neurocrit Care* 2005; 2(2): 124-32.

266. Vajkoczy P, Horn P, Bauhuf C, Munch E, Hubner U, Ing D, *et al.* Effect of intra-arterial papaverine on regional cerebral blood flow in hemodynamically relevant cerebral vasospasm. *Stroke* 2001; 32(2): 498-505.

267. Feng L, Fitzsimmons BF, Young WL, Berman MF, Lin E, Aagaard BD, *et al.* Intra-arterially administered verapamil as adjunct therapy for cerebral vasospasm: safety and 2-year experience. *AJNR Am J Neuroradiol* 2002; 23(8): 1284-90.

268. Keuskamp J, Murali R, Chao KH. High-dose intra-arterial verapamil in the treatment of cerebral vasospasm after aneurysmal subarachnoid hemorrhage. *J Neurosurg* 2008; 108(3): 458-63.

269. Badjatia N, Topcuoglu MA, Pryor JC, Rabinov JD, Ogilvy CS, Carter BS, *et al.* Preliminary experience with intra-arterial nicardipine as a treatment for cerebral vasospasm. *AJNR Am J Neuroradiol* 2004; 25(5): 819-26.

270. Biondi A, Ricciardi GK, Puybasset L, Abdennour L, Longo M, Chiras J, *et al.* Intra-arterial nimodipine for the treatment of symptomatic cerebral vasospasm after aneurysmal subarachnoid hemorrhage: preliminary results. *AJNR Am J Neuroradiol* 2004; 25(6): 1067-76.

271. Eddleman CS, Hurley MC, Naidech AM, Batjer HH, Bendok BR. Endovascular options in the treatment of delayed ischemic neurological deficits due to cerebral vasospasm. *Neurosurg Focus* 2009; 26(3): E6.

Chapter 9

Management of spontaneous intracerebral hemorrhage

Barbara Voetsch MD PhD, Assistant Professor of Neurology
Lahey Clinic Medical Center, Tufts University School of Medicine
Burlington, Massachusetts, USA

Carlos S. Kase MD, Professor of Neurology
Boston Medical Center, Boston University School of Medicine
Boston, Massachusetts, USA

Introduction

Spontaneous intracerebral hemorrhage (ICH) is a major public health problem, accounting for 10-15% of approximately 15 million new strokes worldwide each year [1, 2]. It is the main cause of stroke-related death and disability, with a 30-day mortality rate that approaches 50% [3, 4]. Only 20% of patients are expected to be functionally independent at 6 months [1]. The incidence of ICH is higher among the elderly, among individuals of African and Asian descent, in patients with poorly controlled hypertension, and in those being treated with long-term oral anticoagulation. Hospital admissions for ICH increased by almost 20% between 1990 and 2000 [5] and are expected to continue to do so as the population ages, because of changes in racial demographics, and due to the increasing use of anticoagulants and antiplatelet agents.

Despite the large medical and socioeconomic impact of ICH, when the first American Heart Association (AHA) guidelines for the management of ICH were published in 1999 [6], only nine small randomized trials of ICH existed, while 315 randomized clinical trials for acute ischemic stroke and 78 trials for subarachnoid hemorrhage were available. This dramatically changed over the past decade, and numerous trials were completed or are underway to address the medical and surgical management of ICH. These can be reviewed in detail on the continuously updated online Stroke Trials Registry at http://www.strokecenter.org/trials/. The goal of this chapter is to provide evidence-based recommendations based on a comprehensive review of the ICH literature and existing management guidelines.

Initial assessment

ICH is a medical emergency and mandates prompt diagnosis as any delay in treatment will worsen the outcome. The risk of cardiopulmonary instability and rapid neurological deterioration in the first hours after symptom onset is high [7, 8]. Airway support, blood pressure (BP) control, intracranial pressure (ICP) treatment, reversal of anticoagulation and neurosurgical consultation are often initiated in the emergency department. As in any acutely unstable patient, the initial attention should be directed at the 'ABCs' of emergency therapy. About one third of patients with supratentorial hemorrhage and the majority with brainstem or cerebellar hemorrhage have either decreased consciousness or bulbar muscle dysfunction requiring early endotracheal intubation [9, 10]. Generally, intubation is indicated for patients with a Glasgow Coma Scale (GCS) score ≤8 or in those with rapidly worsening level of consciousness. This is best achieved with short-acting agents such as propofol or etomidate that will prevent transient increases in ICP caused by tracheal stimulation [11], without prolonged effects on the level of consciousness or neurological function. If circulatory resuscitation is required, isotonic fluids should be given. Hypotonic fluids can exacerbate cerebral edema and increase ICP because free water accumulates in the injured brain tissue. Dextrose-containing solutions should be avoided as hyperglycemia is detrimental to ICH patients [12, 13] **(IV/C)**.

Even for patients who do not require ventilatory support, observation in an intensive care unit (ICU) is strongly recommended for at least the first 24 hours after ictus given the need for close monitoring of cardiopulmonary variables and frequent examinations during this period in which the risk of neurologic deterioration is highest [14] **(Ib/A)**. Evidence is rapidly accumulating that outcomes are improved when patients are cared for in a neurologic or neurosurgical (neuro) ICU. Diringer and colleagues retrospectively analyzed mortality rates in over 1000 patients with ICH admitted to 43 neuro, medical or surgical ICUs in the United States [15]. A clear positive impact on outcome was observed in those cared for by a specialized neurocritical care team (OR for mortality in general ICUs of 3.4; 95% CI, 1.65-7.6). In addition, having a full time intensivist on staff was associated with lower mortality rate (OR 0.39; 95% CI, 0.22-0.67). In another retrospective analysis comparing data from patients treated in a new neuroscience ICU to a similar cohort cared for 2 years earlier in a general ICU setting, outcome measures of percent mortality and disposition at discharge, as well as hospital length of stay and total costs of care were significantly better in the specialized care unit [16]. Finally, in a prospective controlled study, 121 patients with ICH were randomly assigned to an acute stroke unit or a general medical ward [17]. The 30-day mortality rate was 39% in the acute stroke unit compared with 63% in the general medical ward (p=0.007); 1-year mortality rates were 52% and 69%, respectively (p=0.013).

Medical management of intracerebral hemorrhage

Blood pressure management

Blood pressure monitoring and management is critical after ICH, yet the exact treatment targets are still a matter of controversy. Hypertension in the acute setting of ICH is common, occurring in about three quarters of cases [18], and in several studies it has been shown to be associated with hematoma enlargement and poor outcome [19-23]. Conversely, a post hoc analysis of clinical and computer tomography (CT) data from patients enrolled in a prospective observational study of ICH found no association between hemodynamic parameters and hematoma expansion [19, 24], suggesting that the pathophysiology of this process is not yet fully understood. While most investigators agree that elevated BP underlies hematoma growth at least to some extent, a hypertensive response may also occur in an attempt to maintain cerebral perfusion pressure (CPP) in the setting of a large ICH. Therefore, the primary goal of BP management is to lower it enough to avoid hematoma expansion yet without compromising cerebral CPP. In addition, there is a theoretical concern that BP reduction may induce ischemia in the immediate perihematomal region. Although imaging studies have demonstrated a rim of reduced cerebral blood flow and MRI diffusion restriction surrounding large hematomas [25, 26], this does not appear to be a clinically relevant phenomenon both in animal models or in humans with ICH [27-30].

Until recently, recommendations regarding BP management in patients with acute ICH were based on data from observational studies and clinical series. Some of these studies have suggested a greater therapeutic benefit with more aggressive BP treatment. In a small, retrospective study, Suri and colleagues showed that aggressive BP reduction in patients with acute ICH was not only safe, but significantly reduced the risk of neurological deterioration in the first 24 hours after admission [31]. In one observational study, hematomas enlarged in 9% of patients with systolic BP maintained below 150mm Hg and in 30% of those with systolic BP above 160mm Hg (p=0.025) [22]. Two recently completed randomized, multicenter trials have provided stronger preliminary data on BP control after ICH. The Intensive Blood Pressure Reduction in Acute Cerebral Hemorrhage Trial (INTERACT) enrolled patients with spontaneous ICH diagnosed by CT and elevated systolic BP (150-220mm Hg), who were eligible to start the assigned treatment within 6 hours of ICH onset [32]. Patients with severe hypertension (systolic BP >200mm Hg), a clear contraindication to intensive reduction of BP, and GCS of 3-5 were excluded. Patients were randomized to early intensive BP treatment (the 'intensive' group, with a target systolic BP of 140mm Hg to be achieved within 1 hour of randomization; n=203) or standard management of BP based on the 1999 American Heart Association guidelines for the management of ICH [6] (the 'guideline' group, with a target systolic BP of 180mm Hg; n=201). Baseline demographic characteristics were similar in both arms, but initial hematoma volumes were smaller in the guideline group (12.7 ± 11.6cc) compared to the intensive group (14.2 ± 14.5cc). Mean proportional hematoma growth was 36.3% in the guideline group and 13.7% in the intensive treatment group at 24 hours (adjusted p=0.06), and a post hoc analysis revealed that patients recruited within 3 hours of symptom onset and patients with initial systolic BP above 180mm Hg seemed to benefit most from intensive BP reduction. There was no difference in the rate of adverse events or in clinical outcomes at 90 days, yet the study was not adequately powered to analyze these results. Overall, the INTERACT trial established that early intensive BP-lowering treatment is clinically feasible, well tolerated, and seems to reduce hematoma growth in ICH. INTERACT-2 is currently underway and plans to enroll 2800 patients to assess the effect of aggressive BP reduction on death and disability after ICH.

The Antihypertensive Treatment of Acute Cerebral Hemorrhage (ATACH) study was a multicenter, prospective, dose-escalation study conducted concurrently with the INTERACT trial to assess the feasibility and safety of three levels of antihypertensive treatment with IV nicardipine in patients with ICH [33, 34]. Patients were enrolled if systolic BP exceeded 170mm Hg on two separate measurements and treatment was started within 12 hours of symptom onset. Comatose patients (GCS ≤8) and those with large hematomas (>60cc) were excluded. Blood pressure treatment targets were: 170-200mm Hg, 140-170mm Hg, and 110-140mm Hg. A total of 18, 20, and 22 patients were enrolled in the respective three tiers of BP target. The observed proportions of the primary safety endpoints of neurologic deterioration and serious adverse events were below the prespecified safety thresholds, and the 90-day mortality was lower than expected (approximately 20%) in all three BP tiers [33]. A post hoc analysis of the ATACH study showed that the more aggressively treated patients developed less hematoma expansion, less perihematomal edema, and had better outcomes; however, none of these results was statistically significant owing to the limited sample size [35]. Given the promising direction of these associations, ATACH-2 is currently underway. This is planned to be a 5-year, international, multicenter, randomized trial to determine the efficacy of early, aggressive antihypertensive treatment using IV nicarpidine in subjects with spontaneous ICH and comorbid hypertension.

Despite the encouraging results of INTERACT and ATACH, the effect of antihypertensive therapy on clinical outcome in acute ICH (the aim of the ongoing INTERACT-2 and ATACH-2 trials) remains to be assessed, and while these trials are underway, the guidelines set forth by the AHA [14] and European Union Stroke Initiative (EUSI) [36] should be followed (IIa/B). The AHA recommends cautious management of severe hypertension with continuous infusion of fast-acting antihypertensive drugs such as labetalol, esmolol, or nicardipine as summarized in Table 1. Use of nitroprusside is not favored as this agent may exacerbate cerebral edema and intracranial pressure [37]. The approach used by the EUSI is somewhat different and takes into consideration the patient's premorbid condition [36, 38]. In patients with known hypertension or with signs of chronic hypertension (e.g. electrocardiogram abnormalities or retinal changes), the recommendation is to start BP treatment when the systolic BP exceeds 180mm Hg and/or diastolic BP exceeds 105mm Hg; the target BP should be 160/100mm Hg (or mean arterial pressure [MAP] of 120mm Hg). If there is no previous history of hypertension, treatment should be initiated for values of 160mm Hg systolic and/or 95mm Hg diastolic with a target BP of 150/90mm Hg (or MAP of 110mm Hg). In either case, the MAP should not be lowered by more than 20% of the baseline value. In comatose patients with an ICP monitor in place, both sets of guidelines recommend that BP management be targeted to maintain cerebral perfusion pressure between 60-70mm Hg. Though no prospective study has addressed the optimal timing of conversion from intravenous to oral antihypertensive management, in stable patients this process can generally be started within 24 to 72 hours [39].

Management of elevated intracranial pressure

Intracerebral hemorrhage can lead to increased intracranial pressure (ICP) not only because of its space-occupying effect *per se*, but also secondary to the development of

Table 1. Intravenous antihypertensive agents for acute intracerebral hemorrhage. *Modified with permission from Springer Science+Business Media B.V. Rincon F, Mayer SA* [46].

Drug	Mechanism	Bolus dose	Continuous infusion rate	Side effects
Nicardipine	Calcium channel blocker	NA	5-15mg/h	Myocardial ischemia, hypotension, caution in severe aortic stenosis
Labetalol	Alpha-1, beta-1, and beta-2 receptor antagonist	20-80mg every 10-15 min	0.5-2mg/min (max 300mg/d)	Bradycardia, congestive heart failure, bronchospasm, hypotension
Esmolol	Beta-1 receptor antagonist	250-500µg/kg loading dose	25-300µg/kg/min	Bradycardia, congestive heart failure, bronchospasm
Enalapril	ACE inhibitor	First dose of 0.625mg, then 1.25-5mg every 6h	NA	Precipitous fall in blood pressure in high-renin states
Hydralazine	Unclear; direct vascular smooth muscle relaxant	5-20mg every 30 min	1.5-5µg/kg/min	Tachycardia, angina, headache, agranulocytosis
Nitroprusside*	Arterial and venous vasodilator	NA	0.1-10µg/kg/min	Increased intracranial pressure, headache, myocardial ischemia, cyanide toxicity, hypotension

* Nitroprusside is not recommended in patients with acute intracerebral hemorrhage given the risk of increasing intracranial pressure
NA = not applicable; ACE = angiotensin-converting enzyme

perihematomal edema and/or hydrocephalus due to alterations of normal cerebrospinal fluid (CSF) flow dynamics. In the initial hours after ICH onset, extravasation of blood causes injury by mechanical disruption of neurons and glia [39]. The clotting blood then extrudes serum that collects around the central hematoma. This serum is rich in thrombin and proteases [40, 41]. As shown in both experimental and human ICH, thrombin has a central role in promoting perihematomal edema, mediated by inflammation, cytotoxicity, and disruption of the blood-brain barrier [42]. This is reflected in the observation that patients with thrombolysis-related ICH have substantially less edema than patients with spontaneous ICH, attributed to a decreased amount of thrombin in the perihematoma region as a result of the thrombolytic effect [43]. Edema increases in volume by about 75% in the first 24 hours after ICH, peaks around 5-6 days, and lasts up to 14 days [42].

The degree of intracranial hypertension (ICP ≥15mm Hg or ≥20cmH$_2$O) depends on the size and location of the ICH, as well as the presence of intraventricular extension of the hemorrhage. Patients with small hematomas often have no ICP issues at all. When ICP does increase, deterioration in consciousness quickly ensues and treatment needs to be instituted promptly. The overall management goal is to achieve normal levels of ICP while maintaining a cerebral perfusion pressure of 60mm Hg or higher [14, 36]. As will be discussed below, there are currently a number of available treatment options, yet most are associated with major side effects and the evidence to support their use is limited. Therefore, the current recommendation is to treat intracranial hypertension with a stepwise approach, beginning with simple measures and progressing to more aggressive therapies as clinically indicated [14] (Figure 1). Patients with large volume ICH, intracranial mass effect, and coma may benefit from ICP monitoring, though this intervention has not been shown to benefit outcome [44, 45]. In addition, because ICH is a focal condition, pressures within the skull may vary, and the patient may undergo a herniation syndrome while the ICP monitor continues to record a value within normal limits. Therefore, when obtainable, the clinical examination should always be used for detection of neurological deterioration and to guide therapy.

Head-of-bed elevation
The most basic measure to reduce ICP is adequate positioning of the patient's head. The head should be midline and, with the exception of patients who are hypotensive or hypovolemic, head-of-bed should be elevated to 30° to promote jugular venous outflow (III/B).

Sedation and analgesia
Continuous, intravenous sedation is necessary in intubated patients to maintain airway control and ventilation. In addition, sedation and analgesia should be used to minimize agitation and pain, both factors that can lead to transient elevations of ICP which, in turn, can precipitate further tissue shifts and neurological deterioration (III/B). The favored regimen is a combination of a short-acting opioid, such as fentanyl, for analgesia and propofol or midazolam for sedation [46]. Bolus injections of opioids should be avoided in patients with intracranial hypertension because they can transiently lower MAP and increase ICP due to autoregulatory vasodilation of cerebral vessels [47]. Propofol has the advantage of a very short half-life that allows for periodic neurological examinations, and in a trial comparing sedation regimens in traumatic brain injury patients, those receiving propofol required fewer ICP-lowering interventions than those sedated with an opioid-based regimen [48]. The drawback of propofol is the uncommon and poorly understood development of the propofol infusion syndrome, a potentially lethal condition manifested by metabolic derangement, multi-organ failure and circulatory collapse [49].

Hyperventilation
Hyperventilation is a very effective method for rapid ICP reduction, as intracerebral vessels are highly sensitive to CO$_2$ levels and extracellular fluid pH. It lowers ICP by the induction of

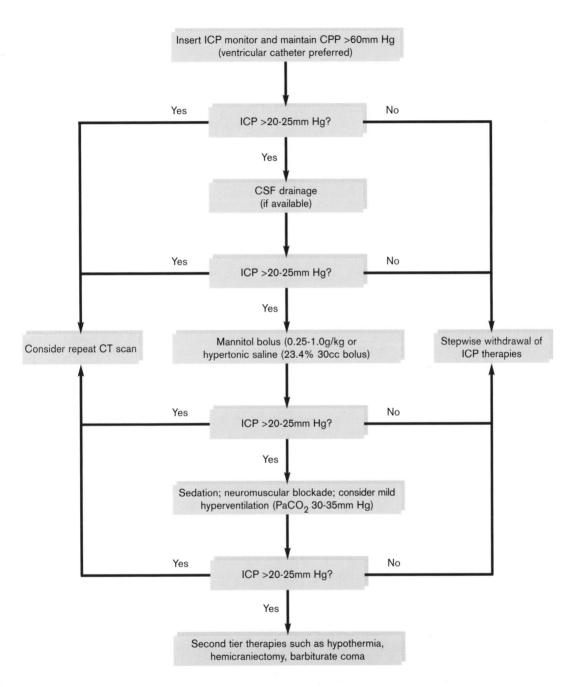

Figure 1. Algorithm outlining a stepwise approach to the management of elevated intracranial pressure (ICP) in patients with intracerebral hemorrhage. CPP = cerebral perfusion pressure; CSF = cerebrospinal fluid. *Reproduced with permission from the Brain Trauma Foundation. Guidelines for Management and Prognosis of Severe Traumatic Brain Injury. New York, NY: Brain Trauma Foundation, 2000. Copyright © 2000, Brain Trauma Foundation.*

cerebral vasoconstriction with a subsequent decrease in cerebral blood volume [50]. While potent, this method has the disadvantage of being short-lived and simultaneously reducing cerebral blood flow, which can lead to regional or global ischemia [51]. In addition, reversal of hyperventilation after use for 6 hours or more poses the risk of a significant rebound effect on ICP. Therefore, hyperventilation is advocated as a temporizing measure in situations of impending herniation before a more definitive therapy, such as ventriculostomy placement or hematoma evacuation, can be instituted (III/B). The target pCO_2 level is 30-35mm Hg. Hyperventilation to pCO_2 levels below 30mm Hg is not recommended, as it may cause excessive vasoconstriction and exacerbation of ischemia during the acute phase of ICH. Controlled hyperventilation therapy can be optimized by monitoring of jugular vein oxygen saturation and partial brain tissue oxygenation.

Osmotic therapy

Mannitol has been used for ICP reduction for several decades [52], and is the preferred osmotic diuretic in most neurocritical care units. It has multiple mechanisms of action, the most relevant of which is shifting of water from the brain parenchyma to the intravascular space [53]. In addition, it increases cardiac preload and CPP, decreases blood viscosity, and reduces CSF production, effects that all culminate in a decrease in brain volume and ICP. Despite its clinical importance, treatment protocols vary from center to center, and the dose-response relationship is not well understood [54]. The usual initial dose of mannitol is between 1-1.5g/kg of a 20% solution, followed by bolus doses of 0.25-1.0g/kg as frequently as once an hour, with the goal of achieving a target serum osmolality of 300-320mOsm/kg [46]. Common adverse effects include intravascular volume depletion, hyperosmolality and electrolytic disturbances. In a recent placebo-controlled trial of mannitol for ICH, 128 patients were randomized to receive low-dose mannitol (100cc of 20% solution) or sham therapy every 4 hours for 5 days with a rapid taper over 48 hours. The mortality rate at 1 month was 25% in both groups and disability scores at 3 months did not differ significantly between groups [55]. Mannitol should only be considered for short-term use in ICH patients with evidence of transtentorial herniation or acute neurological deterioration associated with high ICP or mass effect (IIb/B). A single-center observational study demonstrated that early, aggressive reversal of transtentorial herniation with the combined use of osmotic drugs and hyperventilation improved long-term outcome [56].

Hypertonic saline can be used as an alternative to mannitol, particularly when CPP augmentation is desirable (III/B) [53, 57]. A 23.4% saline solution should be used for emergency situations, at a rate of 0.5-2.0cc/kg. In non-emergent situations, 3% hypertonic saline is an option in cases of systemic hypo-osmolality (<280mOsm/L) or as a resuscitation fluid for patients with significant perihematomal edema and mass effect after ICH [46]. Hypertonic saline has an osmotic effect on the brain because of its high tonicity and ability to effectively remain outside the blood-brain barrier. In animal models with cerebral injury, the maximum benefit is observed within 2 hours of the infusion in situations of focal injury associated with vasogenic edema [58, 59]. Most comparisons with mannitol suggest almost equal efficacy in reducing ICP, but there is a suggestion that mannitol may have a longer duration of action [57]. Nonetheless, hypertonic saline has been shown to be effective even in cases refractory to hyperventilation and mannitol [60]. In a clinical setting, only case reports and small series have been reported, yet the efficacy and safety of hypertonic saline has not been studied in randomized trials. Adverse effects include electrolyte abnormalities, fluid overload in the setting of cardiac or renal failure, bleeding diathesis, and phlebitis.

Ventricular drainage

Hydrocephalus is an independent predictor of poor outcome and mortality from ICH [61, 62]. It results from intraventricular extension of intraparenchymal blood or from direct obstruction of CSF flow as seen, for example, in cerebellar hemorrhages. Extension of the hemorrhage into the ventricles is a common phenomenon, occurring in approximately 40% of patients with ICH. Most secondary intraventricular hemorrhages are the result of hypertensive hemorrhages involving the basal ganglia and thalamus [63]. Epidemiological data show that the amount of intraventricular blood correlates directly with the degree of injury and likelihood of survival [64]. Ventriculostomy drains CSF and blood from the ventricular system, lowering ICP and simultaneously allowing for ICP monitoring. As a general rule, an ICP monitor or external ventricular drain should be placed in all comatose ICH patients (GCS score of 8 or less) with the goal of maintaining ICP below 20cmH$_2$O (<15mm Hg) and CPP greater than 60mm Hg (III/B). Although ventriculostomy can be a life-saving measure for patients with hydrocephalus and intraventricular hemorrhage, observational studies show that outcome remains poor [65]. Morbidity and mortality derive in part from the high risk of complications with ventriculostomy, in particular catheter obstruction and infection [66, 67]. The incidence of ventriculostomy-related infections is reported to be as high as 20% and increases with duration of catheterization. Prophylactic catheter exchange does not appear to modify the risk of developing later ventriculostomy-related infections in retrospective studies [68]. Shortening the length of external ventricular drainage with early ventriculoperitoneal shunt placement or lumbar drainage for communicating hydrocephalus may be more effective in lowering the rate of infections [69, 70]. A recent prospective observational study analyzed the use of a standardized evidence-based ventriculostomy catheter insertion protocol with and without the use of antibiotic-impregnated catheters and found a significant reduction in infection rate with the former when compared to pre-protocol infection rates (1.0% vs. 6.7%; p=0.0005) [71]. Treatment strategies for intraventricular hemorrhage are discussed in the section on surgical management of ICH.

Barbiturate coma

High-dose barbiturate treatment acts by reducing cerebral metabolic activity and blood flow, and should be reserved for cases of severe and refractory intracranial hypertension (IV/C). This is achieved with intravenous pentobarbital given in an initial loading dose of 5-20mg/kg, followed by a continuous infusion of 1-4mg/kg/h [46]. This treatment requires intensive monitoring and is associated with a number of severe complications, the most common being hypotension typically requiring the use of pressors to maintain adequate BP levels [72]. An electroencephalogram should be continuously recorded, and the dose of pentobarbital titrated to produce a burst-suppression pattern, with approximately 6-8 second interbursts, to avoid excessive sedation.

Hypothermia

Elevated cerebral temperature is a strong contributing factor to ischemic brain damage and intracranial pressure [73-75]. In models of ischemia, laboratory data show that hypothermia is a robust neuroprotectant, and its efficacy is critically dependent on the duration, depth and timing of hypothermia relative to the cerebral insult [76]. In ICH, most experimental data derive from rat models of acute subdural hematoma and reveal that thrombin-induced brain edema formation and inflammatory response are significantly reduced with hypothermia [77, 78]. Whether this can be extrapolated to improve outcome in patients with ICH is less clearly established (IV/C). Therapeutic cooling to 32-34°C has been investigated in acute brain injuries and effectively lowers refractory ICP [79, 80]; however, it carries a relatively high risk of medical complications including infections (especially pneumonia), cardiac arrhythmias, coagulopathy, and electrolyte abnormalities [81]. Furthermore, there is a risk of rebound ICP elevation if the hypothermia reversal occurs too rapidly [82]. Because these risks increase with the depth and duration of cooling, particularly with long-term use (24-48 hours), some intensivists advocate the induction of mild hypothermia (34-36°C) if temperature reduction is required for a prolonged period of time to control ICP [81, 83].

Hemostatic therapy

Hematoma growth is a common and early phenomenon in ICH. In the first report of hematoma expansion, Fujii and colleagues described that almost one fifth of patients with ICH presenting within 24 hours of symptom onset showed hematoma expansion when a head CT was repeated within 24 hours of admission [84]. Those who presented earliest were more likely to have hematoma enlargement. Later studies better defined the time course of hematoma expansion and showed that in the majority of cases, it occurs within the first minutes to hours after onset, being uncommon after 6 hours and virtually not occurring after 24 hours [19, 85]. Most importantly, hematoma expansion is associated consistently with clinical deterioration and increased mortality [19, 84]. Several factors were identified as possible predictors of rebleeding, including size and shape of the hematoma (large, irregular hematomas are more likely to expand), BP, and coagulation disorders [19-21]. However, the most consistent predictor of hematoma growth was the interval from onset of symptoms to initial CT; the earlier the first scan is obtained, the higher the likelihood of expansion on follow-up scan, again pointing out that bleeding is an ongoing process in the first hours. This observation, taken together with the lack of success of other medical treatments or surgical interventions, led to interest in the use of hemostatic therapy as a strategy to limit hematoma growth.

Recombinant activated Factor VII (rFVIIa) was initially developed for the treatment of hemorrhagic episodes in patients with hemophilia who carry inhibitors to Factors VIII or IX [86]. It has since been shown to also enhance hemostasis in non-hemophiliac patients [86]. Recombinant FVIIa is a potent initiator of coagulation by directly activating Factor X and ultimately leading to increased thrombin formation [87]. Thrombin in turn converts fibrinogen into fibrin, thereby contributing to clot stabilization. In a phase IIb, placebo-controlled, dose-escalation trial published by Mayer and colleagues in 2005, 399 patients with spontaneous ICH were randomized to treament with rFVIIa at doses of 40, 80, or 160µg/kg, or placebo within 4 hours of symptom onset [88]. There was a dose-dependent reduction in hematoma expansion with rFVIIa when compared to placebo (increase in hematoma volume of 16%, 14% and 11% with doses of 40, 80 and 160µg/kg, respectively, vs. 29% in the placebo group), yet this was significant only in patients treated in the first 3 hours (13% increase in rFVIIa group vs. 34% with placebo; p=0.004). In addition, treatment with rFVIIa was associated with improved functional outcome and reduced mortality rates at 90 days (18% for rFVIIa-treated patients vs. 29% for the placebo group; p=0.02). These positive results were accompanied, however, by predominantly arterial thromboembolic events in the rFVIIa-treated patients (7% vs. 2% for rFVIIa and placebo, respectively, p=0.12), half of which occurred in the group receiving the highest dose of rFVIIa [88, 89].

In light of these findings, a phase III trial was designed using lower doses of rFVIIa (20 and 80μg/kg) compared with placebo, in an attempt to prevent the occurrence of adverse thromboemblic events [90]. The Factor VII for Acute Hemorrhagic Stroke Trial (FAST) enrolled 841 patients with similar inclusion/exclusion criteria and treatment parameters as the previous study. Although a dose-related reduction in hematoma expansion was again observed in the rFVIIa-treated group (mean increase in hematoma volume of 18% with 20μg/kg [p=0.09] and 11% with 80μg/kg vs. 26% in the placebo group [p<0.001]), it did not translate into a beneficial effect on the risk of death or severe disability at 90 days. In addition, while the overall frequency of serious thromboembolic adverse events was similar in the three groups, arterial events occurred significantly more often in the group receiving 80μg/kg of rFVIIa compared to placebo (9% vs. 4%, p=0.04). Therefore, on the basis of this study, routine use of rFVIIa as a hemostatic agent for all patients with ICH within a 4-hour time window cannot be recommended **(Ib/A)**. However, post hoc analysis of the FAST data suggests that rFVIIa might be beneficial in patients ≤70 years of age with a baseline supratentorial ICH volume <60cc and low volume (<5cc) of intraventricular hemorrhage (IVH), if administered within 2.5 hours of the onset of symptoms [91].

Recent studies have identified the presence of contrast extravasation on CT angiography ('spot sign') as a significant, independent predictor of hematoma expansion with good sensitivity and negative predictive value [92-94] (Figure 2). This imaging modality may therefore be a useful strategy to more accurately identify the target population that might benefit most from treatment with rFVIIa. This is being investigated in the STOP-IT (Spot Sign for Predicting and Treating ICH Growth) study, a phase II, randomized, placebo-controlled trial sponsored by the NIH/NINDS. The purpose of this study is two-fold:

- to determine if CT angiography can predict which individuals with ICH will experience significant hematoma growth; and
- to compare the effect of treatment with rFVIIa at a dose of 80μg/kg versus placebo on hemorrhage expansion in those individuals with a positive spot sign.

ICH must be diagnosed by non-contrast CT scan within 5 hours of symptom onset, followed by CT angiogram. The time window for study drug administration is within 90 minutes of the enrolling CT scan. Patients not determined to have a spot sign on CT angiogram will be enrolled into a prospective observational group. Hematoma growth will be determined by comparing the baseline ICH volume with that of a head CT scan performed at 24 hours. Follow-up is planned at 3 months. At the time of this writing, enrollment had not yet begun.

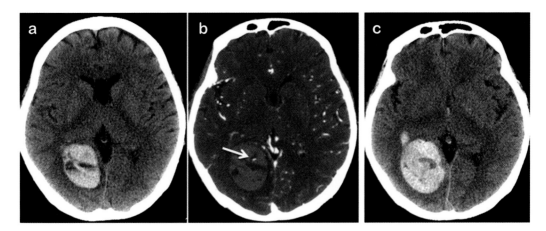

Figure 2. a) Baseline non-contrast head CT showing right posterior intracerebral hemorrhage (initial volume: 34cc). b) CT angiography shows a small area of contrast extravasation (arrow) within the hematoma consistent with a 'spot sign'. c) Repeat head CT after 24 hours shows hematoma expansion (volume: 46cc).

ICH related to coagulation abnormalities

Underlying coagulation abnormalities contribute to ICH and can significantly worsen its outcome if not rapidly corrected. The scenario most commonly encountered are patients on oral or intravenous anticoagulation therapy, yet other primary (congenital) or secondary abnormalities of hemostasis can predispose to or worsen the hemorrhage. Among the primary abnormalities, deficiencies of coagulation Factors I, VII, VIII, IX and XIII as well as von Willebrand Factor have been associated with ICH, and immediate specific factor replacement to normalize the coagulation defect is indicated [14, 95] **(IV/C)**. Among secondary alterations in hemostasis, qualitative or quantitative platelet abnormalities, as well as coagulation factor consumption contribute to the risk of ICH in patients with idiopathic or thrombotic thrombocytopenic purpura, disseminated intravascular coagulation, myeloproliferative or myelodysplastic disorders, hepatic or renal dysfunction, and after exposure to certain medications [14, 95-97]. For severe thrombocytopenia, platelet transfusion is indicated [14, 95] **(IV/C)**. Most importantly, treatment of the underlying cause is usually required.

Warfarin-associated ICH is an increasing problem as more elderly patients, in particular those with atrial fibrillation, are being treated with long-term oral anticoagulation [98] (Figure 3). Patients undergoing treatment with warfarin are reported to account for 12-14% (range 6-18%) of patients with ICH [99], but at a tertiary hospital almost one fourth of ICH patients have been found to be anticoagulated [100]. The main risk factors for warfarin-related ICH include age, hypertension [101], and associated conditions such as cerebral amyloid angiopathy [102]. In addition, the risk of ICH is directly related to the intensity of anticoagulation [100]. The mortality rate in patients with warfarin-associated ICH is over 50% [100], and if the INR at presentation is >3, the outcome is fatal in two thirds of patients [99].

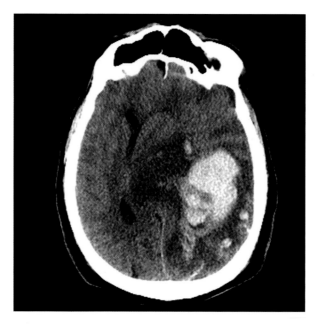

Figure 3. Spontaneous intracerebral hemorrhage with marked edema and midline shift in a patient on long-term warfarin therapy.

As in any patient on oral anticoagulation who has a life-threatening hemorrhage, the cornerstone of treatment is to reverse the International Normalized Ratio (INR) as rapidly as possible [103]. How to best achieve this goal is not entirely defined. There are no randomized trials that have adequately investigated this issue, and management is based on observational data, small clinical series, and the opinion of experts [99]. Vitamin K and fresh frozen plasma (FFP) are standard therapies for the reversal of oral anticoagulation, but neither is ideal in an emergency setting as they take hours to correct the INR (Table 2). Vitamin K (10mg intravenously) takes 6-24 hours to normalize the INR [104] and should, therefore, only be used as an adjunct to a more rapidly acting agent **(III/B)**. FFP replenishes the vitamin K-dependent coagulation factors inhibited by warfarin, but at the recommended dose of 15-20cc/kg has the disadvantage of requiring a large volume infusion that is not only time costly but may lead to volume overload particularly in elderly patients. Additional drawbacks of FFP include the variability in coagulation factor concentration among different batches and the time required for thawing if only frozen units of FFP are available in the blood bank. For both vitamin K and FFP, time to treatment is a major determinant of anticoagulation reversal. A retrospective study correlating the timing of FFP administration in the emergency room with time to reach an INR of 1.4 or less demonstrated that every 30 minutes of delay in the first dose of FFP was associated with a 20% decreased likelihood of INR reversal within 24 hours [105]. In this study, almost one fifth of patients still did not have their INR corrected after 24 hours.

Table 2. Therapies available to reverse anticoagulation in acute intracerebral hemorrhage. Modified with permission from Quadrant HealthCom. Aguilar MI, Hart RG, Kase CS, et al [99].		
Therapeutic option	Time to anticoagulation reversal	Comments
Vitamin K	6-24 h	Replacement of Factors IX and X takes longer than 24 h; risk of anaphylaxis with intravenous injection; warfarin resistance in higher doses up to 1 week
Fresh frozen plasma	3-6 h for infusion, followed by 12-32 h for reversal	Large volume infusion; risk of volume overload; time-consuming thawing process; variable coagulation factor concentration among batches
Prothrombin complex concentrate	15 min after 10 min to 1 h infusion	Variable coagulation factor concentration based on manufacturer; limited availability; cost; risk of thrombotic events (low)
Recombinant Factor VIIa	15 min after bolus infusion	Short half-life; cost; risk of thrombotic events (high); currently not recommended for use by AHA

AHA = American Heart Association

Two alternative potential therapies for anticoagulation reversal in ICH include prothrombin complex concentrates (PCCs) and rFVIIa. PCCs are hemostatic blood products derived from plasma that contain varying amounts of Factors II, VII, IX, and X. They were originally used to treat hemophilia B (Factor IX deficiency), but given the high concentration of other vitamin K-dependent factors, lend themselves to the use for correction of the effects of warfarin [106, 107]. PCCs have the advantage of being easily reconstituted to a small volume and rapidly administered. Although PCC preparations are heterogeneous in terms of factor concentration, they uniformly have a rapid effect on the INR in patients taking warfarin [108, 109]. A number of retrospective series and case-control studies have shown that PCC and vitamin K correct the INR more rapidly than FFP and vitamin K, but without a positive effect on outcome (studies reviewed by Aguilar and colleagues [99]). A small, prospective trial (n=8) randomized patients with warfarin-associated ICH to either PCC supplemented with FFP versus FFP alone [110]. Although in patients receiving PCC the INR was reversed at a faster rate, their neurological outcome did not improve; however, a higher complication rate was observed in the FFP-treated group. There have been some reports that PCCs may increase the risk of thrombotic events [107, 111], but it appears that this risk is relatively low, ranging between 2-3% of patients [107, 109, 112]. Despite the lack of well-designed, prospective, randomized trials, the use of PCCs for the treatment of warfarin-associated ICH or other life-threatening hemorrhages is being advocated in several guidelines [14, 36, 103, 113] (IIa/B). While

PCCs have been used in Europe for INR reversal in patients with ICH for over a decade, they are still limited by availability and cost in the United States and other countries.

Recombinant FVIIa has been considered as a potential alternative for the treatment of warfarin-associated ICH, particularly after the encouraging results described among patients with spontaneous ICH (detailed above). Although correction of the INR with rFVIIa administration is achieved within minutes, the effect on neurological outcome is unclear [114-116]. There is a concern that rFVIIa only corrects the deficiency of FVII without replenishing other factors inhibited by warfarin, and its effect is falsely estimated by the improving INR. A study comparing the hemostatic effects of rFVIIa and PCCs *in vitro* and *in vivo* found that, in fact, thrombin generation is only adequately restored with PCCs [117]. In addition, as the half-life of rFVIIa is short and repeat infusions may be necessary, some investigators believe this may increase the risk of thrombotic complications. Based on these concerns and the limited existing data on the benefit of rFVIIa in ICH associated with oral anticoagulant use, the American Society of Hematology and AHA do not recommend the routine use of rFVIIa for warfarin reversal [14, 118] **(Ib/A)**.

General supportive care

Management of hyperglycemia
Hyperglycemia occurs in 20-40% of patients with ischemic stroke and is well known to be associated with larger infarct size, worse functional outcome and higher mortality [119, 120]. In two series of patients with ICH, elevated glucose levels on admission were correlated with increased 30-day and 3-month mortality rates in both diabetic and non-diabetic patients [12, 13]. Whether hyperglycemia is a manifestation of premorbid abnormal glucose metabolism or a stress response to the cerebral insult is still uncertain; however, data are accumulating to support the latter [12, 121]. While both hypo- and hyperglycemia should be corrected, the targets for glycemic control in ICH are as yet undefined. Therefore, it seems reasonable to follow the guidelines applied to patients with acute ischemic stroke [122]. Based on improved outcome with tight glycemic control in medical ICU patients, the most recent AHA guidelines recommend that glucose values above 140-180mg/dL be corrected [14, 122] **(III/B)**, with close monitoring to avoid hypoglycemia [123]. Intensive insulin therapy in critically ill patients with a range of neurological conditions has been shown to reduce ICP, length of mechanical ventilation and risk of seizures [124].

Temperature control
Fever worsens outcome in experimental models of brain injury and after clinical ICH [125, 126]. Not only does hyperthermia cause direct neuronal damage [127], but it also contributes to cerebral edema and elevated ICP [74]. Fever after ICH is common, particularly in the presence of intraventricular hemorrhage [126, 128]. While there are no prospective randomized trials to support this measure in patients with ICH, there is agreement that fever should be treated aggressively based on findings in other types of neurocritical care patients **(IV/C)**. Acetaminophen and cooling blankets are recommended for patients with a sustained temperature >101°F (38.3°C). Newer adhesive surface cooling systems and endovascular

heat exchange catheters have been shown to be more effective for maintaining normothermia [129, 130]; however, it remains to be seen if these measures improve clinical outcome. Use of induced hypothermia is discussed in the section on ICP management.

Seizure management and prophylaxis

Seizures are common after ICH. In a large series of over 700 consecutive ICH patients, 4.2% had clinical seizures within 24 hours of symptom onset, while the incidence in the first month post-ICH was 8.1% [131]. Status epilepticus occurred in 1-2%. Lobar location and neurologic complications, mainly hematoma expansion, were predictors of early seizures. In addition, in two cohorts of ICH patients undergoing continuous electroencephalogram monitoring, up to 28% developed electrographic seizures during the first 72 hours after admission [132, 133]. These were associated with neurologic worsening as measured by the NIHSS score, increase in midline shift, and a trend toward worse outcome [132].

Seizures should be promptly treated with benzodiazepines followed by an intravenous antiepileptic drug, generally fosphenytoin or levetiracetam (IIa/B). The threshold for obtaining electroencephalographic studies if there is any suspicion of subclinical seizures should be low. The use of prophylactic anticonvulsant medication is controversial and is justified only in the subgroup of patients with lobar ICH based on one observational study showing that in these patients, the risk of early seizures was reduced by prophylactic therapy [131]. No prospective controlled trials have examined the issue. Patients who have a seizure more than 2 weeks after ICH onset might need long-term prophylactic treatment with anticonvulsants.

Prevention of deep venous thrombosis and pulmonary embolism

Deep vein thrombosis and pulmonary embolism are preventable but nonetheless common causes of morbidity and mortality in acute ICH patients. In a retrospective study of almost 2000 patients with ICH and over 15,000 patients with ischemic stroke, the prevalence of venous thromboembolism was almost four times higher in the hemorrhagic stroke group (1.9% vs. 0.5% in the ischemic stroke patients) [134]. This can be explained in part by the higher rate of disability and prolonged immobilization with ICH as well as the concern that early pharmacologic prophylaxis in these patients may lead to ICH extension.

There is consensus that mechanical prophylaxis should be initiated on admission in all ICH patients [135] (Ib/A). The VICTORIAh (Venous Intermittent Compression and Thrombosis Occurrence Related to Intracerebral Acute hemorrhage) trial randomized 151 patients with ICH to compression stockings alone or in combination with intermittent pneumatic compression [136]. While no clinically relevant thromboembolism occurred, asymptomatic deep vein thrombosis of the lower limbs was detected by ultrasonography at day 10 in 15.9% of patients wearing compression stockings alone and in 4.7% in the combined group (relative risk [RR] 0.29; 95% CI, 0.08 to 1.00). Only one small study addressed the risk of early prophylactic therapy with anticoagulants in patients with ICH [137]. Boeer and colleagues randomized 68 patients with spontaneous ICH to low-dose heparin (5000 U of heparin subcutaneously three times per day) beginning on the second, fourth or tenth day after ICH onset. Early treatment (day 2) significantly lowered the incidence of pulmonary embolism. No increase in the number of patients with rebleeding was observed in any of the groups, suggesting that the early use of heparin is safe and effective for the prevention of thromboembolic complications in patients with acute ICH **(Ib/A)**. Treatment with low-molecular-weight heparin (enoxaparin 40mg daily) is a possible alternative if renal function is normal [46].

Surgical management of intracerebral hemorrhage

Craniotomy

Given that the sudden extravasation of blood into the brain parenchyma underlies the clinical manifestations of ICH and triggers the pathophysiological cascade that leads to damage of the surrounding brain tissue, one would intuitively expect the surgical removal or at least reduction in size of the hematoma to be beneficial. This remains a controversial topic. A small number of randomized trials (reviewed by Fernandes and colleagues [138]), the first of which was published as early as 1961 [139], have compared surgery to medical management of ICH and have yielded conflicting results. Most of these trials were small, single-center studies, often with less than 50 patients in each arm and are difficult to compare based on the differences in populations studied, technique and timing of the surgical intervention, and outcome measures used. These studies have been reviewed in a series of meta-analyses over the past years [138, 140-142], the most recent of which failed to show a statistically significant pooled reduction in the odds of death (OR 0.84; 95% CI, 0.67-1.07) in the surgical group compared with standard medical therapy [142].

While these small studies did not show convincing evidence that surgical management of ICH is better than conservative therapy overall, they suggested a beneficial effect of surgery in certain subgroups of patients. One study concluded that for patients presenting with a mild to moderately decreased level of consciousness (GCS score 7 to 10), surgery might reduce the risk of death without, however, improving functional outcome [143]. Another trial found that ultra-early evacuation improved the NIHSS score at 3 months [144]. This set the stage for the first large multicenter trial comparing surgical to non-surgical treatment of ICH, the International Surgical Trial in Intracerebral Hemorrhage (STICH) [145]. This landmark study, performed from 1995 to 2003, randomized 1033 patients with spontaneous supratentorial ICH from 107 centers worldwide to either surgery or standard medical management. Patients were eligible if enrolled within 72 hours of symptom onset and if operated on within 24 hours of randomization. A minimum hematoma diameter of 2cm was required, and patients with underlying lesions such as arteriovenous malformations, aneurysms or tumors were excluded. Patients with cerebellar hemorrhages were also excluded. Importantly, based on the principle of 'clinical equipoise', patients were only randomized if the local investigators were uncertain about the benefit of surgery; hence, patients estimated by the local neurosurgeon to have a better chance of a good outcome with hematoma evacuation or, conversely, those with very poor neurological condition defined as a GCS (Glasgow Coma Score) <5 were not enrolled.

Risk factors, hematoma localization, and size were well distributed between the 503 patients randomized to surgery and the 530 patients in the medical arm. The surgical methods were not standardized, and the choice of surgical technique was left to the neurosurgeon's discretion. Craniotomy was the favored approach in 75% of patients, while minimally invasive techniques were used in the rest. Of note, there was a high rate (26%) of cross-over from the medical to the surgical arm due to neurological deterioration or rebleeding, and 85% of the cross-over patients were then submitted to craniotomy.

Overall, the intention-to-treat analysis showed no statistically significant difference in outcome between the surgical and medical groups at 6 months, both when comparing functional outcome and mortality rates. The trial, however, identified patients in predetermined subgroup analyses that showed a non-significant trend to benefit with surgery. These included patients with lobar hemorrhages located no deeper than 1cm from the cortical surface (29% relative benefit for early surgery), patients with a GCS score between 9 to 12, and those submitted to craniotomy as opposed to other surgical approaches (all pre-defined). In contrast, comatose patients with a GCS score of 5 to 8 did worse with surgical management. Furthermore, the high rate of cross-over begs the question of whether these patients would have done better if operated on early or whether their permanence in the non-surgical arm would have increased mortality in that group, favoring the surgical arm as far as mortality is concerned. Based on these findings, taken together with data from previous observational studies and non-randomized trials, the STICH II trial is currently underway. This study will include patients with lobar hemorrhages of 10-100cc in volume located within 1cm of the cortical surface, with a GCS ≥8. Patients will be randomized within 48 hours of ICH onset, with surgery to follow within 12 hours from randomization, applying the same clinical 'equipoise' principle used in STICH.

In contrast to supratentorial ICH, there is overall consensus regarding surgical intervention for cerebellar hemorrhages. While hemorrhages can occur at any site in the cerebellum, they are typically unilateral and hemispheric, rarely involving the adjacent brainstem directly yet often compressing it. In addition to classic unilateral cerebellar findings often in conjunction with signs of ipsilateral tegmental pontine involvement, these patients may present with variable levels of consciousness and have abrupt and dramatic clinical deterioration secondary to acute obstructive hydrocephalus [146]. Hematoma diameter ≥3cm, hydrocephalus, intraventricular extension of the hemorrhage, and clinical signs of brainstem compression have been identified as reliable predictors of poor outcome [147, 148], and several non-randomized case series have shown better outcomes with surgical evacuation for patients with large hematomas (≥3 cm), or in the presence of brainstem compression or obstruction of the fourth ventricle [146, 147, 149-152] (IIa/B). When surgery is indicated on the basis of the above clinical and surgical criteria, it should be performed emergently to prevent further clinical deterioration.

Minimally invasive surgery

As emergent craniotomy does not improve neurological outcome after ICH for most patients, there has been growing interest in other surgical methods of hematoma removal, particularly minimally invasive surgery. The advantages of this technique include reduced operative time, the possibility of performance under local anesthesia, and reduced surgical trauma [1]. In addition, these methods may allow for safer access to deep-seated hematomas. The procedures consist of either endoscopic or stereotactic aspiration of the hematoma, with or without the use of local thrombolytic instillation to facilitate clot lysis.

Endoscopic aspiration of ICH was studied by Auer and colleagues in a small, single-center, randomized trial over two decades ago [153]. One hundred patients with spontaneous supratentorial hemorrhages at least 10cc in volume were randomized to either continuous neuroendoscopic lavage of the hematoma cavity or medical therapy. All surgical patients had at least a 50% reduction in hematoma size, and in 45% of patients, clot reduction was 70% or greater. At 6 months, the mortality rate in the surgical group (42%) was significantly lower when compared to that of the medical arm (70%; p=0.01), while more surgically treated patients made a good functional recovery (40% vs. 25% in the medical group). When outcome was stratified by size of the ICH, surgical patients with smaller hematomas had the most benefit in terms of quality of life. In addition, surgery was most effective in younger patients (<60 years) and in those with lobar hematomas.

Evacuation by stereotactic guidance was assessed in a randomized trial involving 242 patients with spontaneous putaminal hemorrhage without severe reduction in consciousness [154]. Stereotactic evacuation was associated with better functional outcome and lower mortality when compared to conservative treatment. Two studies then directly compared endoscopic surgery to stereotactic evacuation and found that both methods are effective procedures with low complication and mortality rates [155, 156]; however, endoscopy had the advantage of being more rapidly available, with shorter operating time, higher hematoma evacuation rate and, when tested in a pediatric population [156], with significantly better long-term outcomes.

With the goal of improving the rate of ICH evacuation and outcome of these minimally invasive surgical techniques, some neurosurgeons have instilled thrombolytics into the hematoma prior to aspiration. Initial results using urokinase were promising, with aspiration rates ranging from 30-90% of the initial hematoma volume, rebleeding rates similar to those observed with conventional craniotomy, and favorable outcomes [1, 84, 157, 158]. In a small, single-center, randomized, pilot study of early surgical treatment of ICH (within 24 hours of onset and 3 hours of randomization), patients with deep hemorrhages randomized to the surgical group (four out of nine subjects) were treated with stereotactic aspiration of the clot preceded by infusion of urokinase [144]. All four patients did well, giving impetus for a larger multicenter trial. The SICHPA (Stereotactic Treatment of Intracerebral Hematoma by means of a Plasminogen Activator) trial was a multicenter, randomized, controlled study that assigned 70 patients presenting with supratentorial hematomas at least 10cc in volume and a GCS score ≥5 to either urokinase infusion followed by stereotactic clot removal or medical therapy [159]. Patients were treated within 72 hours of onset with 5000 IU of local urokinase every 6 hours for a maximum of 48 hours. Reduction in ICH volume was significantly higher in the surgical group (median reduction of 40% from baseline vs 18% in the medical group) and mortality rates were slightly lower, but with higher rates of rebleeding (35% vs 17% in the medically treated patients). Importantly, there was no difference in functional outcome at 6 months between the two groups.

Due to a temporary lack of availability of urokinase in the United States, the encouraging experimental results with hematoma aspiration after fibrinolysis with recombinant tissue plasminogen activator (rt-PA) in animal models of ICH [160], and the observation that rt-PA was more effective than urokinase in clearing intraventricular hemorrhage in humans [161], the use of rt-PA as an adjunct to stereotactic evacuation began to be investigated. In small pilot series, daily treatment with rt-PA administered into the bed of the ICH resulted in a 70-80% average hematoma reduction by 2-4 days after onset [162-164]. There was no hemorrhage expansion, and no major neurological or systemic complications were reported. Surgical technique and drug dosing were slightly different in each study. These findings laid the ground for the MISTIE (Minimally-Invasive Surgery plus rt-PA for Intracerebral Hemorrhage Evacuation) trial, a phase II, multicenter, randomized, controlled study designed to compare the effect of minimally invasive surgery plus rt-PA with best medical management in patients with spontaneous supratentorial ICH of a volume ≥25cc [165]. Patients enrolled into the surgical arm underwent stereotactic catheter placement and clot aspiration, followed by infusion of 0.3mg rt-PA into the hematoma cavity every 8 hours for a maximum of 3 days. After each rt-PA injection the system was closed for 60 minutes prior to opening for gravitational drainage. Preliminary results of the first 21 patients of the dose-finding phase of the trial were published in 2008 [165]. On average, 20% of the hematoma was removed through surgical aspiration alone, while administration of rt-PA reduced the clot to almost 50% of its volume at presentation. Adverse events were within safety limits (30-day mortality, 8%; symptomatic rebleeding, 8%). Patients randomized to medical management showed 6% hematoma resolution at 7 days. An additional important finding was that clot resolution rates are greatly dependent on precise catheter positioning within the hematoma. The MISTIE trial is currently completing its dose-finding phase which will be followed by a safety study.

Intraventricular thrombolytic therapy

As previously discussed, intraventricular extension is a common occurrence in ICH and directly impacts the outcome [64]. Although ventriculostomy allows for the drainage of blood and cerebrospinal fluid, this process is often slow and hampered by catheter obstruction. Therefore, recent efforts have focused on the use of intraventricular thrombolytic agents as an adjunct to external ventricular drainage in an attempt to expedite clot lysis and the clearance of intraventricular blood. A number of small clinical series and case-control studies investigated the effect of intraventricular delivery of urokinase [166, 167] or rt-PA [161, 168, 169], and most have suggested a reduction in morbidity and mortality with a fairly low complication rate. Two systematic literature reviews addressing the use of fibrinolytic agents concluded that this treatment modality might be of therapeutic value, but that the design of most studies was not appropriate, and randomized trials were, therefore, necessary to definitively confirm its safety and efficacy [65, 170]. In a pilot randomized study, Naff and colleagues demonstrated that treatment with intraventricular urokinase given at 12-hour intervals until discontinuation of the ventriculostomy led to faster resolution of intraventricular hemorrhage when compared to treatment with ventricular drainage alone [171].

This was followed by the recently completed Clear IVH (Clot Lysis: Evaluating Accelerated Resolution of Intraventricular Hemorrhage) trial, a phase II, multicenter, prospective study to evaluate the safety of open-label doses of intraventricular recombinant rt-PA in patients with intraventricular extension of a spontaneous ICH ≤30cc that required ventriculostomy as the standard of care [172]. The first dose of rt-PA had to be given within 48 hours of diagnosis of intraventricular hemorrhage by CT scan. The trial was performed in two phases. Phase A focused on the pharmacokinetics of intraventricular injections of rt-PA and determined that the safest and most effective dose of rt-PA was 1mg. This dose was then used every 8 hours in 36 patients in phase B. Adverse events were within predetermined safety limits. Preliminary analyses show that low-dose rt-PA can be safely administered to stable intraventricular clots and may increase lysis rates, particularly in areas closest to the drug-delivering external ventricular drain. The effect on outcome is currently being evaluated in a phase III trial (CLEAR III) that plans to enroll 500 participants.

Conclusions

ICH is a devastating condition with a long history of poor outcomes driven in part by the lack of consensus regarding its optimal management. This has changed quite dramatically in the past decade, when new insights into the pathophysiology of ICH, better understanding of mechanisms of hematoma expansion, and the results of both medical and surgical trials propelled our knowledge and increased optimism towards the potential efficacy of treatment. Blood pressure, hyperglycemia, fever and DVT prophylaxis have become the goal of targeted medical management strategies. Measures to prevent and reduce elevated intracranial pressure have been adopted as part of routine practice in the intensive care of the critically ill ICH patient. Recent radiological findings have promoted the use of CT angiography as a tool for recognizing patients with increased risk of hematoma expansion in the initial hours after ICH onset. Finally, ongoing randomized, controlled trials are attempting to identify patients that might benefit from surgical intervention, including minimally invasive surgical techniques to achieve maximal hematoma removal with limited damage to normal tissue. Recommendations based on a comprehensive review of the current ICH literature as well as their levels of evidence are summarized in the table below. Hopefully this will serve as a guide to help replace the nihilism in treating ICH patients with the realization that aggressive management in the acute phase can translate into improved outcomes.

Key points	Evidence level
◆ Observation in an intensive care unit with neurologic expertise is strongly recommended for at least the first 24 hours after ICH onset.	Ib/A
◆ While clinical trials of BP management in ICH are ongoing, the guidelines set forth by the AHA [14] and EUSI [36], recommending cautious management of severe hypertension with fast-acting intravenous antihypertensive drugs, should be followed.	IIa/B
◆ In patients with intracranial hypertension, sedation and analgesia should be used to minimize agitation and pain.	III/B
◆ Hyperventilation is advocated as a temporizing measure in situations of impending herniation before a more definitive therapy can be instituted.	III/B
◆ Mannitol should be considered for short-term use in ICH patients with evidence of transtentorial herniation or acute neurological deterioration associated with high ICP or mass effect.	IIb/B
◆ Hypertonic saline can be used as an alternative to mannitol, particularly when CPP augmentation is desirable.	III/B
◆ Placement of an ICP monitor or external ventricular drain should be considered in comatose ICH patients (GCS score of 8 or less).	III/B
◆ Routine use of rFVIIa as a hemostatic agent in ICH patients cannot be recommended.	Ib/A
◆ Patients with a severe coagulation factor deficiency or severe thrombocytopenia should receive immediate specific factor replacement or platelet transfusion, respectively.	IV/C
◆ Patients with warfarin-associated ICH should receive vitamin K as an adjunct to rapid replacement of vitamin-K-dependent factors (FFP or PCCs).	III/B
◆ Despite the lack of randomized trials, the use of PCCs for the treatment of warfarin-associated ICH is being advocated.	IIa/B
◆ Based on safety concerns and limited evidence of benefit, the routine use of rFVIIa for warfarin reversal is not recommended.	Ib/A
◆ Glucose management should target normoglycemia, with close monitoring to avoid hypoglycemia.	III/B
◆ Dextrose-containing and hypotonic solutions should be avoided.	IV/C
◆ Fever should be treated aggressively.	IV/C
◆ Clinical and electrographic seizures should be promptly treated with antiepileptic drugs.	IIa/B
◆ Mechanical venous thromboembolism prophylaxis should be initiated on admission in all ICH patients.	Ib/A

Continued

Key points *continued*	Evidence level
◆ Early use of subcutaneous heparin may be considered for the prevention of thromboembolic complications after 2 days from ICH onset.	Ib/A
◆ For most patients with ICH, craniotomy cannot be recommended.	Ib/A
◆ Patients with cerebellar hemorrhage ≥3cm in diameter, who have brainstem compression or hydrocephalus, or who are deteriorating neurologically should be submitted to surgical removal promptly.	IIa/B
◆ The benefit of minimally invasive (stereotactic or endoscopic) surgery with or without use of thrombolysis is currently being investigated in clinical trials, and these procedures are considered investigational.	IIa/B

References

1. Broderick J, Connolly S, Feldmann E, *et al.* Guidelines for the Management of Spontaneous Intracerebral Hemorrhage in Adults: 2007 update: a Guideline from the American Heart Association/American Stroke Association Stroke Council, High Blood Pressure Research Council, and the Quality of Care and Outcomes in Research Interdisciplinary Working Group. *Stroke* 2007; 38: 2001-23.

2. American Heart Association. International Cardiovascular Disease Statistics. http://wwwamericanheartorg/downloadable/heart/1236204012112INTLpdf 2009.

3. Fogelholm R, Murros K, Rissanen A, Avikainen S. Long-term survival after primary intracerebral haemorrhage: a retrospective population-based study. *J Neurol Neurosurg Psychiatry* 2005; 76: 1534-8.

4. Broderick JP, Brott T, Tomsick T, Miller R, Huster G. Intracerebral hemorrhage more than twice as common as subarachnoid hemorrhage. *J Neurosurg* 1993; 78: 188-91.

5. Qureshi AI, Suri MF, Nasar A, *et al.* Changes in cost and outcome among US patients with stroke hospitalized in 1990 to 1991 and those hospitalized in 2000 to 2001. *Stroke* 2007; 38: 2180-4.

6. Broderick JP, Adams HP, Jr., Barsan W, *et al.* Guidelines for the Management of Spontaneous Intracerebral Hemorrhage: a Statement for Healthcare Professionals from a Special Writing Group of the Stroke Council, American Heart Association. *Stroke* 1999; 30: 905-15.

7. Mayer SA, Sacco RL, Shi T, Mohr JP. Neurologic deterioration in noncomatose patients with supratentorial intracerebral hemorrhage. *Neurology* 1994; 44: 1379-84.

8. Moon JS, Janjua N, Ahmed S, *et al.* Prehospital neurologic deterioration in patients with intracerebral hemorrhage. *Crit Care Med* 2008; 36: 172-5.

9. Roch A, Michelet P, Jullien AC, *et al.* Long-term outcome in intensive care unit survivors after mechanical ventilation for intracerebral hemorrhage. *Crit Care Med* 2003; 31: 2651-6.

10. Gujjar AR, Deibert E, Manno EM, Duff S, Diringer MN. Mechanical ventilation for ischemic stroke and intracerebral hemorrhage: indications, timing, and outcome. *Neurology* 1998; 51: 447-51.

11. Reynolds SF, Heffner J. Airway management of the critically ill patient: rapid-sequence intubation. *Chest* 2005; 127: 1397-412.

12. Fogelholm R, Murros K, Rissanen A, Avikainen S. Admission blood glucose and short-term survival in primary intracerebral haemorrhage: a population-based study. *J Neurol Neurosurg Psychiatry* 2005; 76: 349-53.

13. Passero S, Ciacci G, Ulivelli M. The influence of diabetes and hyperglycemia on clinical course after intracerebral hemorrhage. *Neurology* 2003; 61: 1351-6.

14. Morgenstern LB, Hemphill JC, 3rd, Anderson C, *et al.* Guidelines for the management of spontaneous intracerebral hemorrhage: a guideline for healthcare professionals from the American Heart Association/American Stroke Association. *Stroke* 2010; 41: 2108-29.

15. Diringer MN, Edwards DF. Admission to a neurologic/neurosurgical intensive care unit is associated with reduced mortality rate after intracerebral hemorrhage. *Crit Care Med* 2001; 29: 635-40.

16. Mirski MA, Chang CW, Cowan R. Impact of a neuroscience intensive care unit on neurosurgical patient outcomes and cost of care: evidence-based support for an intensivist-directed specialty ICU model of care. *J Neurosurg Anesthesiol* 2001; 13: 83-92.

17. Ronning OM, Guldvog B, Stavem K. The benefit of an acute stroke unit in patients with intracranial haemorrhage: a controlled trial. *J Neurol Neurosurg Psychiatry* 2001; 70: 631-4.

18. Qureshi AI, Ezzeddine MA, Nasar A, *et al.* Prevalence of elevated blood pressure in 563,704 adult patients with stroke presenting to the ED in the United States. *Am J Emerg Med* 2007; 25: 32-8.

19. Brott T, Broderick J, Kothari R, *et al.* Early hemorrhage growth in patients with intracerebral hemorrhage. *Stroke* 1997; 28: 1-5.

20. Fujii Y, Takeuchi S, Sasaki O, Minakawa T, Tanaka R. Multivariate analysis of predictors of hematoma enlargement in spontaneous intracerebral hemorrhage. *Stroke* 1998; 29: 1160-6.

21. Kazui S, Minematsu K, Yamamoto H, Sawada T, Yamaguchi T. Predisposing factors to enlargement of spontaneous intracerebral hematoma. *Stroke* 1997; 28: 2370-5.

22. Ohwaki K, Yano E, Nagashima H, Hirata M, Nakagomi T, Tamura A. Blood pressure management in acute intracerebral hemorrhage: relationship between elevated blood pressure and hematoma enlargement. *Stroke* 2004; 35: 1364-7.

23. Davis SM, Broderick J, Hennerici M, *et al.* Hematoma growth is a determinant of mortality and poor outcome after intracerebral hemorrhage. *Neurology* 2006; 66: 1175-81.

24. Jauch EC, Lindsell CJ, Adeoye O, *et al.* Lack of evidence for an association between hemodynamic variables and hematoma growth in spontaneous intracerebral hemorrhage. *Stroke* 2006; 37: 2061-5.

25. Kidwell CS, Saver JL, Mattiello J, *et al.* Diffusion-perfusion MR evaluation of perihematomal injury in hyperacute intracerebral hemorrhage. *Neurology* 2001; 57: 1611-7.

26. Rosand J, Eskey C, Chang Y, Gonzalez RG, Greenberg SM, Koroshetz WJ. Dynamic single-section CT demonstrates reduced cerebral blood flow in acute intracerebral hemorrhage. *Cerebrovasc Dis* 2002; 14: 214-20.

27. Qureshi AI, Wilson DA, Hanley DF, Traystman RJ. Pharmacologic reduction of mean arterial pressure does not adversely affect regional cerebral blood flow and intracranial pressure in experimental intracerebral hemorrhage. *Crit Care Med* 1999; 27: 965-71.

28. Qureshi AI, Wilson DA, Hanley DF, Traystman RJ. No evidence for an ischemic penumbra in massive experimental intracerebral hemorrhage. *Neurology* 1999; 52: 266-72.

29. Powers WJ, Zazulia AR, Videen TO, *et al.* Autoregulation of cerebral blood flow surrounding acute (6 to 22 hours) intracerebral hemorrhage. *Neurology* 2001; 57: 18-24.

30. Hirano T, Read SJ, Abbott DF, *et al.* No evidence of hypoxic tissue on 18F-fluoromisonidazole PET after intracerebral hemorrhage. *Neurology* 1999; 53: 2179-82.

31. Suri MF, Suarez JI, Rodrigue TC, *et al.* Effect of treatment of elevated blood pressure on neurological deterioration in patients with acute intracerebral hemorrhage. *Neurocrit Care* 2008; 9: 177-82.

32. Anderson CS, Huang Y, Wang JG, *et al.* Intensive Blood Pressure Reduction in Acute Cerebral Haemorrhage Trial (INTERACT): a randomised pilot trial. *Lancet Neurol* 2008; 7: 391-9.

33. Antihypertensive Treatment of Acute Cerebral Hemorrhage. *Crit Care Med* 2010; 38: 637-48.

34. Qureshi AI. Antihypertensive Treatment of Acute Cerebral Hemorrhage (ATACH): rationale and design. *Neurocrit Care* 2007; 6: 56-66.

35. Qureshi AI, Palesch YY, Martin R, *et al.* Effect of systolic blood pressure reduction on hematoma expansion, perihematomal edema, and 3-month outcome among patients with intracerebral hemorrhage: results from the Antihypertensive Treatment of Acute Cerebral Hemorrhage study. *Arch Neurol* 2010; 67: 570-6.

36. Steiner T, Kaste M, Forsting M, *et al.* Recommendations for the management of intracranial haemorrhage - part I: spontaneous intracerebral haemorrhage. The European Stroke Initiative Writing Committee and the Writing Committee for the EUSI Executive Committee. *Cerebrovasc Dis* 2006; 22: 294-316.

37. Rose JC, Mayer SA. Optimizing blood pressure in neurological emergencies. *Neurocrit Care* 2004; 1: 287-99.

38. Steiner T, Juttler E. American guidelines for the management of spontaneous intracerebral hemorrhage in adults: European perspective. *Pol Arch Med Wewn* 2008; 118: 181-2.

39. Qureshi AI, Tuhrim S, Broderick JP, Batjer HH, Hondo H, Hanley DF. Spontaneous intracerebral hemorrhage. *N Engl J Med* 2001; 344: 1450-60.

40. Wagner KR, Xi G, Hua Y, *et al.* Lobar intracerebral hemorrhage model in pigs: rapid edema development in perihematomal white matter. *Stroke* 1996; 27: 490-7.
41. Xi G, Wagner KR, Keep RF, *et al.* Role of blood clot formation on early edema development after experimental intracerebral hemorrhage. *Stroke* 1998; 29: 2580-6.
42. Qureshi AI, Mendelow AD, Hanley DF. Intracerebral haemorrhage. *Lancet* 2009; 373: 1632-44.
43. Gebel JM, Brott TG, Sila CA, *et al.* Decreased perihematomal edema in thrombolysis-related intracerebral hemorrhage compared with spontaneous intracerebral hemorrhage. *Stroke* 2000; 31: 596-600.
44. Unwin DH, Giller CA, Kopitnik TA. Central nervous system monitoring. What helps, what does not. *Surg Clin North Am* 1991; 71: 733-47.
45. Schwab S, Aschoff A, Spranger M, Albert F, Hacke W. The value of intracranial pressure monitoring in acute hemispheric stroke. *Neurology* 1996; 47: 393-8.
46. Rincon F, Mayer SA. Clinical review: critical care management of spontaneous intracerebral hemorrhage. *Crit Care* 2008; 12: 237.
47. Albanese J, Durbec O, Viviand X, Potie F, Alliez B, Martin C. Sufentanil increases intracranial pressure in patients with head trauma. *Anesthesiology* 1993; 79: 493-7.
48. Kelly DF, Goodale DB, Williams J, *et al.* Propofol in the treatment of moderate and severe head injury: a randomized, prospective double-blinded pilot trial. *J Neurosurg* 1999; 90: 1042-52.
49. Cremer OL. The propofol infusion syndrome: more puzzling evidence on a complex and poorly characterized disorder. *Crit Care* 2009; 13: 1012.
50. Raichle ME, Plum F. Hyperventilation and cerebral blood flow. *Stroke* 1972; 3: 566-75.
51. Stocchetti N, Maas AI, Chieregato A, van der Plas AA. Hyperventilation in head injury: a review. *Chest* 2005; 127: 1812-27.
52. Shenkin HA, Goluboff B, Haft H. The use of mannitol for the reduction of intracranial pressure in intracranial surgery. *J Neurosurg* 1962; 19: 897-901.
53. Diringer MN, Zazulia AR. Osmotic therapy: fact and fiction. *Neurocrit Care* 2004; 1: 219-33.
54. Sorani MD, Manley GT. Dose-response relationship of mannitol and intracranial pressure: a meta-analysis. *J Neurosurg* 2008; 108: 80-7.
55. Misra UK, Kalita J, Ranjan P, Mandal SK. Mannitol in intracerebral hemorrhage: a randomized controlled study. *J Neurol Sci* 2005; 234: 41-5.
56. Qureshi AI, Geocadin RG, Suarez JI, Ulatowski JA. Long-term outcome after medical reversal of transtentorial herniation in patients with supratentorial mass lesions. *Crit Care Med* 2000; 28: 1556-64.
57. Qureshi AI, Suarez JI. Use of hypertonic saline solutions in treatment of cerebral edema and intracranial hypertension. *Crit Care Med* 2000; 28: 3301-13.
58. Qureshi AI, Wilson DA, Traystman RJ. Treatment of elevated intracranial pressure in experimental intracerebral hemorrhage: comparison between mannitol and hypertonic saline. *Neurosurgery* 1999; 44: 1055-63; discussion 1063-6.
59. Qureshi AI, Wilson DA, Traystman RJ. Treatment of transtentorial herniation unresponsive to hyperventilation using hypertonic saline in dogs: effect on cerebral blood flow and metabolism. *J Neurosurg Anesthesiol* 2002; 14: 22-30.
60. Suarez JI, Qureshi AI, Bhardwaj A, *et al.* Treatment of refractory intracranial hypertension with 23.4% saline. *Crit Care Med* 1998; 26: 1118-22.
61. Diringer MN, Edwards DF, Zazulia AR. Hydrocephalus: a previously unrecognized predictor of poor outcome from supratentorial intracerebral hemorrhage. *Stroke* 1998; 29: 1352-7.
62. Phan TG, Koh M, Vierkant RA, Wijdicks EF. Hydrocephalus is a determinant of early mortality in putaminal hemorrhage. *Stroke* 2000; 31: 2157-62.
63. Hallevi H, Albright KC, Aronowski J, *et al.* Intraventricular hemorrhage: anatomic relationships and clinical implications. *Neurology* 2008; 70: 848-52.
64. Hanley DF. Intraventricular hemorrhage: severity factor and treatment target in spontaneous intracerebral hemorrhage. *Stroke* 2009; 40: 1533-8.
65. Nieuwkamp DJ, de Gans K, Rinkel GJ, Algra A. Treatment and outcome of severe intraventricular extension in patients with subarachnoid or intracerebral hemorrhage: a systematic review of the literature. *J Neurol* 2000; 247: 117-21.
66. Lozier AP, Sciacca RR, Romagnoli MF, Connolly ES, Jr. Ventriculostomy-related infections: a critical review of the literature. *Neurosurgery* 2002; 51: 170-81; discussion 181-2.

67. Schade RP, Schinkel J, Visser LG, Van Dijk JM, Voormolen JH, Kuijper EJ. Bacterial meningitis caused by the use of ventricular or lumbar cerebrospinal fluid catheters. *J Neurosurg* 2005; 102: 229-34.

68. Holloway KL, Barnes T, Choi S, *et al*. Ventriculostomy infections: the effect of monitoring duration and catheter exchange in 584 patients. *J Neurosurg* 1996; 85: 419-24.

69. Yilmazlar S, Abas F, Korfali E. Comparison of ventricular drainage in poor grade patients after intracranial hemorrhage. *Neurol Res* 2005; 27: 653-6.

70. Huttner HB, Nagel S, Tognoni E, *et al*. Intracerebral hemorrhage with severe ventricular involvement: lumbar drainage for communicating hydrocephalus. *Stroke* 2007; 38: 183-7.

71. Harrop JS, Sharan AD, Ratliff J, *et al*. Impact of a standardized protocol and antibiotic-impregnated catheters on ventriculostomy infection rates in cerebrovascular patients. *Neurosurgery* 2010; 67: 187-91; discussion 191.

72. Schwab S, Spranger M, Schwarz S, Hacke W. Barbiturate coma in severe hemispheric stroke: useful or obsolete? *Neurology* 1997; 48: 1608-13.

73. Reith J, Jorgensen HS, Pedersen PM, *et al*. Body temperature in acute stroke: relation to stroke severity, infarct size, mortality, and outcome. *Lancet* 1996; 347: 422-5.

74. Rossi S, Zanier ER, Mauri I, Columbo A, Stocchetti N. Brain temperature, body core temperature, and intracranial pressure in acute cerebral damage. *J Neurol Neurosurg Psychiatry* 2001; 71: 448-54.

75. Stocchetti N, Protti A, Lattuada M, *et al*. Impact of pyrexia on neurochemistry and cerebral oxygenation after acute brain injury. *J Neurol Neurosurg Psychiatry* 2005; 76: 1135-9.

76. Krieger DW, Yenari MA. Therapeutic hypothermia for acute ischemic stroke: what do laboratory studies teach us? *Stroke* 2004; 35: 1482-9.

77. Kawai N, Nakamura T, Okauchi M, Nagao S. Effects of hypothermia on intracranial hemodynamics and ischemic brain damage-studies in the rat acute subdural hematoma model. *Acta Neurochir Suppl* 2000; 76: 529-33.

78. Kawai N, Nakamura T, Okauchi M, Nagao S. Effects of hypothermia on intracranial pressure and brain edema formation: studies in a rat acute subdural hematoma model. *J Neurotrauma* 2000; 17: 193-202.

79. Krieger DW, De Georgia MA, Abou-Chebl A, *et al*. Cooling for acute ischemic brain damage (cool aid): an open pilot study of induced hypothermia in acute ischemic stroke. *Stroke* 2001; 32: 1847-54.

80. Shiozaki T, Sugimoto H, Taneda M, *et al*. Effect of mild hypothermia on uncontrollable intracranial hypertension after severe head injury. *J Neurosurg* 1993; 79: 363-8.

81. Schwab S, Georgiadis D, Berrouschot J, Schellinger PD, Graffagnino C, Mayer SA. Feasibility and safety of moderate hypothermia after massive hemispheric infarction. *Stroke* 2001; 32: 2033-5.

82. Steiner T, Friede T, Aschoff A, Schellinger PD, Schwab S, Hacke W. Effect and feasibility of controlled rewarming after moderate hypothermia in stroke patients with malignant infarction of the middle cerebral artery. *Stroke* 2001; 32: 2833-5.

83. Rincon F, Mayer SA. Therapeutic hypothermia for brain injury after cardiac arrest. *Semin Neurol* 2006; 26: 387-95.

84. Fujii Y, Tanaka R, Takeuchi S, Koike T, Minakawa T, Sasaki O. Hematoma enlargement in spontaneous intracerebral hemorrhage. *J Neurosurg* 1994; 80: 51-7.

85. Kazui S, Naritomi H, Yamamoto H, Sawada T, Yamaguchi T. Enlargement of spontaneous intracerebral hemorrhage. Incidence and time course. *Stroke* 1996; 27: 1783-7.

86. Roberts HR, Monroe DM, White GC. The use of recombinant Factor VIIa in the treatment of bleeding disorders. *Blood* 2004; 104: 3858-64.

87. Allen GA, Hoffman M, Roberts HR, Monroe DM, 3rd. Recombinant activated Factor VII: its mechanism of action and role in the control of hemorrhage. *Can J Anaesth* 2002; 49: S7-14.

88. Mayer SA, Brun NC, Begtrup K, *et al*. Recombinant activated Factor VII for acute intracerebral hemorrhage. *N Engl J Med* 2005; 352: 777-85.

89. Diringer MN, Skolnick BE, Mayer SA, *et al*. Risk of thromboembolic events in controlled trials of rFVIIa in spontaneous intracerebral hemorrhage. *Stroke* 2008; 39: 850-6.

90. Mayer SA, Brun NC, Begtrup K, *et al*. Efficacy and safety of recombinant activated Factor VII for acute intracerebral hemorrhage. *N Engl J Med* 2008; 358: 2127-37.

91. Mayer SA, Davis SM, Skolnick BE, *et al*. Can a subset of intracerebral hemorrhage patients benefit from hemostatic therapy with recombinant activated Factor VII? *Stroke* 2009; 40: 833-40.

92. Goldstein JN, Fazen LE, Snider R, *et al.* Contrast extravasation on CT angiography predicts hematoma expansion in intracerebral hemorrhage. *Neurology* 2007; 68: 889-94.

93. Thompson AL, Kosior JC, Gladstone DJ, *et al.* Defining the CT angiography 'spot sign' in primary intracerebral hemorrhage. *Can J Neurol Sci* 2009; 36: 456-61.

94. Wada R, Aviv RI, Fox AJ, *et al.* CT angiography 'spot sign' predicts hematoma expansion in acute intracerebral hemorrhage. *Stroke* 2007; 38: 1257-62.

95. del Zoppo GJ, Mori E. Hematologic causes of intracerebral hemorrhage and their treatment. *Neurosurg Clin N Am* 1992; 3: 637-58.

96. Niizuma H, Suzuki J, Yonemitsu T, Otsuki T. Spontaneous intracerebral hemorrhage and liver dysfunction. *Stroke* 1988; 19: 852-6.

97. Oppenheim-Eden A, Glantz L, Eidelman LA, Sprung CL. Spontaneous intracerebral hemorrhage in critically ill patients: incidence over six years and associated factors. *Intensive Care Med* 1999; 25: 63-7.

98. Flaherty ML, Kissela B, Woo D, *et al.* The increasing incidence of anticoagulant-associated intracerebral hemorrhage. *Neurology* 2007; 68: 116-21.

99. Aguilar MI, Hart RG, Kase CS, *et al.* Treatment of warfarin-associated intracerebral hemorrhage: literature review and expert opinion. *Mayo Clin Proc* 2007; 82: 82-92.

100. Rosand J, Eckman MH, Knudsen KA, Singer DE, Greenberg SM. The effect of warfarin and intensity of anticoagulation on outcome of intracerebral hemorrhage. *Arch Intern Med* 2004; 164: 880-4.

101. Hart RG, Aguilar MI. Anticoagulation in atrial fibrillation: selected controversies including optimal anticoagulation intensity, treatment of intracerebral hemorrhage. *J Thromb Thrombolysis* 2008; 25: 26-32.

102. Rosand J, Hylek EM, O'Donnell HC, Greenberg SM. Warfarin-associated hemorrhage and cerebral amyloid angiopathy: a genetic and pathologic study. *Neurology* 2000; 55: 947-51.

103. Ansell J, Hirsh J, Hylek E, Jacobson A, Crowther M, Palareti G. Pharmacology and management of the vitamin K antagonists: American College of Chest Physicians Evidence-Based Clinical Practice Guidelines (8th Edition). *Chest* 2008; 133: 160S-98.

104. Watson HG, Baglin T, Laidlaw SL, Makris M, Preston FE. A comparison of the efficacy and rate of response to oral and intravenous Vitamin K in reversal of over-anticoagulation with warfarin. *Br J Haematol* 2001; 115: 145-9.

105. Goldstein JN, Thomas SH, Frontiero V, *et al.* Timing of fresh frozen plasma administration and rapid correction of coagulopathy in warfarin-related intracerebral hemorrhage. *Stroke* 2006; 37: 151-5.

106. Samama CM. Prothrombin complex concentrates: a brief review. *Eur J Anaesthesiol* 2008; 25: 784-9.

107. Bershad EM, Suarez JI. Prothrombin complex concentrates for oral anticoagulant therapy-related intracranial hemorrhage: a review of the literature. *Neurocrit Care* 2010; 12: 403-13.

108. Gilmore R, Harmon S, Keane G, Gannon C, O'Donnell JS. Variation in anticoagulant composition regulates differential effects of prothrombin complex concentrates on thrombin generation. *J Thromb Haemost* 2009; 7: 2154-6.

109. Leissinger CA, Blatt PM, Hoots WK, Ewenstein B. Role of prothrombin complex concentrates in reversing warfarin anticoagulation: a review of the literature. *Am J Hematol* 2008; 83: 137-43.

110. Boulis NM, Bobek MP, Schmaier A, Hoff JT. Use of Factor IX complex in warfarin-related intracranial hemorrhage. *Neurosurgery* 1999; 45: 1113-8; discussion 1118-9.

111. Bertram M, Bonsanto M, Hacke W, Schwab S. Managing the therapeutic dilemma: patients with spontaneous intracerebral hemorrhage and urgent need for anticoagulation. *J Neurol* 2000; 247: 209-14.

112. Preston FE, Laidlaw ST, Sampson B, Kitchen S. Rapid reversal of oral anticoagulation with warfarin by a prothrombin complex concentrate (Beriplex): efficacy and safety in 42 patients. *Br J Haematol* 2002; 116: 619-24.

113. Baglin TP, Cousins D, Keeling DM, Perry DJ, Watson HG. Safety indicators for inpatient and outpatient oral anticoagulant care: [corrected] Recommendations from the British Committee for Standards in Haematology and National Patient Safety Agency. *Br J Haematol* 2007; 136: 26-9.

114. Sorensen B, Johansen P, Nielsen GL, Sorensen JC, Ingerslev J. Reversal of the International Normalized Ratio with recombinant activated Factor VII in central nervous system bleeding during warfarin thromboprophylaxis: clinical and biochemical aspects. *Blood Coagul Fibrinolysis* 2003; 14: 469-77.

115. Freeman WD, Brott TG, Barrett KM, *et al.* Recombinant Factor VIIa for rapid reversal of warfarin anticoagulation in acute intracranial hemorrhage. *Mayo Clin Proc* 2004; 79: 1495-500.

116. Ilyas C, Beyer GM, Dutton RP, Scalea TM, Hess JR. Recombinant Factor VIIa for warfarin-associated intracranial bleeding. *J Clin Anesth* 2008; 20: 276-9.

117. Tanaka KA, Szlam F, Dickneite G, Levy JH. Effects of prothrombin complex concentrate and recombinant activated Factor VII on vitamin K antagonist-induced anticoagulation. *Thromb Res* 2008; 122: 117-23.

118. Rosovsky RP, Crowther MA. What is the evidence for the off-label use of recombinant Factor VIIa (rFVIIa) in the acute reversal of warfarin? ASH evidence-based review 2008. *Hematology Am Soc Hematol Educ Program* 2008: 36-8.

119. Baird TA, Parsons MW, Phanh T, *et al.* Persistent post-stroke hyperglycemia is independently associated with infarct expansion and worse clinical outcome. *Stroke* 2003; 34: 2208-14.

120. Williams LS, Rotich J, Qi R, *et al.* Effects of admission hyperglycemia on mortality and costs in acute ischemic stroke. *Neurology* 2002; 59: 67-71.

121. Capes SE, Hunt D, Malmberg K, Pathak P, Gerstein HC. Stress hyperglycemia and prognosis of stroke in nondiabetic and diabetic patients: a systematic overview. *Stroke* 2001; 32: 2426-32.

122. Adams HP, Jr., del Zoppo G, Alberts MJ, *et al.* Guidelines for the Early Management of Adults with Ischemic Stroke: a Guideline from the American Heart Association/American Stroke Association Stroke Council, Clinical Cardiology Council, Cardiovascular Radiology and Intervention Council, and the Atherosclerotic Peripheral Vascular Disease and Quality of Care Outcomes in Research Interdisciplinary Working Groups: the American Academy of Neurology affirms the value of this guideline as an educational tool for neurologists. *Stroke* 2007; 38: 1655-711.

123. Oddo M, Schmidt JM, Carrera E, *et al.* Impact of tight glycemic control on cerebral glucose metabolism after severe brain injury: a microdialysis study. *Crit Care Med* 2008; 36: 3233-8.

124. Van den Berghe G, Schoonheydt K, Becx P, Bruyninckx F, Wouters PJ. Insulin therapy protects the central and peripheral nervous system of intensive care patients. *Neurology* 2005; 64: 1348-53.

125. Turaj W, Slowik A, Szczudlik A. Factors related to the occurrence of hyperthermia in patients with acute ischaemic stroke and with primary intracerebral haemorrhage. *Neurol Neurochir Pol* 2008; 42: 316-22.

126. Schwarz S, Hafner K, Aschoff A, Schwab S. Incidence and prognostic significance of fever following intracerebral hemorrhage. *Neurology* 2000; 54: 354-61.

127. Baena RC, Busto R, Dietrich WD, Globus MY, Ginsberg MD. Hyperthermia delayed by 24 hours aggravates neuronal damage in rat hippocampus following global ischemia. *Neurology* 1997; 48: 768-73.

128. Commichau C, Scarmeas N, Mayer SA. Risk factors for fever in the neurologic intensive care unit. *Neurology* 2003; 60: 837-41.

129. Mayer SA, Kowalski RG, Presciutti M, *et al.* Clinical trial of a novel surface cooling system for fever control in neurocritical care patients. *Crit Care Med* 2004; 32: 2508-15.

130. Diringer MN. Treatment of fever in the neurologic intensive care unit with a catheter-based heat exchange system. *Crit Care Med* 2004; 32: 559-64.

131. Passero S, Rocchi R, Rossi S, Ulivelli M, Vatti G. Seizures after spontaneous supratentorial intracerebral hemorrhage. *Epilepsia* 2002; 43: 1175-80.

132. Vespa PM, O'Phelan K, Shah M, *et al.* Acute seizures after intracerebral hemorrhage: a factor in progressive midline shift and outcome. *Neurology* 2003; 60: 1441-6.

133. Claassen J, Jette N, Chum F, *et al.* Electrographic seizures and periodic discharges after intracerebral hemorrhage. *Neurology* 2007; 69: 1356-65.

134. Gregory PC, Kuhlemeier KV. Prevalence of venous thromboembolism in acute hemorrhagic and thromboembolic stroke. *Am J Phys Med Rehabil* 2003; 82: 364-9.

135. Albers GW, Amarenco P, Easton JD, Sacco RL, Teal P. Antithrombotic and thrombolytic therapy for ischemic stroke: the Seventh ACCP Conference on Antithrombotic and Thrombolytic Therapy. *Chest* 2004; 126: 483S-512.

136. Lacut K, Bressollette L, Le Gal G, *et al.* Prevention of venous thrombosis in patients with acute intracerebral hemorrhage. *Neurology* 2005; 65: 865-9.

137. Boeer A, Voth E, Henze T, Prange HW. Early heparin therapy in patients with spontaneous intracerebral haemorrhage. *J Neurol Neurosurg Psychiatry* 1991; 54: 466-7.

138. Fernandes HM, Gregson B, Siddique S, Mendelow AD. Surgery in intracerebral hemorrhage. The uncertainty continues. *Stroke* 2000; 31: 2511-6.

139. McKissock W, Richardson A, Taylor J. Primary intracerebral haemorrhage: a controlled trial of surgical and conservative treatment in 180 unselected cases. *Lancet* 1961; 2: 221-6.

140. Hankey GJ, Hon C. Surgery for primary intracerebral hemorrhage: is it safe and effective? A systematic review of case series and randomized trials. *Stroke* 1997; 28: 2126-32.

141. Prasad K, Browman G, Srivastava A, Menon G. Surgery in primary supratentorial intracerebral hematoma: a meta-analysis of randomized trials. *Acta Neurol Scand* 1997; 95: 103-10.

142. Teernstra OP, Evers SM, Kessels AH. Meta-analyses in treatment of spontaneous supratentorial intracerebral haematoma. *Acta Neurochir* 2006; 148: 521-8; discussion 528.

143. Juvela S, Heiskanen O, Poranen A, *et al*. The treatment of spontaneous intracerebral hemorrhage. A prospective randomized trial of surgical and conservative treatment. *J Neurosurg* 1989; 70: 755-8.

144. Zuccarello M, Brott T, Derex L, *et al*. Early surgical treatment for supratentorial intracerebral hemorrhage: a randomized feasibility study. *Stroke* 1999; 30: 1833-9.

145. Mendelow AD, Gregson BA, Fernandes HM, *et al*. Early surgery versus initial conservative treatment in patients with spontaneous supratentorial intracerebral haematomas in the International Surgical Trial in Intracerebral Haemorrhage (STICH): a randomised trial. *Lancet* 2005; 365: 387-97.

146. Ott KH, Kase CS, Ojemann RG, Mohr JP. Cerebellar hemorrhage: diagnosis and treatment. A review of 56 cases. *Arch Neurol* 1974; 31: 160-7.

147. Little JR, Tubman DE, Ethier R. Cerebellar hemorrhage in adults. Diagnosis by computerized tomography. *J Neurosurg* 1978; 48: 575-9.

148. St Louis EK, Wijdicks EF, Li H, Atkinson JD. Predictors of poor outcome in patients with a spontaneous cerebellar hematoma. *Can J Neurol Sci* 2000; 27: 32-6.

149. Da Pian R, Bazzan A, Pasqualin A. Surgical versus medical treatment of spontaneous posterior fossa haematomas: a cooperative study on 205 cases. *Neurol Res* 1984; 6: 145-51.

150. Firsching R, Huber M, Frowein RA. Cerebellar haemorrhage: management and prognosis. *Neurosurg Rev* 1991; 14: 191-4.

151. Kirollos RW, Tyagi AK, Ross SA, van Hille PT, Marks PV. Management of spontaneous cerebellar hematomas: a prospective treatment protocol. *Neurosurgery* 2001; 49: 1378-86; discussion 1386-7.

152. Morioka J, Fujii M, Kato S, *et al*. Surgery for spontaneous intracerebral hemorrhage has greater remedial value than conservative therapy. *Surg Neurol* 2006; 65: 67-72; discussion 72-3.

153. Auer LM, Deinsberger W, Niederkorn K, *et al*. Endoscopic surgery versus medical treatment for spontaneous intracerebral hematoma: a randomized study. *J Neurosurg* 1989; 70: 530-5.

154. Hattori N, Katayama Y, Maya Y, Gatherer A. Impact of stereotactic hematoma evacuation on activities of daily living during the chronic period following spontaneous putaminal hemorrhage: a randomized study. *J Neurosurg* 2004; 101: 417-20.

155. Cho DY, Chen CC, Chang CS, Lee WY, Tso M. Endoscopic surgery for spontaneous basal ganglia hemorrhage: comparing endoscopic surgery, stereotactic aspiration, and craniotomy in noncomatose patients. *Surg Neurol* 2006; 65: 547-55; discussion 555-6.

156. Nishihara T, Morita A, Teraoka A, Kirino T. Endoscopy-guided removal of spontaneous intracerebral hemorrhage: comparison with computer tomography-guided stereotactic evacuation. *Childs Nerv Syst* 2007; 23: 677-83.

157. Mohadjer M, Braus DF, Myers A, Scheremet R, Krauss JK. CT-stereotactic fibrinolysis of spontaneous intracerebral hematomas. *Neurosurg Rev* 1992; 15: 105-10.

158. Niizuma H, Shimizu Y, Yonemitsu T, Nakasato N, Suzuki J. Results of stereotactic aspiration in 175 cases of putaminal hemorrhage. *Neurosurgery* 1989; 24: 814-9.

159. Teernstra OP, Evers SM, Lodder J, Leffers P, Franke CL, Blaauw G. Stereotactic treatment of IntraCerebral Hematoma by means of a Plasminogen Activator: a multicenter randomized controlled trial (SICHPA). *Stroke* 2003; 34: 968-74.

160. Wagner KR, Xi G, Hua Y, *et al*. Ultra-early clot aspiration after lysis with tissue plasminogen activator in a porcine model of intracerebral hemorrhage: edema reduction and blood-brain barrier protection. *J Neurosurg* 1999; 90: 491-8.

161. Rohde V, Schaller C, Hassler WE. Intraventricular recombinant tissue plasminogen activator for lysis of intraventricular haemorrhage. *J Neurol Neurosurg Psychiatry* 1995; 58: 447-51.

162. Lippitz BE, Mayfrank L, Spetzger U, Warnke JP, Bertalanffy H, Gilsbach JM. Lysis of basal ganglia haematoma with recombinant tissue plasminogen activator (rtPA) after stereotactic aspiration: initial results. *Acta Neurochir* 1994; 127: 157-60.

163. Schaller C, Rohde V, Meyer B, Hassler W. Stereotactic puncture and lysis of spontaneous intracerebral hemorrhage using recombinant tissue-plasminogen activator. *Neurosurgery* 1995; 36: 328-33; discussion 333-5.

164. Vespa P, McArthur D, Miller C, *et al*. Frameless stereotactic aspiration and thrombolysis of deep intracerebral hemorrhage is associated with reduction of hemorrhage volume and neurological improvement. *Neurocrit Care* 2005; 2: 274-81.

165. Morgan T, Zuccarello M, Narayan R, Keyl P, Lane K, Hanley D. Preliminary findings of the Minimally-Invasive Surgery plus rtPA for Intracerebral Hemorrhage Evacuation (MISTIE) clinical trial. *Acta Neurochir Suppl* 2008; 105: 147-51.

166. Murry KR, Rhoney DH, Coplin WM. Urokinase in the treatment of intraventricular hemorrhage. *Ann Pharmacother* 1998; 32: 256-8.

167. Naff NJ, Carhuapoma JR, Williams MA, *et al*. Treatment of intraventricular hemorrhage with urokinase: effects on 30-day survival. *Stroke* 2000; 31: 841-7.

168. Fountas KN, Kapsalaki EZ, Parish DC, *et al*. Intraventricular administration of rt-PA in patients with intraventricular hemorrhage. *South Med J* 2005; 98: 767-73.

169. Huttner HB, Tognoni E, Bardutzky J, *et al*. Influence of intraventricular fibrinolytic therapy with rt-PA on the long-term outcome of treated patients with spontaneous basal ganglia hemorrhage: a case-control study. *Eur J Neurol* 2008; 15: 342-9.

170. Lapointe M, Haines S. Fibrinolytic therapy for intraventricular hemorrhage in adults. *Cochrane Database Syst Rev* 2002: CD003692.

171. Naff NJ, Hanley DF, Keyl PM, *et al*. Intraventricular thrombolysis speeds blood clot resolution: results of a pilot, prospective, randomized, double-blind, controlled trial. *Neurosurgery* 2004; 54: 577-83; discussion 583-4.

172. Morgan T, Awad I, Keyl P, Lane K, Hanley D. Preliminary report of the Clot Lysis Evaluating Accelerated Resolution of Intraventricular Hemorrhage (CLEAR-IVH) clinical trial. *Acta Neurochir Suppl* 2008; 105: 217-20.

Chapter 10

Cerebral venous sinus thrombosis

José M. Ferro MD PhD, Chairman and Full Professor
Patrícia Canhão MD PhD, Assistant Professor and Consultant Neurologist
Department of Neurosciences, Hospital de Santa Maria
University of Lisbon, Lisboa, Portugal

Introduction

Thrombosis of the dural sinus and of the cerebral veins (CVT) is less common (0.5-1% of all strokes), has a more varied clinical presentation and is more difficult to diagnose than other types of stroke [1-3]. CVT is more frequent in children, young adults and females. CVT can have an acute, subacute or less often chronic presentation. The most frequent symptoms are headaches, seizures, motor, sensory or language deficits, and altered mental status or decreased consciousness. Symptoms and signs can be grouped into three major presentation syndromes: isolated intracranial hypertension (headache +/- vomiting, papilloedema and visual symptoms), focal syndrome (focal deficits, seizures or both) and encephalopathy (multifocal signs, mental status changes, stupor/coma) [4]. Clinical symptoms and signs depend on the site and number of occluded sinus and veins, on the presence and type of parenchymal lesions, on the age [5, 6] and gender [7] of the patient, and on the interval from onset to presentation [3].

CVT can be secondary to multiple predisposing conditions and precipitants (Table 1). Multiple risk factors may be found in about half of patients, while in less that 15% no underlying cause can be found [8].

CVT has a variable prognosis, with more than 80% of patients achieving a good outcome. The death or dependency rate in adults is 15% [8] and the 30-day case mortality rate is 4-15% [9-11]. Long-term complications include seizures, headaches, visual loss and arteriovenous fistulae.

Table 1. Risk factors and associated conditions for CVT.

Transient risk factors

Pregnancy and puerperium (or post-abortion)
Oral contraceptives
Post-menopausal hormonal therapy
Other drugs with prothrombotic effect
Intracranial infection, including meningitis
Infection of neighbouring structure (eye, sinus, ear, tooth, skin of face, scalp)
Other infections
Mechanical causes (head trauma, lumbar puncture)
Severe dehydration
Severe anemia
Neurosurgery

Permanent risk factors

Genetic prothrombotic conditions (protein C, protein S and antithrombin deficiencies; Factor V Leiden and prothrombin G20210A mutations)
Malignancies
Hematological diseases (polycythemia, thrombocythemia)
Systemic lupus erythematosus and other connective tissue disease
Antiphospholipid antibody syndrome
Behçet's disease
Other vasculitis
Other inflammatory systemic conditions (e.g. inflammatory bowel disease)
Intracranial causes (meningioma, brain vascular malformations)

Confirmation of the diagnosis

Confirmation of the diagnosis of CVT is based on the neuroimaging demonstration of an occluded sinus/vein and of the thrombus. In clinical practice, computed tomography (CT) is usually the first investigation to be performed. It is useful to rule out other acute cerebral disorders, but may be normal in up to 30% of cases, and most of the findings are non-specific. CT may show direct signs such as the cord sign due to the hyperdensity of a thrombosed cortical vein and/or dural sinus, the cord sign and the dense triangle sign, or indirect signs of CVT, dilated transcerebral veins, small ventricles and parenchymal abnormalities [4] (Figure 1). Parenchymal abnormalities may occur in 60-80% of cases and comprise: intracerebral hematomas, hemorrhagic infarct, subarachnoid hemorrhage (<1%) usually in the convexity, areas of hypodensity due to focal edema or venous infarction, usually

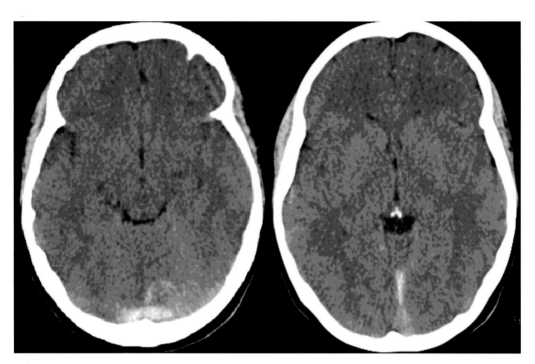

Figure 1. Non-contrast cerebral computed tomography scan showing spontaneous hyperdensity of the torculae and the straight sinus.

not respecting the arterial boundaries and diffuse brain edema. After contrast injection, the occluded superior sagittal sinus (SSS) appears as the empty delta sign and there may be an intense contrast enhancement of falx and tentorium or areas of gyral enhancement. In serial CT the parenchymal lesions may disappear ('vanishing infarcts') or new lesions may appear. CT venography demonstrates the filling defects in the occluded sinus or veins [12-14] and is at least equivalent to MR venography in the diagnosis of CVT [15, 16]. However, drawbacks to CT venography include radiation exposure, contrast allergy and the possibility of aggravating poor renal function.

Magnetic resonance imaging (MRI) combined with magnetic resonance angiography (MRA) is the most sensitive examination technique for the diagnosis of CVT [17, 18] (Figure 2). Direct visualization of the thrombus confirms the diagnosis of CVT. The characteristics of the signal depend on the age of the thrombus: in the first 5 days they are isointense on T1-weighted images and hypointense on T2-weighted images due to increased deoxyhemoglobin; after this time the diagnosis becomes easier due to an increased signal on both T1- and T2-weighted images due to methemoglobin; after the first month there is a variable pattern of signal, which may become isointense [17, 19]. The combination of an abnormal signal in a sinus and a corresponding absence of flow on MRA supports the diagnosis of CVT. Gradient echo T2*-weighted images improve the diagnosis of CVT, enabling the identification of isolated cortical venous thrombosis as an hypointense area [20-24]. Non-thrombosed hypoplastic sinus will not have an abnormal low signal in the sinus on gradient echo (GRE) and/or susceptibility-weighted imaging (SWI). After contrast (gadolinium)

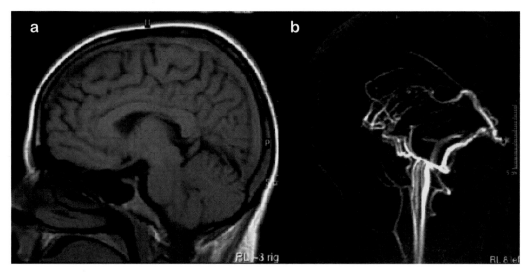

Figure 2. a) T1-weighted image shows extensive isointense thrombus in the superior sagittal sinus; b) venoMR confirms the absence of flow in the superior sagittal sinus.

injection the thrombus appears as a central isodense lesion in a venous sinus with surrounding enhancement. MRI is also useful in showing the parenchymal lesions secondary to venous occlusion, in particular in differentiating vasogenic oedema from a venous infarct, where there is increased signal in diffusion-weighted MRI (DWI) (Figure 3). Turbulent, slow sinus flow and flow gaps are commonly seen on time-of-flight (TOF) MR venographic images, and may be misdiagnosed as thrombosis.

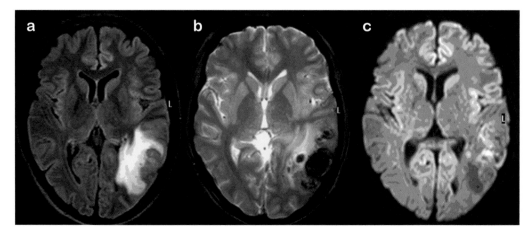

Figure 3. Hemorrhagic venous infarcts in a patient with left lateral sinus thrombosis, showed as: a) hyperintense lesions on FLAIR sequence; and b) hypointense on gradient echo T2*; c) diffusion-weighted MRI (DWI) which does not show a hyperintense signal in the corresponding area of the brain oedema.

Intra-arterial angiography has a spatial resolution superior to CT or MR venography but is nowadays rarely performed and is reserved for cases with inconclusive or contradictory findings from other imaging modalities or when intervention is planned [25].

Independently of the modality (CT, MR or IA), venography has limitations related to anatomical venous variations, such as hypoplasia of the anterior part of the SSS, duplication of the SSS, intrasinus septa, giant arachnoid granulations and hypo- or aplasia of the transverse sinuses [4], which may be misdiagnosed as thrombosis [26-29].

The inter-observer agreement on CVT diagnosis is not perfect. The proportion of agreement is 62% for angiography and 94% for MR plus angiography [30]. Agreement is lower in cortical vein thrombosis and left transverse sinus occlusion [31].

As the diagnosis of CVT requires neuroimaging investigations which are not always immediately accessible, it would be of great clinical interest to have access to a test that is easy to perform in the emergency care setting that could confidently rule out CVT. Unfortunately such a test does not yet exist. Measurement of D-dimer levels, a product of fibrin degradation, may be helpful to identify patients with a low probability of CVT, who will have a level <500ug/L or equivalent using sensitive immunoassay or ELISA [32-34]. However, false negatives can occur, for instance, CVT patients presenting with isolated headache, those with a subacute or chronic presentation and those with a lesser clot burden may have normal D-dimer levels [32-38].

Identification of the causes of CVT

Many predisposing conditions and precipitating factors have been described in association with CVT, but for the majority of them no causality can be established (Table 1), as the association relies on case or case-series reports and less often on case-control studies [39]. These associated conditions and precipitating factors are better labelled risk factors than causes. CVT patients can be grouped in:

- those who only have transient risk factors;
- those with only permanent risk factors;
- patients with both transient and permanent risk factors;
- patients without identifiable risk factors (cryptogenic CVT) [40].

The more frequent risk factors are prothrombotic conditions, either genetic or acquired, oral contraceptives, puerperium or pregnancy, malignancy and infection [8]. Infections and pregnancy/puerperium-related cases are more frequent in developing countries. In more than 85% of patients, at least one risk factor can be identified [8]. Multiple risk factors may be found in about half of patients, including a prothrombotic condition which can be identified in a third of patients, being genetically determined in a quarter of patients and acquired in the remaining, mainly antiphospholipid antibody syndrome (APL) [8]. The genetic background probably determines the inherent individual risk. In the presence of some genetic prothrombotic conditions (e.g. antithrombin, protein C or protein S deficiency; Factor V Leiden mutation; prothrombin gene mutation), patients are at increased risk of developing a CVT when exposed to transient risk factors such as oral contraceptives, pregnancy/puerperium, infections, head trauma, lumbar puncture, surgery or prothrombotic drugs. Therefore, testing for APL and for genetic prothrombotic conditions is recommended in all CVT patients, even when another associated condition is already identified. The diagnosis of APL requires abnormal high titers of lupus anticoagulant, anticardiolipin IgG or anti-β2-glycoprotein IgG antibodies, on two or more occasions at least 12 weeks apart. Testing for deficiencies of protein C, S, and antithrombin must be performed at least 6 weeks after a thrombotic event, cannot be performed during warfarin treatment and should be confirmed with repeat testing and family studies. Cerebrospinal fluid examination through a lumbar puncture is only indicated if there is a clinical suspicion of meningitis.

In elderly CVT patients, the proportion of cases with malignancies and hematological disorders such as polycythemia is higher [6]. In almost 15% of adult CVT patients, extensive search reveals no underlying cause. Sometimes, the cause (e.g. vasculitis, antiphospholipid antibody syndrome, malignancy, polycythemia, thrombocythemia) is revealed only weeks or months after the acute phase or after repeated testing. Therefore, in the elderly patient and in cryptogenic CVT, search for an occult neoplasm is recommended.

Outcome and prognosis

Only a few cohort studies analyzed the prognostic factors for the short- [9] and long-term outcome of CVT patients [8, 41-45]. In the largest cohort study (ISCVT) [8], complete recovery at last follow-up (median 16 months) was observed in 79% of patients, the overall death rate was 8.3% and there was a 5.1% dependency rate (mRS ≥3) at the end of follow-up (12.6%, for patients surviving with a mRS ≥2). In a systematic review including both retrospective and prospective studies, overall mortality was 9.4% and the proportion of dependency (mRS ≥3 or Glasgow Outcome Scale [GOS] ≥3) was 9.7% [10]. Considering only cohort studies (including the prospective part of retrospective-prospective studies where information can be analyzed separately), the overall death and dependency rate was 15% (95% CI, 13-18) [8].

Around a quarter of CVT patients experience a neurologic worsening featuring depressed consciousness, mental status disturbance, new seizure, worsening of or a new focal deficit, increase in headache intensity, or visual loss. This worsening may occur even several days after diagnosis. About one third of patients with neurologic deterioration will have new parenchymal lesions if neuroimaging is repeated [46]. Four to 15% of patients die in the acute phase of CVT [9-11]. The main cause of acute death with CVT is transtentorial herniation secondary to a large hemorrhagic lesion [9], followed by herniation due to multiple lesions or to diffuse brain edema. Status epilepticus, medical complications, and pulmonary embolism are among other causes of early death [44, 47]. Deaths after the acute phase are mainly due to the underlying conditions, in particular, malignancies [8].

Risk factors for poor long-term prognosis in the ISCVT cohort were central nervous system infection, any malignancy, thrombosis of the deep venous system, intracranial hemorrhage on the admission CT/MR, Glasgow Coma Scale score (GCS) <9, mental status disturbance, age >37 years and male gender [8, 48]. Brain herniation leading to early death was more frequent in young patients, while late deaths due to malignancies and less favorable functional outcome were more frequent in elderly patients [6, 9].

Risk stratification scores might improve the ability to inform CVT patients on their individual prognosis and to select those who might benefit most from intensive monitoring and invasive treatments [48-50]. The ISCVT study group developed a risk score for poor outcomes (mRS Scale >2)(Table 2), which was tested in two validation samples of CVT patients. Using the risk score (range from 0 to 9) with a cut-off of ≥3 points, overall efficiency was 85.4%, 84.4% and 90.1% in the derivation and validation samples, respectively. Sensitivity and specificity in the three samples combined was 96.1% and 13.6%.

Table 2. CVT risk score.

Prognostic variable	HR (95%CI)	Risk points
Malignancy	4.53 (2.52-8.15)	2
Coma	4.19 (2.20-6.28)	2
Thrombosis of the deep venous system	3.03 (1.76-5.23)	2
Mental status disturbance	2.18 (1.37-3.46)	1
Male gender	1.60 (1.01-5.23)	1
Intracranial haemorrhage	1.42 (0.88-2.27)	1

The risk score model ranges from 0 (lowest risk) to 9 (highest risk) with a cut-off of ≥3 points indicating a higher risk of death or dependency at 6 months

Long-term complications of CVT include seizures, headaches, visual loss, dural arteriovenous fistulae and recurrent venous thrombosis of the brain, limbs, abdomen or pelvis.

Treatment

Treatment of CVT includes:

◆ treatment of the associated condition/risk factors;
◆ antithrombotic treatment;
◆ symptomatic treatment; and
◆ prevention/treatment of complications.

Treatment of the associated conditions

Because of the multitude of conditions that have been described in association with CVT, the treatment of these conditions is obviously beyond the scope of this chapter. However, we would like to stress the importance of antibiotic treatment, whenever there is a sepsis, meningitis or other intracranial infection or an infection of a neighbouring structure (e.g. otitis, mastoiditis).

Antithrombotic treatment

Heparins

Currently, there is a large consensus on the use of either IV heparin or subcutaneous low-molecular-weight heparin (LMWH) in acute CVT to prevent thrombus propagation and pulmonary embolism and to increase the chances of recanalisation. The use of heparin in acute CVT is supported by four clinical trials [51-53] and a meta-analysis of two of these trials [54], which showed a non-significant relative risk of 0.33 (95% CI, 0.08-1.21) for death and 0.46 (95% CI, 0.16-1.31) for death or dependency after anticoagulant therapy as compared to placebo. Two other trials performed in India were excluded from the meta-analysis, because one was performed only in puerperal CVT [53] and in the other the diagnosis of CVT was based only on CT. If these trials are included, the relative risk of death would be 0.33 and significant (95% CI, 0.14-0.78) **(Ia/A)**.

Concerning safety for the use of heparin in CVT with intracranial hemorrhagic lesions, several observational series showed that heparin is safe and can be used in acute CVT patients with intracranial hemorrhagic lesions **(III/B)**.

Thrombocytopenia occurs commonly with IV heparin. LMWHs have a longer half-life, more predictable clinical response and less interaction with platelets compared with standard heparin. If lumbar puncture or other interventions are planned to be performed, heparin should be stopped to attain a normalised activated partial thromboplastin time (APTT) and then restarted. A non-matched case control study of cases treated with IV heparin and LMWH in the ISCVT showed that death or dependency was more frequent in IV heparin treated patients (16% vs. 9%; p=0.05). Inclusion of patients who received both IV and

LMWH (n=96), based on the therapy they received first, yielded similar results, although the difference in poor outcome was no longer statistically significant (15% vs. 9%; p=0.1; OR 1.7; p=0.2). These results indicate that LMWH is at least equally effective and possibly superior to IV heparin for the treatment of CVT [55] **(IIb/B)**.

Endovascular thrombolysis

Direct endovascular thrombolysis aiming to dissolve the venous clot and reopen the occluded sinus or vein is used as an alternative to heparin in severe cases or in patients who fail to improve or deteriorate despite anticoagulation or if there is an elevation in intracranial pressure that increases despite conventional treatment. Catheterization of the sigmoid, transverse and superior sagittal sinuses via the femoral venous or jugular approach is followed by local injection of rt-PA or urokinase. Mechanical thrombolysis by disruption (guiding catheter), removal (balloon catheter) or suction (rheolytic catheter) may also be performed **(IV/C)**.

No randomized trials of endovascular treatment for sinus thrombosis have been performed. The published literature consists of case reports or uncontrolled case series. A systematic review including 169 patients with CVT treated with local thrombolysis, suggested a possible benefit for severe CVT cases, indicating that thrombolytics may reduce case fatality in critically ill patients. Intracranial hemorrhage after thrombolysis was reported in 17% of cases, and was associated with clinical worsening in 5% [56]. However, the possibility of publication bias must be kept in mind. In a recent Dutch series of 20 patients treated with IV local thrombolysis, 12 recovered to independent living while 6 died [57], but local thrombolysis was not useful in patients with large infarcts and impending herniation. A randomized trial to compare endovascular treatment vs. heparin in acute CVT has been recently launched. Pending the results of this trial, endovascular thrombolysis should be considered a treatment option and can be routinely recommended for CVT patients who worsen despite anticoagulant therapy, in particular those with thrombosis of the cerebral deep venous system and without large hemispheric lesions with mass effect **(III/B)**.

Oral anticoagulation

Prolonged oral anticoagulation with warfarin is recommended after the acute phase of CVT to prevent further venous thrombotic events, including the recurrence of CVT. The risk of all venous thrombotic events after the initial CVT was 4·1 per 100 person-years and the rate of recurrence was 1·5 per 100 person-years in the ISCVT [40].

In the Rochester Mayo Clinic series, the likelihood of recurrent venous thrombosis was the same after CVT and lower extremity deep venous thrombosis. Recurrence of CVT was not influenced by warfarin therapy [58]. In children, age at CVT onset (after 2 years), persistent venous occlusion, the G20210A mutation and non-administration of anticoagulation predict recurrent CVT or systemic venous thrombosis [59]. In the ISCVT, recurrence of venous thrombosis (all territories) after CVT was more frequent among men and in patients with polycythemia/thrombocythemia [40]. In the Martinelli *et al* series [60], males and patients with severe thrombophilias (or combined defects) had an increased risk of further venous thrombotic events. Such risk was not increased in mild thrombophilia. APL and the rare hereditary deficiencies of antithrombin, protein C and protein S are considered as severe thrombophilias, while the more common Factor V Leiden and prothrombin 20210GA mutations are classified as mild thrombophilia [61].

The optimal duration of anticoagulation has not yet been addressed in any randomized controlled trials, although such a study is in the planning phase. Oral anticoagulation is usually maintained for 6-12 months after acute CVT, aiming at an International Normalized Ratio (INR) of 2-3. If CVT is related to a transient risk factor, current recommendations suggest anticoagulants for 6 months. In patients with cryptogenic CVT, the period of anticoagulation must be extended for 6-12 months. In CVT associated with 'mild' thrombophilia, the guideline recommends 6-12 months and in patients with 'severe' thrombophilia, anticoagulants should be given for life [62] **(III/B)**.

Treatment of intracranial hypertension

In patients presenting with a syndrome of isolated increased intracranial pressure, featuring severe headache and papilloedema, intracranial hypertension can be reduced and symptoms relieved through a therapeutic lumbar puncture. Despite the lack of randomised trials, acetazolamide is also used in some centres **(IV/C)**.

Despite their potential to reduce vasogenic oedema, corticosteroids do not improve outcome in the acute phase of CVT, as shown by a large case-control study [63] **(IIa/B)**. Measures to control acutely increased ICP include elevating the head of the bed, osmotic diuretics such as mannitol, intensive care unit admission with sedation, hyperventilation to a target $PaCO_2$ of 30-35mm Hg, and ICP monitoring **(IV/C)**.

Decompressive surgery

Herniation due to a unilateral mass effect is the major cause of death in CVT [9]. Decompressive surgery is life-saving in these patients. Recent case-series, a retrospective registry [64] and a systematic review of 68 cases of CVT [65], who were treated by decompressive surgery (hemicraniectomy or hematoma drainage), showed that in CVT patients with large parenchymal lesions causing herniation, decompressive surgery was life-saving and often resulted in good functional outcome, irrespective of age, coma, aphasia, bilateral lesions or bilateral fixed pupils **(III/B)**. At the last follow-up (median 13 months), 26 (38%) patients had a mRS 0-1, 29 (43%) a mRs ≥3, and only 4 (6%) were alive with a mRS >3. Eleven (16%) patients died. A prospective registry is underway to confirm these encouraging results.

Shunting

Except in the rare occurrence of hydrocephalus, ventriculostomy or ventriculo-peritoneal shunts are not indicated in acute CVT **(IV/C)**. In patients presenting a syndrome of isolated increased intracranial pressure, a lumbo-peritoneal shunt may be indicated if severe headaches and /or visual loss develop or do not improve with repeated lumbar punctures and other medical measures to reduce intracranial pressure **(IV/C)**.

Headache

Headache is a common complaint during the follow-up of CVT patients: severe headaches requiring bed rest or hospital admission were reported in 14% of patients in the ISCVT [14] and 11% in the VENOPORT [44]. In general, headaches are primary and not related to CVT [8, 45, 66]. In patients with persistent or severe headaches, MR with veno-MR should be completed to rule out recurrent CVT. These MR results should be compared to a 'baseline' follow-up MR obtained 3 months following CVT diagnosis, looking for CVT at a new site or an increase in size of a previous thrombus. Occasionally, MRV may show stenosis of a previously occluded sinus, but the clinical significance of this is unclear. If headache persists and MRI is normal, lumbar puncture may be needed to exclude elevated intracranial pressure.

Visual loss

Severe visual loss due to CVT rarely occurs (2-4%) [8, 44, 45, 67]. Patients with papilledema or visual complaints should have a complete neuro-ophthalmological study, including visual acuity and formal visual field testing. Rapid diagnosis of CVT [3] **(III/B)** and treatment of intracranial hypertension are the main measures to prevent visual loss **(IV/C)**. Surgical fenestration of the optic nerve is rarely required **(IV/C)**.

Treatment and prevention of seizures

Focal or generalized post-CVT seizures can be divided into early (discussed above) or remote (occurring more than 2 weeks after diagnosis) [68-70]. In general, routine prescription of anti-epileptic drugs is not indicated to prevent seizures and should be reserved for high-risk patients. Concerning early seizures, seizures prior to or at admission and supratentorial lesions are the risk factors for subsequent early seizures. Patients with both risk factors should be prescribed anti-epileptic drugs in the acute phase **(IIa/B)**. This may also be considered in patients with a single seizure in the absence of parenchymal lesions **(IIa/B)**.

Remote seizures affect 5-32% of patients. Most of these seizures occur in the first year of follow-up [69, 70]. Risk factors for remote seizures are haemorrhagic lesions on admission CT/MR, early seizure and paresis. Five percent of patients have post-CVT epilepsy (more than one remote seizure). Post-CVT epilepsy is also associated with haemorrhagic lesions on admission CT/MR, early seizure and paresis [70]. Prophylactic anti-epileptics for a defined duration usually (1 year) should be prescribed in patients with early seizure and parenchymal lesions and in those with post-CVT epilepsy [62] **(III/B)**. It may also be considered in patients with a single seizure in the absence of parenchymal lesions.

Contraception, future pregnancies, and related matters

Oral contraception and hormonal replacement therapy should be stopped. Emergency contraception is also contraindicated [71]. Contraceptive methods other than oral or parental contraceptives should be used (III/B).

CVT and pregnancy or puerperium-related CVT is not a contraindication for future pregnancy (III/B). A comprehensive search for associated conditions and for prothrombotic genetic conditions and APL syndrome should be pursued. Although pregnancy and the puerperium are risk factors for CVT, the risk of complications during subsequent pregnancy among women who have a history of CVT is low. There is information in the literature of 83 women who became pregnant after a CVT, resulting in 101 pregnancies; 88% terminated in normal births. There were only two cases of deep venous thrombosis and none of recurrent CVT. However, a high proportion of spontaneous abortion was noticed [8, 42, 44, 72-74].

CVT occurring during pregnancy should be preferentially treated with LMWH and this treatment should be continued for at least 6 weeks post-partum (IV/C). Warfarin is teratogenic and should not be given in the first trimester of pregnancy. Oral anticoagulants may also induce foetal or placental haemorrhage, mainly in the last trimester of pregnancy and at delivery, because they cross the placenta.

Special aspects of management of CVT in children

The incidence of CVT is higher than in adults, in particular among neonates [5]. Neonates have a non-specific presentation with seizures or lethargy, whereas older infants and children have a clinical presentation similar to adults. Concerning risk factors, perinatal complications and dehydration are frequently present in neonates with CVT. The confirmation of the diagnosis can be made by MR and MRV or CTV. Transfontanellar ultrasound and transcranial Doppler may also be useful for supporting the diagnosis of CVT [75].

Given the frequency of epileptic seizures in children with an acute CVT, continuous electroencephalography monitoring may be considered for children who are unconscious and/or mechanically ventilated.

As in adults, the mainstay of treatment is anticoagulation [76] (III/B). The AHA/ASA guidelines [77-79] recommend treating children with acute CVT diagnosed beyond the first 28 days of life with full-dose LMWH even in the presence of intracranial hemorrhage and to continue LMWH or oral vitamin K antagonists for 3-6 months or to stop earlier if recanalization is documented (III/B). In neonates with acute CVT, treatment with LMWH or UFH may also be considered as well as continuation of LMWH for 6 weeks to 3 months, with earlier discontinuation if full recanalization is documented (III/B). As in adults, the efficacy and safety of endovascular intervention is uncertain in pediatric patients. Its use may only be considered in selected patients with progressive neurological deterioration despite intensive care and therapeutic levels of anticoagulant treatment (IV/C).

Conclusions

A high suspicion rate is necessary to detect CVT and to select the patients who should have MR in combination with MR venography or other type of venography performed to confirm or rule out the diagnosis of CVT. A comprehensive search for the risk factors and associated conditions should be pursued, including laboratorial prothrombotic screening in all patients. Essentials of treatment include LMWH or IV heparin for almost all patients during the acute phase, followed by oral anticoagulation for a variable period, depending on the inherent thrombotic risk. Hemicraniectomy or local thrombolysis is used only in a few selected patients. Antiepileptic drugs are reserved for patients with seizures and supratentorial lesions.

Ongoing and future multicentre cooperative clinical research will increase the evidence-based management of CVT, focusing in particular on the efficacy of hemicraniectomy and local thrombolysis. The appropriateness of current guidelines should also be evaluated. Searching for novel genes and conditions associated with an increased risk of CVT will be an additional research priority.

Key points	Evidence level
◆ Patients with acute CVT without contraindications for anticoagulation should be treated either with subcutaneous low-molecular-weight heparin or intravenous heparin.	Ia/A
◆ If acute CVT patients deteriorate despite adequate anticoagulation, local IV thrombolysis may be a therapeutic option in those without impending herniation from large haemorrhagic infarcts.	III/B
◆ Oral anticoagulants may be given for 3 months if CVT was secondary to a transient risk factor, for 6-12 months in patients with idiopathic CVT and in those with 'mild' thrombophilia. Indefinite oral anticoagulation should be considered in patients with two or more episodes of CVT and in those with one episode of CVT and 'severe' thrombophilia.	III/B
◆ In patients with acute CVT and a single seizure with parenchymal lesions, early initiation of anti-epileptic drugs is recommended to prevent further seizures.	IIa/B
◆ In patients with acute CVT and a single seizure without parenchymal lesions, early initiation of anti-epileptic drugs for a defined duration is probably recommended to prevent further seizures.	IIa/B
◆ Steroids seem not to be useful and should be avoided to reduce an elevated intracranial pressure in patients with CVT, unless they are needed to treat an underlying disease.	IIa/B
◆ In patients with severe CVT and impending herniation attributable to large haemorrhagic infarcts, decompressive craniectomy can be life-saving.	III/B

References

1. Bousser MG, Ferro JM. Cerebral venous thrombosis: an update. *Lancet Neurol* 2007; 6: 162-70.
2. Stam J. Thrombosis of the cerebral veins and sinuses. *N Engl J Med* 2005; 352: 1791-8.
3. Ferro JM, Canhão P, Stam J, *et al*; ISCVT Investigators. Delay in the diagnosis of cerebral vein and dural sinus thrombosis: influence on outcome. *Stroke* 2009; 40: 3133-8.
4. Bousser MG, Russell RR. Cerebral venous thrombosis. In: *Major Problems in Neurology*. Warlow CP, Van Gijn J, Eds. London, UK: WB Saunders, 1997; Vol 33.
5. deVeber G, Andrew M, Adams C, *et al* and the Canadian Pediatric Ischemic Stroke Study Group. Cerebral sinovenous thrombosis in children. *N Engl J Med* 2001; 345: 417-23.
6. Ferro JM, Canhão P, Bousser MG, Stam J, Barinagarrementeria F; ISCVT Investigators. Cerebral vein and dural sinus thrombosis in elderly patients. *Stroke* 2005; 36: 1927-32.
7. Coutinho JM, Ferro JM, Canhão P, *et al.* Cerebral venous and sinus thrombosis in women. *Stroke* 2009; 40: 2356-61.
8. Ferro JM, Canhão P, Stam J, Bousser MG, Barinagarrementeria F; ISCVT Investigators. Prognosis of cerebral vein and dural sinus thrombosis: results of the International Study on Cerebral Vein and Dural Sinus Thrombosis (ISCVT). *Stroke* 2004; 35: 664-70.
9. Canhão P, Ferro JM, Lindgren AG, Bousser MG, Stam J, Barinagarrementeria F; ISCVT Investigators. Causes and predictors of death in cerebral venous thrombosis. *Stroke* 2005; 36:1720-5.
10. Dentali F, Gianni M, Crowther MA, Ageno W. Natural history of cerebral vein thrombosis: a systematic review. *Blood* 2006; 108: 1129-34.
11. Khealani BA, Wasay M, Saadah M, *et al*; Sultana E, Mustafa S, Khan FS, Kamal AK. Cerebral venous thrombosis. A descriptive multicenter study of patients in Pakistan and Middle East. *Stroke* 2008; 39: 2707-11.
12. Casey SO, Alberico RA, Patel M, *et al.* Cerebral CT venography. *Radiology* 1996; 198: 163-70.
13. Majoie CB, van Straten M, Venema HW, den Heeten GJ. Multisection CT venography of dural sinuses and cerebral veins by using matched mask bone elimination. *AJNR Am J Neuroradiol* 2004; 25: 787-91.
14. Wetzel SG, Kirsch E, Stock KW. Cerebral veins: comparative study of CT venography with intra-arterial digital subtraction angiography. *Am J Neuroradiol* 1999; 20: 249-55.
15. Rodallec MH, Krainik A, Feydy A, Hélias A, Colombani J-M, Jullès M-C, Marteau V, Zins M. Cerebral venous thrombosis and multidetector CT angiography: tips and tricks. *RadioGraphics* 2006; 26: S5-18.
16. Linn J, Erti-Wagner B, Seelos KC, *et al.* Diagnostic value of multidetector-row CT angiography in the evaluation of thrombosis in the cerebral venous sinuses. *AJNR Am J Neuroradiol* 2007; 28: 946-52.
17. Dormont D, Anxionnat R, Evrard S, Louaille C, Chiras J, Marsault C. MRI in cerebral venous thrombosis. *J Neuroradiol* 1994; 21: 81-99.
18. Lafitte F, Boukobza M, Guichard JP, *et al.* MRI and MRA for diagnosis and follow-up of cerebral venous thrombosis (CVT). *Clin Radiol* 1997; 52: 672-9.
19. Isensee C, Reul J, Thron A. Magnetic resonance imaging of thrombosed dural sinuses. *Stroke* 1994; 25: 29-34.
20. Cakmak S, Hermier M, *et al.* T2*-weighted MRI in cortical venous thrombosis. *Neurology* 2004; 63: 1698.
21. Selim M, Fink J, Linfante I, Kumar S, Schlaug G, Caplan LR. Diagnosis of cerebral venous thrombosis with echo-planar T2*-weighted magnetic resonance imaging. *Arch Neurol* 2002; 59: 1021-6.
22. Fellner FA, Fellner C, Aichner FT, Mölzer G. Importance of T2*-weighted gradient-echo MRI for diagnosis of cortical vein thrombosis. *Eur J Neurol* 2005; 56: 235-9.
23. Idbaih A, Boukobza M, Crassard I, Porcher R, Bousser MG, Chabriat H. MRI of clot in cerebral venous thrombosis: high diagnostic value of susceptibility-weighted images. *Stroke* 2006; 37: 991-5.
24. Leach JL, Strub WM, Gaskill-Shipley MF. Cerebral venous thrombus signal intensity and susceptibility effect on gradient recalled-echo MR imaging. *AJNR Am J Neuroradiol* 2007; 28: 940-5.
25. Janjua N. Cerebral angiography and venography for evaluation of cerebral venous thrombosis. *J Pak Med Assoc* 2006; 56: 527-30.
26. Liang L, Korogi Y, Sugahara T, *et al.* Normal structures in the intracranial dural sinuses: delineation with 3D contrast-enhanced magnetization prepared rapid acquisition gradient-echo imaging sequence. *AJNR Am J Neuroradiol* 2002; 23: 1739-46.
27. Zouaoui A, Hidden G. Cerebral venous sinuses: anatomical variants or thrombosis? *Acta Anat* (Basel) 1988; 133: 318-24.
28. Ayanzen RH, Bird CR, Keller PJ, McCully FJ, Theobald MR, Heiserman JE. Cerebral MR venography: normal anatomy and potential diagnostic pitfalls. *AJNR Am J Neuroradiol* 2000; 21: 74-8.

29. Leach JL, Fortuna RB, Jones BV, Gaskill-Shipley MF. Imaging of cerebral venous thrombosis: current techniques, spectrum of findings, and diagnostic pitfalls. *Radiographics* 2006; 26 (Suppl 1): S19-41.
30. de Bruijn SF, Majoie CB, Koster PA, *et al*. Interobserver agreement for MR-imaging and conventional angiography in the diagnosis of cerebral venous thrombosis. In: *Cerebral Venous Sinus Thrombosis. Clinical and Epidemiological Studies*. de Bruijn SF, Ed. Amsterdam: Thesis Publishers, 1998: 23-33.
31. Ferro JM, Morgado C, Sousa R, Canhão P. Interobserver agreement in the magnetic resonance location of cerebral vein and dural sinus thrombosis. *Eur J Neurol* 2007; 14: 353-6.
32. Tardy B, Tardy-Poncet B, Viallon A, *et al*. D-dimer levels in patients with suspected acute cerebral venous thrombosis. *Am J Med* 2002; 113: 238-41.
33. Lalive PH, de Moerloose P, Lovblad K, Sarasin FP, Mermillod B, Sztajzel R. Is measurement of D-dimer useful in the diagnosis of cerebral venous thrombosis? *Neurology* 2003; 61: 1057-60.
34. Kosinski CM, Mull M, Schwarz M, *et al*. Do normal D-dimer levels reliably exclude cerebral sinus thrombosis. *Stroke* 2004; 35: 2820-5.
35. Cucchiara B, Messe S, Taylor R, Clarke J, Pollak E. Utility of D-dimer in the diagnosis of cerebral venous sinus thrombosis. *J Thromb Haemost* 2005; 3: 387-9.
36. Wildberger JE, Mull M, Kilbinger M, Schön S, Vorwerk D. Cerebral sinus thrombosis: rapid test diagnosis by demonstration of increased plasma D-dimer levels (SimpliRED). *Rofo* 1997; 167: 527-9.
37. Talbot K, Wright M, Keeling D. Normal d-dimer levels do not exclude the diagnosis of cerebral venous sinus thrombosis. *J Neurol* 2002; 249: 1603-4.
38. Crassard I, Soria C, Tzourio C, *et al*. A negative D-dimer assay does not rule out cerebral venous thrombosis: a series of seventy-three patients. *Stroke* 2005; 36: 1716-9.
39. Saadatnia M, Fatehi F, Basiri K, Mousavi SA, Mehr GK. Cerebral venous thrombosis risk factors. *Int J Stroke* 2009; 4: 111-23.
40. Miranda B, Ferro JM, Canhão P, Stam J, Bousser MG, Barinagarrementeria F, Scoditti U and the ISCVT Investigators. Venous thromboembolic events after cerebral vein thromboembolic events after cerebral vein thrombosis. *Stroke* 2010; 41: 1901-6.
41. Rondepierre P, Hamon M, Leys D, *et al*. Thromboses veineuses cérébrales: étude de l'évolution. *Rev Neurol* (Paris) 1995; 151: 100-4.
42. Preter M, Tzourio CH, Ameri A, Bousser MG. Long-term prognosis in cerebral vein thrombosis: a follow-up of 77 patients. *Stroke* 1996; 27: 243-6.
43. de Bruijn SF, de Haan RJ, Stam J, for the Cerebral Venous Sinus Thrombosis Study Group. Clinical features and prognostic factors of cerebral venous sinus thrombosis in a prospective series of 59 patients. *J Neurol Neurosurg Psychiatry* 2001; 70: 105-8.
44. Ferro JM, Lopes MG, Rosas MJ, Ferro MA, Fontes J; Cerebral Venous Thrombosis Portugese Collaborative Study Group (VENOPORT). Long-term prognosis of cerebral vein and dural sinus thrombosis: results of the VENOPORT Study. *Cerebrovasc Dis* 2002; 13: 272-8.
45. Breteau G, Mounier-Vehier F, Godefroy O, *et al*. Cerebral venous thrombosis: 3-year clinical outcome in 55 consecutive patients. *J Neurol* 2003; 250: 29-35.
46. Crassard I, Canhão P, Ferro JM, Bousser MG, Barinagarrementeria F, Stam J. Neurological worsening in the acute phase of cerebral venous thrombosis in ISCVT (International Study on Cerebral Venous Thrombosis). *Cerebrovasc Dis* 2003; 16(suppl 4): 60.
47. Diaz JM, Schiffman JS, Urban ES, Maccario M. Superior sagittal sinus thrombosis and pulmonary embolism: a syndrome rediscovered. *Acta Neurol Scand* 1992; 86: 390-6.
48. Ferro JM, Bacelar-Nicolau H, Rodrigues T, *et al*; ISCVT and VENOPORT investigators. Risk score to predict the outcome of patients with cerebral vein and dural sinus thrombosis. *Cerebrovasc Dis* 2009; 28: 39-44.
49. Barrinagarrementeria F, Cantú C, Arredondo H. Aseptic cerebral venous thrombosis: proposed prognostic scale. *J Stroke Cerebrovasc Dis* 1992; 2: 34-9.
50. Koopman K, Uyttenboogaart M, Vroomen PC, van der Meer J, De Keyser J, Luijckx GJ. Development and validation of a predictive outcome score of cerebral venous thrombosis. *J Neurol Sci* 2009; 276: 66-8.
51. Einhäupl KM, Villringer A, Meister W, *et al*. Heparin treatment in sinus venous thrombosis. *Lancet* 1991; 338: 597-600.
52. de Bruijn SF, Stam J, CVST study group. Randomized, placebo-controlled trial of anticoagulant treatment with low-molecular-weight heparin for cerebral sinus thrombosis. *Stroke* 1999; 30: 484-8.
53. Nagaraja D, Rao B, Taly AB, Subhash MN. Randomized controlled trial of heparin in puerperal cerebral venous/sinus thrombosis. *Nimhans Journal* 1995; 13: 111-5.
54. Stam J, de Bruijn SF, deVeber G. Anticoagulation for cerebral sinus thrombosis. *Cochrane Database Syst Rev* 2002; 4: CD002005.

55. Coutinho JM, Ferro JM, Canhão P, Barinagarrementeria F, Bousser MG, Stam J; ISCVT Investigators. Unfractionated or low-molecular-weight heparin for the treatment of cerebral venous thrombosis. *Stroke* 2010; 41: 2575-80.

56. Canhão P, Falcão F, Ferro JM. Thrombolytics for cerebral sinus thrombosis: a systematic review. *Cerebrovasc Dis* 2003; 15: 159-66.

57. Stam J, Majoie BLM, van Delden OM, van Lienden KP, Reekers JA. Endovascular thrombectomy and thrombolysis for severe cerebral sinus thrombosis: a prospective study. *Stroke* 2008; 39: 1487-90.

58. Gosk-Bierska I, Wysokinski W, Brown RD Jr, Karnicki K, Grill D, Wiste H, Wysokinska E, McBane RD 2nd. Cerebral venous sinus thrombosis: incidence of venous thrombosis recurrence and survival. *Neurology* 2006; 67: 814-9.

59. Kenet G, Kirkham F, Niederstadt T, European Thromboses Study Group. Risk factors for recurrent venous thromboembolism in the European collaborative paediatric database on cerebral venous thrombosis: a multicentre cohort study. *Lancet Neurol* 2007; 6: 595-603.

60. Martinelli I, Bucciarelli P, Passamonti SM, Battaglioli T, Previtali E, Mannucci PM. Long-term evaluation of the risk of recurrence after cerebral sinus-venous thrombosis. *Circulation* 2010; 121: 2740-6.

61. Makris M. Thrombophilia: grading the risk. *Blood* 2009; 113: 5038-9.

62. Einhäupl K, Stam J, Bousser MG, *et al*. EFNS guideline on the treatment of cerebral venous and sinus thrombosis in adult patients. *Eur J Neurol* 2010; 17: 1229-35.

63. Canhão P, Cortesão A, Cabral M, *et al*, for the ISCVT investigators. Are steroids useful to treat cerebral venous thrombosis? *Stroke* 2008; 39: 105-10.

64. Ferro JM, Bousser M-G, Stam J, *et al*. Decompressive surgery in cerebrovenous thrombosis (CVT). A retrospective multicentre registry (ISCVT 2). *Cerebrovasc Dis* 2010; 29(suppl 2): 46

65. Crassard I, Bousser M-G, Canhão P, Coutinho J, Stam J, Ferro JM. Decompressive surgery in cerebrovenous thrombosis (CVT). A systematic review of individual patient data. *Cerebrovasc Dis* 2010; 29(suppl 2): 286.

66. Cumurciuc R, Crassard I, Sarov M, Valade D, Bousser MG. Headache as the only neurological sign of cerebral venous thrombosis: a series of 17 cases. *J Neurol Neurosurg Psychiatry* 2005; 76: 1084-7.

67. Biousse V, Ameri A, Bousser MG. Isolated intracranial hypertension as the only sign of cerebral venous thrombosis. *Neurology* 1999; 53: 1537-42.

68. Ferro JM, Canhão P, Bousser MG, Stam J, Barinagarrementeria F; ISCVT Investigators. Early seizures in cerebral vein and dural sinus thrombosis. Risk factors, and role of antiepileptics *Stroke* 2008; 39: 1152-8.

69. Ferro JM, Correia M, Rosas MJ, Pinto AN, Neves G; Cerebral Venous Thrombosis Portuguese Collaborative Study Group [Venoport]. Seizures in cerebral vein and dural sinus thrombosis. *Cerebrovasc Dis* 2003; 15: 78-83.

70. Ferro JM, Vasconcelos J, Canhão P, Bousser MG, Stam J, Barinagarrementeria F, ISCVT Investigators. Remote seizures in acute cerebral vein and dural sinus thrombosis (CVT). Incidence and associated conditions. *Cerebrovasc Dis* 2007; 23(suppl 2): 48.

71. Horga A, Santamaria E, Quinlez A, de Francisco J, Garcia-Martinez R, Alvarez-Sabin J. Cerebral venous thrombosis associated with repeated use of emergency contraception. *Eur J Neurol* 2007; 14: e-5.

72. Srinivasan K. Cerebral venous and arterial thrombosis in pregnancy and puerperium. A study of 135 patients. *Angiology* 1983; 34: 731-46.

73. Lamy C, Hamon JB, Coste J, Mas JL. Ischemic stroke in young women: risk of recurrence during subsequent pregnancies. French Study Group on Stroke in Pregnancy. *Neurology* 2000; 55: 269-74.

74. Merhraein S, Ortwein H, Busch M, Weih M, Einhäupl K, Masuhr F. Risk of recurrence of cerebral venous and sinus thrombosis during subsequent pregnancy and puerperium. *J Neurol Neurosurg Psychiatry* 2003; 74: 814-6.

75. Tsao PN, Lee WT, Peng SF, Lin JH, Yau KI. Power Doppler ultrasound imaging in neonatal cerebral venous sinus thrombosis. *Pediatr Neurol* 1999; 21: 652-5.

76. deVeber G, Chan A, Monagle P, *et al*. Anticoagulation therapy in pediatric patients with sinovenous thrombosis: a cohort study. *Arch Neurol* 1998; 55: 1533-7.

77. Roach ES, Golomb MR, Adams R, *et al*; American Heart Association Stroke Council; Council on Cardiovascular Disease in the Young. Management of Stroke in Infants and Children: a Scientific Statement from a Special Writing Group of the American Heart Association Stroke Council and the Council on Cardiovascular Disease in the Young. *Stroke* 2008; 39: 2644-91.

78. Paediatric Stroke Working Group. Stroke in Childhood: Clinical Guidelines for Diagnosis, Management and Rehabilitation, 2004. www.replondon.ac.uk/pubs/books/childstroke.

79. Monagle P, Chalmers E, Chan A, *et al*; American College of Chest Physicians. Antithrombotic Therapy in Neonates and Children. American College of Chest Physicians Evidence-Based Clinical Practice Guidelines (8th Edition). *Chest* 2008; 133(suppl 6): 887S-968.

Chapter 11

Ischemic stroke in children

E. Steve Roach MD, Professor and Chief
Division of Child Neurology
Ohio State University School of Medicine
Nationwide Children's Hospital
Columbus, Ohio, USA

Introduction

Few randomized clinical trials have been completed in children with stroke. Consequently, it is difficult to compile exacting evidence-based recommendations for the diagnosis and management of stroke in these individuals. There are several reasons for this paucity of clinical stroke trials in children. Although stroke probably occurs more often among children than once suspected, the low incidence of childhood stroke and the diverse pathophysiology of stroke in these individuals make it difficult to identify children with the specific characteristics needed for a clinical trial. Despite increasing awareness of childhood stroke by physicians and the public in the last two decades, the diagnosis of stroke in children is often delayed by several hours, hindering the study of thrombolytic agents and other time-sensitive treatments.

Despite these limitations, progress is being made. Several randomized clinical trials have been completed or are ongoing in children with sickle cell disease (SCD), a relatively common disease with near-complete hematological expressivity and a high stroke risk among affected individuals. There is also an ongoing study of the effects of systemic infection on stroke in children and a recently funded multicenter safety trial of recombinant tissue plasminogen activator (rt-PA) in ischemic stroke in children. The Canadian Pediatric Ischemic Stroke Registry now contains data on hundreds of children with stroke, allowing more precise retrospective analysis of the etiology and outcome of childhood stroke. Several published series summarize large numbers of children with specific cerebrovascular abnormalities, such as cerebral hemorrhage or ischemic infarction due to moyamoya disease. Other topics, however, are represented only in case reports and small case series. Any evidence-based management recommendations for childhood stroke must reflect this unevenness of the available evidence, and, for this reason, topics for which more evidence is available are presented in more detail than others in this chapter. We will also focus on the aspects of stroke that are relatively unique to children.

Ischemic stroke in children

Risk factors for ischemic stroke

The most obvious difference between ischemic stroke in children and those in adults is the great variety of conditions that cause stroke in children. Close to half of children with acute ischemic stroke are already known to have a stroke risk factor at the time of presentation, and two thirds of these children have one or more vascular risk factor after a thorough diagnostic evaluation. Congenital heart disease and SCD are common causes of ischemic stroke in children. In most large series, congenital heart lesions are responsible for 20-25% of the ischemic strokes that occur in children [1]. However, SCD may be the most common cause of pediatric stroke in centers with a large at-risk population. Even after a thorough diagnostic investigation, however, no specific cause can be pinpointed in up to a third of the children with ischemic stroke. Treatment of the risk factors is essential if subsequent strokes are to be prevented, and it is sometimes the underlying condition that determines the patient's eventual outcome. A complete discussion of the known or suspected pediatric stroke risk factors is beyond the scope of this chapter, but additional information is available elsewhere [2].

Sickle cell disease

Of all the causes of ischemic stroke in children, SCD provides the strongest evidence to support management recommendations [1]. There are several completed and ongoing clinical trials investigating stroke due to SCD. These trials are possible in individuals with SCD because the condition is relatively common and almost always diagnosed early in life before the occurrence of a stroke. Affected individuals have a high stroke risk, and transcranial Doppler (TCD) provides a means of identifying a subgroup of patients who have an even higher stroke risk. All of these factors combine to make clinical trials more feasible with SCD than with other stroke risk factors.

Data from the Baltimore-Washington Cooperative Young Stroke Study indicate a stroke incidence in individuals with SCD of 238 per 100,000 per year and 47.5 per 100,000 per year for ischemic stroke and intracerebral hemorrhage, respectively [3]. In sharp contrast, the childhood stroke incidence in this study was 1.29 per 100,000 per year for all types of stroke, 0.58 per 100,000 per year for ischemic stroke, and 0.71 per 100,000 per year for intracerebral hemorrhage [3]. The cumulative stroke risk due to SCD increases over time: 11% by age 20, 15% by age 30, and 24% by age 45 [4]. After having one SCD-related stroke, an individual's risk of having a second stroke soars to over 50%. Silent infarction, shown with magnetic resonance imaging in an individual without a defined neurological deficit, occurs in another 22% of children homozygous for SCD [5, 6]. Compounding risk factors for stroke in individuals with SCD include a high white blood cell count, systemic hypertension, previous silent brain infarction, and a history of chest crisis [4].

Children with SCD who have an elevated (time-averaged mean velocity 200cm/s) cerebral blood flow velocity on TCD have a stroke rate of about 10% per year [7, 8]. Coupled with the high incidence of SCD, the typically early diagnosis, and the high stroke rate of affected individuals, the ability to use TCD to identify a subset of patients with an even higher stroke risk makes it easier to enroll sufficient numbers of patients to complete clinical trials. It is appropriate to monitor younger children and individuals with relatively high flow velocities on prior TCD studies more often [8-10] **(IIb/B)**. Wang suggested that children with a normal TCD (≤170cm/s) be re-examined yearly, that those with an abnormal TCD (≥200cm/s) be re-examined in a month, that individuals with borderline study results (170-184cm/s) be restudied in 6 months, and that patients with velocities of 185-199cm/s be restudied in 3 months [11].

Standard acute treatment of ischemic symptoms due to SCD include hydration, correction of hypoxemia, treatment of hypotension, and exchange transfusion, although there are no controlled studies to prove the value of this approach [1] **(IV/C)**.

Given the exceedingly high risk of additional infarctions after an initial stroke due to SCD, regular blood transfusions designed to lower the percent of sickle hemoglobin to less than 30% have been used for several years after the first stroke due to SCD [12]. These authors estimated that the likelihood of stroke-free survival while receiving chronic transfusions for SCD was 80% after 50 months compared to only 30% without transfusion therapy [12]. Scothorn and colleagues estimated an annual stroke recurrence rate of about 2% despite ongoing transfusion [13]. Thus, a chronic transfusion program to lower the percentage of sickle hemoglobin is usually recommended after a stroke due to SCD **(III/B)**.

A randomized trial (Stroke Prevention Trial in Sickle Cell Anemia, the STOP study) compared periodic blood transfusion to standard care in 130 children with SCD who were selected for high stroke risk based on their TCD results [8]. This study showed that prophylactic blood transfusion reduces the occurrence of first stroke in high-risk (based on abnormal TCD readings) children with SCD by over 90% [8]. STOP was halted 16 months early after 11 strokes occurred in the standard-care arm compared to only 1 stroke in the group receiving transfusions. Prophylactic red cell transfusions are now recommended for children with SCD who have abnormal flow velocities on TCD **(Ib/A)**. There are no data to justify the use of chronic transfusion to prevent recurrent intracranial hemorrhage in SCD.

Chronic transfusion carries a risk of iron overload, alloimmunization, and infection, as well as considerable expense and lifestyle disruption, so a strategy to limit the duration of transfusions to high-risk intervals would be valuable. In the STOP trial, abnormal TCD readings sometimes reverted to normal after several months of transfusion, so a second randomized trial (STOP II) was devised to investigate whether these individuals could safely discontinue transfusions after 30 months [14]. Children in STOP II were randomly assigned to either continue receiving regular transfusions or to halt transfusions in favor of close TCD monitoring and standard SCD care. This trial too was halted before it reached its projected enrollment number. Among the 41 children who ceased transfusion therapy, two individuals had an ischemic stroke and in 14 others the TCD reverted to abnormal. In contrast, no strokes or TCD conversions occurred in the subjects who continued to receive transfusions. Unfortunately, there is currently no basis for discontinuing transfusion therapy in high-risk individuals.

The feasibility of switching some high-risk individuals from transfusion therapy to hydroxyurea is now being investigated. Hydroxyurea may lessen painful episodes due to SCD [15]. One non-randomized clinical series suggests that hydroxyurea lowers the stroke risk due to SCD and that this agent might be an alternative to chronic transfusions [16]. Another study suggested a benefit from hydroxyurea in individuals with SCD who first received transfusion therapy after a stroke then switched to hydroxyurea in an open-label trial with historical controls [17].

Table 1. Summary of recommendations for sickle cell disease.

◆ Acute management of ischemic stroke due to SCD should include optimal hydration, correction of hypoxemia, and correction of systemic hypotension.	IV/C
◆ It is appropriate to monitor children with sickle cell disease with periodic TCD.	IIb/B
◆ Children with SCD and a confirmed cerebral infarction should begin regular red cell transfusions to reduce the percentage of sickle hemoglobin.	III/B
◆ Periodic transfusions to reduce the percentage of sickle hemoglobin are recommended for children with persistently abnormal TCD results.	Ib/A
◆ Exchange transfusion designed to reduce Hb S to <30% total hemoglobin is reasonable after an acute cerebral infarction due to SCD.	IV/C
◆ Hydroxyurea may be considered in individuals with a high stroke risk due to SCD who cannot maintain a long-term transfusion program.	IIb/B
◆ Bone marrow transplantation may be considered for children with SCD.	IV/C
◆ Surgical revascularization procedures may be considered in children with SCD who continue to have cerebrovascular dysfunction even after optimal medical management.	IV/C

Hydroxyurea with phlebotomy is now being tested in a randomized clinical trial (the SWITCH study, see http://www.clinicaltrials.gov/ct/show/NCT00122980?order=1) [18]. While the definitive study has yet to be completed, it seems reasonable to begin hydroxyurea in individuals who, for whatever reason, cannot start or continue transfusion therapy **(IIb/B)**.

Bone marrow transplantation reportedly may limit the progression of cerebrovascular disease due to SCD, but data are limited [19] **(IV/C)**. Bone marrow transplantation is not always possible due to the unavailability of suitable donors and other issues.

Occasional children with moyamoya syndrome related to SCD undergo surgical bypass procedures [20, 21]. In one report, four of the six children undergoing encephaloduroarterio-synangiosis had already had a stroke, and two of these occurred while the patient was on a chronic transfusion program. One of the two patients who was initially free of cerebrovascular symptoms had an infarction 2 weeks after surgery [21]. The risks and benefits of bypass surgery in this setting should be evaluated in a randomized trial. Despite these limitations, it may be reasonable to consider revascularization surgery as a last resort for SCD patients who continue to have brain infarctions despite medical therapy **(IV/C)**. Recommendations for the management of stroke due to SCD are summarized in Table 1.

Moyamoya disease

Moyamoya disease is characterized by progressive stenosis of the internal carotid arteries with secondary distal telangiectatic collateral vessels. Other cranial arteries are sometimes affected as well. When moyamoya occurs in isolation it is classified as moyamoya disease, while individuals with an accepted risk factor have moyamoya syndrome. Among the clinical conditions reported in conjunction with moyamoya are cranial radiotherapy, neurofibromatosis type 1, sickle cell disease, and Down syndrome [1].

Moyamoya is more common in individuals of Asian heritage, but it occurs in all populations. The incidence rate ratios versus white individuals were 4.6 (95% CI, 3.4-6.3) for Asian Americans, 2.2 (95% CI, 1.3-2.4) for African Americans, and 0.5 (95% CI, 0.3-0.8) for Hispanic individuals [22]. Moyamoya disease has a bimodal age distribution, with one peak in the first decade and a second peak in adults of 30-40 years of age [23]. Affected family members can be identified 6-20% of the time, and autosomal dominant inheritance with variable expressivity has been suggested [24, 25]. Genetic heterogeneity is likely, and moyamoya has been linked to 3p24.2-26. 17q25, and other sites [26-28].

The clinical features of moyamoya depend on the rapidity of vascular occlusion, the availability of collateral flow, the age of the patient, and the location of the ischemia. Children with moyamoya usually present with signs of cerebral ischemia [29]. Half or more of untreated children with moyamoya develop mental retardation and 20-30% develop seizures [30, 31]. Individuals whose symptoms begin before age 4 years are particularly prone to cognitive impairment [31]. Adults can also have ischemic signs but commonly present with hemorrhage [30, 32].

Catheter angiography remains the most precise method of diagnosing moyamoya disease, but the initial diagnosis is usually made with magnetic resonance imaging of the brain and arteries [33-35]. Computed tomographic angiography is accurate but does not lend itself to the repeated imaging that is often required. Transcranial Doppler offers a non-invasive way to track changes in blood flow velocities in the larger cerebral vessels [36, 37]. Positron emission tomography, single photon emission tomography (SPECT), and computed tomography perfusion studies can reveal poor blood flow reserves before treatment and show the extent of improvement of perfusion after therapy [38, 39]. There are no data to justify routine vascular screening for moyamoya syndrome in most individuals, including those with an affected family member. Non-invasive screening may be considered in individuals with multiple affected family members and those with underlying disorders with a substantial risk of moyamoya syndrome [1].

Various surgical revascularization techniques are used for moyamoya disease (IIb/B). These are typically divided into direct bypass procedures (in which the superficial temporal artery is sewn to the middle cerebral artery) and indirect procedures that place an extracranial artery in close proximity to the intracerebral vessels in the hope that collateral channels will develop over time [40]. Direct anastomosis is often technically more difficult in children because of their small arteries. For this reason, small children usually undergo one of the indirect revascularization procedures such as encephaloduroarteriosynangiosis and encephalomyo-arteriosynangiosis [41, 42] (IIb/B). Two large long-term follow-up studies indicated that surgical treatment of moyamoya is reasonably safe (4% risk of stroke within 30 days of surgery per hemisphere) and effective (a 96% probability of remaining stroke-free over a 5-year follow-up period) [25, 43]. A meta-analysis of 1156 surgically treated pediatric moyamoya patients concluded that 87% (1003 individuals) benefited from surgical revascularization, but that there was no difference between the groups undergoing indirect and those undergoing direct/combined procedures [40]. There is little evidence that revascularization procedures are useful in individuals presenting with intracranial hemorrhage, but further studies are now underway [29].

Few studies compare medical and surgical therapy for moyamoya. A large retrospective survey from Japan found no difference in outcome between medically and surgically treated individuals with moyamoya [44]. In another report, however, 38.4% of 651 moyamoya patients who were not initially treated with surgery eventually came to surgery because of new or progressive symptoms [45]. Aspirin is sometimes administered to patients who are poor operative risks or those who have relatively mild and stable disease, but there are few data demonstrating either short- or long-term efficacy. Antiplatelet agents are also used in many individuals after surgery and in patients with suspected emboli arising from the site of arterial stenosis, and routinely for all patients in many operative series [25] (IV/C). Anticoagulants such as warfarin are rarely recommended because of the risk of hemorrhage from moyamoya and the risk of bleeding after inadvertent trauma in children, but low-dose low-molecular-weight heparin (LMWH) has been used on occasion [46].

Moyamoya patients are at additional risk of ischemic symptoms during the peri-operative period. Crying and hyperventilation, common occurrences in children during hospitalization, can lower $PaCO_2$ and induce ischemia secondary to cerebral vasoconstriction [47]. Hyperventilation should be avoided during electroencephalography. Adequate postoperative

Table 2. Summary of moyamoya recommendations in children.

◆ Various revascularization techniques reduce the stroke risk due to moyamoya disease.	IIb/B
◆ Indirect revascularization is preferred for children, whose small caliber vessels make direct anastomosis difficult, but direct bypass is preferable in older individuals.	IIb/B
◆ Indications for moyamoya revascularization include progressive ischemic symptoms or insufficient blood flow or cerebral perfusion reserve.	IIb/B
◆ Measurement of cerebral perfusion and blood flow reserve may assist in the evaluation and follow-up of individuals with moyamoya.	IV/C
◆ Transcranial Doppler may be useful in the evaluation and follow-up of individuals with moyamoya.	IV/C
◆ Aspirin may be useful after moyamoya revascularization or in asymptomatic individuals for whom surgery is not anticipated.	IV/C
◆ Avoiding hyperventilation and minimizing anxiety and pain during procedures may lower the risk of ischemic symptoms due to moyamoya.	IV/C
◆ Anticoagulation is not usually recommended for individuals with moyamoya disease.	IV/C

pain control and procedures to reduce the discomfort and anxiety related to venipuncture, dressing changes, suture removal, and other noxious stimuli may reduce the risk of ischemic symptoms and shorten the hospitalization [48] **(IV/C)**. Diagnostic and treatment recommendations for moyamoya disease are summarized in Table 2.

Cardiogenic embolism and stroke

About 20-25% of ischemic strokes in children result from emboli arising from the heart. Most congenital cardiac lesions that cause stroke are already known to exist before the stroke occurs, and complex congenital heart lesions with right-to-left shunting and cyanosis are more likely to cause stroke. As in adults, the stroke risk in children with a patent foramen ovale is still uncertain. Stroke is more common in individuals with uncorrected congenital heart lesions and in children with congestive heart failure. Surgical repair of the defect lowers but may not completely eliminate the stroke risk. Thromboembolic stroke may complicate cardiac catheterization or surgery.

Table 3. Recommendations for children at risk for stroke from heart disease.	
◆ Treatment of congestive heart failure and arrhythmia may lower the risk of cardiogenic embolism in children with congenital or acquired cardiac lesions.	IV/C
◆ Resection of an atrial myxoma is indicated given its substantial long-term risk of cerebrovascular complications.	IV/C
◆ Congenital heart lesions should be optimally corrected as soon as it is feasible both to improve cardiac function and to reduce the stroke risk.	IV/C
◆ For children with a cardiogenic embolism unrelated to a PFO who are judged to have a high recurrence risk, it is reasonable to initially introduce UFH or LMWH while warfarin therapy is initiated and adjusted.	IV/C
◆ As an alternative to warfarin conversion, it is reasonable to use long-term LMWH in patients with cardiogenic embolism.	IV/C
◆ For children with a suspected cardiac embolism (unrelated to a PFO) with an unknown or lower stroke risk, it is reasonable to begin aspirin and continue it for a year or even indefinitely.	IV/C
◆ In children with a risk of cardiogenic embolism, it is reasonable to continue either LMWH or warfarin until the responsible lesion has been corrected or indefinitely in individuals whose lesion cannot be corrected.	IV/C
◆ Surgical removal of a cardiac rhabdomyoma is not indicated in asymptomatic children without a prior stroke.	IV/C
◆ Anticoagulant therapy is not recommended for individuals with native valve endocarditis.	IV/C

Rheumatic heart disease occurs less often in developed countries because of widespread antibiotic use, but affected individuals with mitral stenosis have a 20% lifetime risk of systemic thromboembolism. Individuals with valvular heart disease or artificial valves have the added burden of infectious embolism related to endocarditis. Cardiomyopathy, myocardial infarction, and cardiac arrhythmia can promote cerebral embolism in children. Myocardial infarction is uncommon in children but occurs in individuals with polyarteritis nodosa, homozygous type II hyperlipoproteinemia, or Kawasaki disease. Cardiomyopathy has been documented with mitochondrial disorders, various forms of muscular dystrophy, Friedreich's ataxia, and Fabry's disease (alpha-galactosidase deficiency). Cardiac myxomas are uncommon in children but carry a significant embolism risk in affected individuals [49]. In contrast, cardiac rhabdomyomas occur in up to two thirds of children with tuberous sclerosis complex and occasionally as an isolated lesion, but few of these children develop a stroke [50].

There are few data to guide stroke prevention efforts in children with heart disease [1]. Treatment of congestive heart failure, cardiac arrhythmia, and endocarditis is advisable **(IV/C)**. The role of anticoagulant therapy in children with cardiac disease is unclear, but the consensus is to use these agents only in children who are judged to have a high risk of embolism [1] **(IV/C)**. Anticoagulation is not usually recommended for cardiac lesions complicated by endocarditis because of the risk of bleeding from infectious aneurysm formation **(IV/C)**. Optimal correction of structural cardiac anomalies probably lowers the long-term stroke risk, so early repair of such lesions should be considered when feasible **(IV/C)**. This recommendation does not yet apply to patent foramen ovale [1]. Surgical resection is recommended for children with atrial myxomas **(IV/C)** but not usually those with a typical cardiac rhabdomyoma. Table 3 summarizes recommendations for the care of children at risk for stroke due to heart disease.

Stroke due to arterial dissection

Cervicocephalic arterial dissection (CCAD) is probably under-recognized as a cause of stroke in children. Dissection accounted for stroke in 16 of 213 children (7.5%) in one series [51-53]. The recurrence rate of CCADs is estimated to be 1% per year [54]. However, young patients and individuals with a family history of arterial dissections seem to have a higher recurrence rate, as do individuals with specific CCAD risk factors such as fibromuscular dysplasia, coarctation of the aorta, or cystic medial necrosis.

Most dissections occur in the extracranial internal carotid artery, typically in its pharyngeal portion. However, children seem to have a higher frequency of intracranial dissection than do adults [55]. CCAD can occur spontaneously or after blunt or penetrating trauma. Intra-oral trauma after falling onto a popsicle stick or similar object is a well-recognized cause of internal carotid artery dissection. Children with a spontaneous CCAD have an underlying defect of the affected artery, as do many of the individuals who develop a dissection following a minor trauma. The diagnosis of CCAD can be made most reliably with catheter angiography (which variably shows a 'string sign', a double-lumen, or a short, tapered stenosis or occlusion of the artery) [55]. Increasingly, the diagnosis is made with computed tomographic angiography or high-resolution MRI.

Ischemic stroke can occur immediately after the CCAD, because of interruption of distal arterial flow without adequate collateral flow, or up to several months later, probably because of a distal embolism from the dissection site. In the absence of an effective agent to limit the damage from an acute infarction, therapy for CCAD aims to prevent stroke due to delayed embolism until the dissection site has healed or recanalized. In one consecutive cohort study, the risk of recurrent stroke or TIA in children with CCAD is 12% (2 of 16 children) [53]. Management of CCAD (Table 4) draws heavily on information gleaned from adult series, although these data are none too robust. The typical approach is immediate anticoagulation with intravenous unfractionated heparin (UFH) or low-molecular-weight heparin (LMWH) followed by a 3-6-month course of warfarin with a target International Normalized Ratio (INR) of 2-3 or continued LMWH [1]. Alternatively, it is acceptable to administer aspirin for 3-6 months or to convert to longer-term aspirin therapy following a course of warfarin or LMWH [1]. Children with an intracranial dissection should probably avoid anticoagulation due to the added risk of subarachnoid hemorrhage. Patients who do not respond to medical management sometimes benefit from proximal ligation of the dissected artery, trapping procedures, or extracranial-intracranial bypass procedures.

Table 4. Recommendations for CCAD in children.

◆ In children with extracranial CCAD, it is reasonable to begin either UFH or LMWH as a bridge to oral anticoagulation.	IV/C
◆ A child with an extracranial CCAD may be treated with either subcutaneous LMWH or warfarin for 3-6 months. Alternatively, aspirin may be substituted for anticoagulation.	IV/C
◆ Continuing anticoagulant therapy beyond 6 months is reasonable for individuals who have recurrent symptoms.	IV/C
◆ Antiplatelet agents may be continued beyond 6 months, especially when there are symptoms or radiographic evidence of a residual abnormality of the dissected artery.	IV/C
◆ Anticoagulation is not recommended for children with an intracranial dissection or those with a subarachnoid hemorrhage CCAD.	IV/C

Drug treatments for stroke in children

Antiplatelet agents

Aspirin is often recommended for children to prevent recurrent stroke or TIA, but there is little age-specific information to support efficacy or on which to base dosing recommendations [1] **(IV/C)**. An aspirin dose of 3-5mg/kg per day is commonly recommended for prevention of stroke in children, with a dose reduction of 1-3mg/kg in the event of gastric distress, frequent or prolonged epistaxis, or other concerns. Retrospective case series suggest that aspirin is reasonably safe in children at the usually recommended doses. No major complications occurred among 49 children with arterial ischemic stroke who were treated with 2-5mg/kg of aspirin each day for 36 months [56]. Aspirin may exacerbate the symptoms of asthma. There have been no reports of Reye's syndrome in children taking the aspirin for stroke prevention, but given the increased threat of Reye's syndrome after influenza and varicella, it is reasonable to vaccinate for these infections and to cease using aspirin during suspected influenza or varicella infections [1] **(IV/C)**.

Although aspirin is often recommended, the data supporting its efficacy in children at risk for stroke are sparse. Non-randomized studies show little difference in the stroke or TIA recurrence rate in children taking aspirin versus those given anticoagulants, although these same studies also hint that either agent may be slightly superior to continued observation without medication [56-58]. Based on these studies, the robust data showing that aspirin is helpful for prevention of some types of infarction in adults, and its relative safety in children, aspirin use is reasonable in children with acute ischemic stroke due to vasculopathy, arterial dissection, and other chronic risk factors that do not require the use of anticoagulation. Aspirin therapy is typically suggested for 3-5 years or even longer in children believed to remain at risk for recurrent stroke. This recommendation is also based largely on an expert consensus [1].

There is even less information about the use of other antiplatelet agents in children. There are inadequate data on the safety or efficacy in children of clopidogrel, ticlopidine, or the combination of low-dose aspirin plus extended-release dipyridamole. Occasional reports document the use of clopidogrel (at about 1mg/kg per day) in children. Two children developed a subdural hemorrhage while taking both aspirin and clopidogrel [59]. Table 5 summarizes the recommendations for various drugs used in the treatment of stroke in children.

Table 5. Summary of recommendations for drug therapy of childhood stroke.	
◆ Aspirin may be considered for secondary prevention of ischemic stroke in children whose infarction is not due to SCD and in individuals without a high risk of recurrent embolism or a severe hypercoagulable disorder.	IV/C
◆ In children taking aspirin for stroke prevention, it is reasonable to vaccinate for varicella and to administer an annual influenza vaccine in an effort to reduce the risk of Reye's syndrome.	IV/C
◆ UFH or LMWH may be used in children for up to a week after an ischemic stroke during the evaluation to determine the stroke's cause.	IV/C
◆ Anticoagulation with warfarin or LMWH is reasonable for the long-term treatment of children with a substantial risk of recurrent cardiac embolism, arterial dissection, or a severe hypercoagulable state.	IV/C
◆ It is reasonable to consider rt-PA administration in older children and adolescents provided that the adult exclusion guidelines are strictly followed.	IV/C

Heparin and unfractionated heparin

Short-term anticoagulation with unfractionated heparin (UFH) or low-molecular-weight heparin (LMWH) is sometimes begun in children after acute ischemic stroke pending evaluation of the etiology of the stroke [1]. Although acute anticoagulation with heparin is ineffective in most elderly stroke patients, some physicians argue that children have a greater likelihood of having an underlying risk factor that might benefit from anticoagulation than older adults, such as arterial dissection, vasculopathy, undiagnosed cardiac disease, or a hypercoagulable state. It can take a few days to rule out these conditions, so it is acceptable to consider giving heparin or LMWH until the reasons for longer-term anticoagulation have been eliminated [1] (IV/C). Although this approach is acceptable based on a consensus of experts, there is insufficient objective evidence to mandate it.

When a reason to continue anticoagulation for several weeks or months is discovered, the patient either continues to receive LMWH or is converted to warfarin. Both warfarin and LMWH have advantages and disadvantages. Warfarin is much cheaper and is often better accepted by children and their parents because it is given orally. LMWH provides predictable pharmacokinetics and requires less frequent monitoring than unfractionated heparin [60].

However, the effects of LMWH cannot be rapidly and completely reversed with protamine sulphate or fresh frozen plasma, a potential problem in situations where acute anticoagulation may need to be rapidly reversed. Although there is no proof of a therapeutic benefit for either LMWH or unfractionated heparin in acute ischemic stroke in children, there are data supporting the safety of these agents in children with cerebrovascular disease [56, 61, 62].

Children are given 1mg/kg of LMWH subcutaneously every 12 hours. However, neonates typically require a dose of 1.5mg/kg every 12 hours [60]. Anti-factor Xa levels reflect the treatment effect (the therapeutic range for anti-factor Xa levels is 0.5-1.0U/mL in a sample drawn 4-6 hours after the dose). Once a therapeutic level is achieved, anti-factor Xa level testing is usually done weekly at first and 3-4 weeks longer-term in uncomplicated individuals.

Warfarin

Age-specific data on the effectiveness or optimal dosing of warfarin for the treatment of cerebrovascular disease in children are sparse. In adults with arterial stroke, warfarin provides no advantage over aspirin except for the prevention of cardiogenic embolism. Warfarin is typically utilized in children who need prolonged anticoagulation, although LMWH by subcutaneous injection is sometimes used instead in these children (IV/C). Long-term warfarin administration is reasonable in children with a substantial risk of cardiogenic embolism, in individuals with a cervical arterial dissection, and in patients with a severe hypercoagulable state [1] (IV/C). Some physicians avoid anticoagulation in individuals with a large brain infarction and those with a history of gastrointestinal bleeding. Anticoagulation may also be more challenging in small children and others who may be prone to frequent falls. The likelihood of a major hemorrhagic complication is <3.2% per patient-year in children receiving warfarin for mechanical heart valves [63]. The risk of hemorrhagic complications has not been established for children receiving warfarin for stroke prevention. With long-term warfarin use, monitoring for bone demineralization may be appropriate [63].

The suggested International Normalized Ratio (INR) in children of 2-3 is based primarily on data from adults with stroke and children with systemic thromboses. The warfarin dosage required to achieve and maintain this INR is based largely on clinical experience. Michelson and colleagues recommend a starting warfarin dose of 0.2mg/kg for 2 days followed by a half this amount for another 2 days with further adjustments determined by the child's INR [64]. Breast milk contains low and potentially variable levels of vitamin K, making accurate dosing of warfarin more difficult in breast-fed infants [1].

Thrombolytic agents

Several case reports document the use of recombinant tissue plasminogen activator (rt-PA) in children with ischemic stroke [65-68]. However, safety and efficacy data for rt-PA in children are largely lacking, both for intravenous or intra-arterial use [69]. It has been suggested that rt-PA effectively dissolves the clot but causes more complications in children than in adults. One report noted that 85% of the 80 children treated with rt-PA had complete or partial clot dissolution, but 70% of the children had complications, 40% of them described as major [70]. Some of the published reports document administration of rt-PA well after the time interval usually recommended in adult stroke patients, and the likelihood of hemorrhagic complications also increases in adults when the drug is administered late.

A consensus panel recommended that rt-PA might be reasonable in older children and adolescents provided that the adult exclusion guidelines were strictly followed in the children [1] **(IV/C)**. These time limitations pose a serious obstacle to the use of rt-PA in children because the diagnosis of stroke is frequently delayed in children [71, 72]. This same consensus group suggested that rt-PA be administered to smaller children only in the context of a clinical trial. Some physicians feel that a lower rt-PA dose might be effective in children and that the lower dose might improve the drug's safety [73]. As is evident from this discussion, there are few age-specific data confirming either the safety or efficacy of rt-PA for acute ischemic stroke in children. However, a multicenter trial is planned that should begin to clarify some of these questions [74].

Conclusions

Few controlled clinical trials have focused on the diagnosis and management of stroke in children, and, except in a few situations, recommendations for these individuals are based largely on expert consensus. Several trials have been completed or are underway in children with sickle cell disease, and the use of TCD to assess stroke risk in these children and the use of periodic red cell transfusions for both primary and secondary stroke prevention are now accepted. Multiple large case series collected over several decades allow reasonably precise recommendations in favor of various revascularization techniques in selected individuals with moyamoya disease. Large cohort series of children with ischemic stroke suggest that drugs such as heparin, LMWH, and aspirin are reasonably safe in children at risk for stroke, although the current data are insufficient to completely establish efficacy of any of these agents in children. Expert consensus based on clinical experience, published case series, and extrapolation from adult clinical trials suggest that these drugs may be used in selected children with cerebrovascular dysfunction.

Key points	Evidence level
♦ It is appropriate to monitor children with SCD with periodic TCD.	IIb/B
♦ Children with SCD and a confirmed cerebral infarction should begin regular red cell transfusions to reduce the percentage of sickle hemoglobin.	III/B
♦ Periodic transfusions to reduce the percentage of sickle hemoglobin are recommended for children with persistently abnormal TCD results.	Ib/A
♦ Hydroxyurea may be considered in individuals with a high stroke risk due to SCD who cannot maintain a long-term transfusion program.	IIb/B
♦ Indirect revascularization is preferred for children with moyamoya disease because their small caliber vessels make direct anastomosis difficult. Direct bypass is preferable in older individuals.	IIb/B
♦ Measurement of cerebral perfusion and blood flow reserve may assist in the evaluation and follow-up of individuals with moyamoya disease.	IV/C
♦ Anticoagulation is not usually recommended for individuals with moyamoya disease.	IV/C
♦ Resection of an atrial myxoma is indicated given its substantial long-term risk of cerebrovascular complications.	IV/C
♦ Congenital heart lesions should be optimally corrected as soon as it is feasible both to improve cardiac function and to reduce the stroke risk.	IV/C
♦ For children with a cardiogenic embolism unrelated to a PFO who are judged to have a high recurrence risk, it is reasonable to initially introduce UFH or LMWH while warfarin therapy is initiated and adjusted.	IV/C
♦ As an alternative to warfarin conversion, it is reasonable to use long-term LMWH in patients with cardiogenic embolism.	IV/C
♦ For children with a suspected cardiac embolism (unrelated to a PFO) with an unknown or lower stroke risk, it is reasonable to begin aspirin and continue it for a year or even indefinitely.	IV/C
♦ In children with a risk of cardiogenic embolism, it is reasonable to continue either LMWH or warfarin until the responsible lesion has been corrected or indefinitely in individuals whose lesion can not be corrected.	IV/C
♦ Aspirin may be considered for secondary prevention of ischemic stroke in children whose infarction is not due to SCD and in individuals without a high risk of recurrent embolism or a severe hypercoagulable disorder.	IV/C
♦ Anticoagulation with warfarin or LMWH is reasonable for the long-term treatment of children with a substantial risk of recurrent cardiac embolism, arterial dissection, or a severe hypercoagulable state.	IV/C
♦ It is reasonable to consider rt-PA administration in older children and adolescents provided that the adult exclusion guidelines are strictly followed.	IV/C

References

1. Roach ES, Golomb MR, Adams RJ, *et al*. Management of stroke in infants and children. A scientific statement for healthcare professionals from a special writing group of the Stroke Council, American Heart Association. *Stroke* 2008; 39: 2644-91.

2. Roach ES. Etiology of stroke in children. *Semin Pediatr Neurol* 2000; 7: 244-60.

3. Earley CJ, Kittner SJ, Feeser BR, *et al*. Stroke in children and sickle-cell disease: Baltimore-Washington Cooperative Young Stroke Study. *Neurology* 1998; 51: 169-76.

4. Ohene-Frempong K, Weiner SJ, Sleeper LA, *et al*. Cerebrovascular accidents in sickle cell disease: rates and risk factors. *Blood* 1998; 91: 288-94.

5. Pegelow CH, Macklin EA, Moser FG, *et al*. Longitudinal changes in brain magnetic resonance imaging findings in children with sickle cell disease. *Blood* 2002; 99: 3014-8.

6. Wang WC. Central nervous system complications of sickle cell disease in children: an overview. *Child Neuropsychol* 2007; 13: 103-19.

7. Adams RJ, Nichols FT, Figueroa R, McKie V, Lott T. Transcranial Doppler correlation with cerebral angiography in sickle cell disease. *Stroke* 1992; 23: 1073-7.

8. Adams RJ, McKie VC, Brambilla D, *et al*. Stroke Prevention Trial in Sickle Cell Anemia. *Control Clin Trials* 1998; 19: 110-29.

9. Adams RJ, Brambilla DJ, Granger S, *et al*. Stroke and conversion to high risk in children screened with transcranial Doppler ultrasound during the STOP study. *Blood* 2004; 103: 3689-94.

10. Armstrong-Wells J, Grimes B, Sidney S, *et al*. Utilization of TCD screening for primary stroke prevention in children with sickle cell disease. *Neurology* 2009; 72: 1316-21.

11. Wang WC. The pathophysiology, prevention, and treatment of stroke in sickle cell disease. *Curr Opin Hematol* 2007; 14: 191-7.

12. Pegelow CH, Adams RJ, McKie V, *et al*. Risk of recurrent stroke in patients with sickle cell disease treated with erythrocyte transfusions. *J Pediatr* 1995; 126: 896-9.

13. Scothorn DJ, Price C, Schwartz D, *et al*. Risk of recurrent stroke in children with sickle cell disease receiving blood transfusion therapy for at least five years after initial stroke. *J Pediatr* 2002; 140: 348-54.

14. Adams RJ, Brambilla D. Discontinuing prophylactic transfusions used to prevent stroke in sickle cell disease. *N Engl J Med* 2005; 353: 2769-78.

15. Charache S, Terrin ML, Moore RD, *et al*. Effect of hydroxyurea on the frequency of painful crises in sickle cell anemia. *N Engl J Med* 1995; 332: 1317-22.

16. Gulbis B, Haberman D, Dufour D, *et al*. Hydroxyurea for sickle cell disease in children and for prevention of cerebrovascular events: the Belgian experience. *Blood* 2005; 105: 2685-90.

17. Ware RE, Zimmerman SA, Sylvestre PB, *et al*. Prevention of secondary stroke and resolution of transfusional iron overload in children with sickle cell anemia using hydroxyurea and phlebotomy. *J Pediatr* 2004; 145: 346-52.

18. Aygun B, McMurray MA, Schultz WH, *et al*. Chronic transfusion practice for children with sickle cell anaemia and stroke. *Br J Haematol* 2009; 145: 524-8.

19. Walters MC, Storb R, Patience M, *et al*. Impact of bone marrow transplantation for symptomatic sickle cell disease: an interim report. Multicenter investigation of bone marrow transplantation for sickle cell disease. *Blood* 2000; 95: 1918-24.

20. Vernet O, Montes JL, O'Gorman AM, Baruchel S, Farmer J-P. Encephaloduroarteriosynangiosis in a child with sickle cell anemia and moyamoya disease. *Pediatr Neurol* 1996; 14: 226-30.

21. Fryer RH, Anderson RC, Chiriboga CA, Feldstein NA. Sickle cell anemia with moyamoya disease: outcomes after EDAS procedure. *Pediatr Neurol* 2003; 29: 124-30.

22. Uchino K, Johnston SC, Becker KJ, Tirschwell DL. Moyamoya disease in Washington State and California. *Neurology* 2005; 65: 956-8.

23. Ikezaki K, Han DH, Kawano T, Inamura T, Fukui M. Epidemiological survey of moyamoya disease in Korea. *Clin Neurol Neurosurg* 1997; 99 Suppl 2: S6-10.

24. Yamauchi T, Houkin K, Tada M, Abe H. Familial occurrence of moyamoya disease. *Clin Neurol Neurosurg* 1997; 99 Suppl 2: S162-7.

25. Scott RM, Smith JL, Robertson RL, Madsen JR, Soriano SG, Rockoff MA. Long-term outcome in children with moyamoya syndrome after cranial revascularization by pial synangiosis. *J Neurosurg* 2004; 100: 142-9.

26. Ikeda H, Sasaki T, Yoshimoto T, Fukui M, Arinami T. Mapping of a familial moyamoya disease gene to chromosome 3p24.2-p26. *Am J Hum Genet* 1999; 64: 533-7.

27. Yamauchi T, Tada M, Houkin K, *et al*. Linkage of familial moyamoya disease (spontaneous occlusion of the circle of Willis) to chromosome 17q25. *Stroke* 2000; 31: 930-5.

28. Inoue TK, Ikezaki K, Sasazuki T, Matsushima T, Fukui M. Linkage analysis of moyamoya disease on chromosome 6. *J Child Neurol* 2000; 15: 179-82.

29. Han DH, Kwon OK, Byun BJ, *et al*. A co-operative study: clinical characteristics of 334 Korean patients with moyamoya disease treated at neurosurgical institutes (1976-1994). The Korean Society for Cerebrovascular Disease. *Acta Neurochir* (Wien) 2000; 142: 1263-73.

30. Yonekawa Y, Kahn N. Moyamoya disease. *Adv Neurol* 2003; 92: 113-8.

31. Moritake K, Handa H, Yonekawa Y, Taki W, Okuno T. [Follow-up study on the relationship between age at onset of illness and outcome in patients with moyamoya disease]. *No Shinkei Geka* 1986; 14: 957-63.

32. Yilmaz EY, Pritz MB, Bruno A, Lopez-Yunez A, Biller J. Moyamoya: Indiana University Medical Center experience. *Arch Neurol* 2001; 58: 1274-8.

33. Yamada I, Nakagawa T, Matsushima Y, Shibuya H. High-resolution turbo magnetic resonance angiography for diagnosis of moyamoya disease. *Stroke* 2001; 32: 1825-31.

34. Yamada I, Suzuki S, Matsushima Y. Moyamoya disease: diagnostic accuracy of MRI. *Neurorad* 1995; 37: 356-61.

35. Yamada I, Suzuki S, Matsushima Y. Moyamoya disease: comparison of assessment with MR angiography and MR imaging versus conventional angiography. *Radiology* 1995; 196: 211-8.

36. Takase K, Kashihara M, Hashimoto T. Transcranial Doppler ultrasonography in patients with moyamoya disease. *Clin Neurol Neurosurg* 1997; 99 Suppl 2: S101-5.

37. Morgenstern C, Griewing B, Muller-Esch G, Zeller JA, Kessler C. Transcranial power-mode duplex ultrasound in two patients with moyamoya syndrome. *J Neuroimaging* 1997; 7: 190-2.

38. Tanaka Y, Nariai T, Nagaoka T, *et al*. Quantitative evaluation of cerebral hemodynamics in patients with moyamoya disease by dynamic susceptibility contrast magnetic resonance imaging - comparison with positron emission tomography. *J Cereb Blood Flow Metab* 2006; 26: 291-300.

39. Ikezaki K, Matsushima T, Kuwabara Y, Suzuki SO, Nomura T, Fukui M. Cerebral circulation and oxygen metabolism in childhood moyamoya disease: a perioperative positron emission tomography study. *J Neurosurg* 1994; 81: 843-50.

40. Fung LW, Thompson D, Ganesan V. Revascularisation surgery for paediatric moyamoya: a review of the literature. *Childs Nerv Syst* 2005; 21: 358-64.

41. Matsushima T, Inoue T, Suzuki SO, Fujii K, Fukui M, Hasuo K. Surgical treatment of moyamoya disease in pediatric patients - comparison between the results of indirect and direct revascularization procedures. *Neurosurgery* 1992; 31: 401-5.

42. Matsushima T, Inoue T, Katsuta T, *et al*. An indirect revascularization method in the surgical treatment of moyamoya disease - various kinds of indirect procedures and a multiple combined indirect procedure. *Neurol Med Chir* (Tokyo) 1998; 38 Suppl: 297-302.

43. Choi JU, Kim DS, Kim EY, Lee KC. Natural history of moyamoya disease: comparison of activity of daily living in surgery and non-surgery groups. *Clin Neurol Neurosurg* 1997; 99 Suppl 2: S11-8.

44. Fukui M. Current state of study on moyamoya disease in Japan. *Surg Neurol* 1997; 47: 138-43.

45. Ikezaki K. A rational approach to treatment of moyamoya disease in childhood. *J Child Neurol* 2000; 15: 350-6.

46. Bowen MD, Burak CR, Barron TF. Childhood ischemic stroke in a nonurban population. *J Child Neurol* 2005; 20: 194-7.

47. Kim HY, Chung CS, Lee J, Han DH, Lee KH. Hyperventilation-induced limb shaking TIA in moyamoya disease. *Neurology* 2003; 60: 137-9.

48. Nomura S, Kashiwagi S, Uetsuka S, Uchida T, Kubota H, Ito H. Perioperative management protocols for children with moyamoya disease. *Childs Nerv Syst* 2001; 17: 270-4.

49. Al-Mateen M, Hood M, Trippel D, Insalaco SJ, Otto RK, Vitikainen KJ. Cerebral embolism from atrial myxoma in pediatric patients. *Pediatrics* 2003; 112: e162-7.

50. Kandt RS, Gebarski SS, Goetting MG. Tuberous sclerosis with cardiogenic cerebral embolism: magnetic resonance imaging. *Neurology* 1985; 35: 1223-5.

51. Fullerton HJ, Johnston SC, Smith WS. Arterial dissection and stroke in children. *Neurology* 2001; 57: 1155-60.

52. Chabrier S, Lasjaunias P, Husson B, Landrieu P, Tardieu M. Ischaemic stroke from dissection of the craniocervical arteries in childhood: report of 12 patients. *Eur J Paediatr Neurol* 2003; 7: 39-42.

53. Rafay MF, Armstrong D, deVeber G, Domi T, Chan A, MacGregor DL. Craniocervical arterial dissection in children: clinical and radiographic presentation and outcome. *J Child Neurol* 2006; 21: 8-16.

54. Touze E, Gauvrit JY, Moulin T, Meder JF, Bracard S, Mas JL. Risk of stroke and recurrent dissection after a cervical artery dissection: a multicenter study. *Neurology* 2003; 61: 1347-51.

55. Schievink WI, Mokri B, Piepgras DG. Spontaneous dissections of the cervicocephalic arteries in childhood and adolescence. *Neurology* 1994; 44: 1607-12.

56. Strater R, Kurnik K, Heller C, Schobess R, Luigs P, Nowak-Gottl U. Aspirin versus low-dose low-molecular-weight heparin: antithrombotic therapy in pediatric ischemic stroke patients: a prospective follow-up study. *Stroke* 2001; 32: 2554-8.

57. Ganesan V, Prengler M, Wade A, Kirkham FJ. Clinical and radiological recurrence after childhood arterial ischemic stroke. *Circulation* 2006; 114: 2170-7.

58. Lanthier S, Kirkham FJ, Mitchell LG, et al. Increased anticardiolipin antibody IgG titers do not predict recurrent stroke or TIA in children. *Neurology* 2004; 62: 194-200.

59. Soman T, Rafay MF, Hune S, Allen A, MacGregor D, deVeber G. The risks and safety of clopidogrel in pediatric arterial ischemic stroke. *Stroke* 2006; 37: 1120-2.

60. Massicotte P, Adams M, Marzinotto V, Brooker LA, Andrew M. Low-molecular-weight heparin in pediatric patients with thrombotic disease: a dose finding study. *J Pediatr* 1996; 128: 313-8.

61. deVeber G, Andrew M, Adams C, et al. Cerebral sinovenous thrombosis in children. *N Engl J Med* 2001; 345: 417-23.

62. Burak CR, Bowen MD, Barron TF. The use of enoxaparin in children with acute, nonhemorrhagic ischemic stroke. *Pediatr Neurol* 2003; 29: 295-8.

63. Monagle P, Chan A, Massicotte P, Chalmers E, Michelson AD. Antithrombotic therapy in children: the Seventh ACCP Conference on Antithrombotic and Thrombolytic Therapy. *Chest* 2004;126: 645S-87.

64. Michelson AD, Bovill E, Andrew M. Antithrombotic therapy in children. *Chest* 1995; 108: 506S-22.

65. Kirton A, Wong JH, Mah J, et al. Successful endovascular therapy for acute basilar thrombosis in an adolescent. *Pediatrics* 2003; 112: e248-51.

66. Carlson MD, Leber S, Deveikis J, Silverstein FS. Successful use of rt-PA in pediatric stroke. *Neurology* 2001; 57: 157-8.

67. Thirumalai SS, Shubin RA. Successful treatment for stroke in a child using recombinant tissue plasminogen activator. *J Child Neurol* 2000; 15: 558.

68. Benedict SL, Ni OK, Schloesser P, White KS, Bale JF, Jr. Intra-arterial thrombolysis in a 2-year-old with cardioembolic stroke. *J Child Neurol* 2007; 22: 225-7.

69. Amlie-Lefond C, Fullerton HJ. Thrombolytics for hyperacute stroke in children. *Pediatr Hematol Oncol* 2009; 26: 103-7.

70. Gupta AA, Leaker M, Andrew M, et al. Safety and outcomes of thrombolysis with tissue plasminogen activator for treatment of intravascular thrombosis in children. *J Pediatr* 2001; 139: 682-8.

71. Gabis LV, Yangala R, Lenn NJ. Time lag to diagnosis of stroke in children. *Pediatrics* 2002; 110: 924-8.

72. Rafay MF, Pontigon AM, Chiang J, et al. Delay to diagnosis in acute pediatric arterial ischemic stroke. *Stroke* 2009; 40: 58-64.

73. Wang M, Hays T, Balasa V, et al. Low-dose tissue plasminogen activator thrombolysis in children. *J Pediatr Hematol Oncol* 2003; 25: 379-86.

74. Amlie-Lefond C, Chan AK, Kirton A, et al. Thrombolysis in acute childhood stroke: design and challenges of the thrombolysis in pediatric stroke clinical trial. *Neuroepidemiology* 2009; 32: 279-86.

Chapter 12

Stroke in pregnancy and puerperium

Rima M. Dafer MD MPH FAHA
Associate Professor of Neurology
Loyola University Chicago
Stritch School of Medicine
Maywood, Illinois, USA

Introduction

Stroke during pregnancy and puerperium is a rare but potentially devastating cause of perinatal morbidity and mortality. The majority of pregnancy-related stroke are ischemic, often occurring in the third trimester, during delivery, or puerperium. Predisposing factors include normal physiologic hemodynamic changes associated with pregnancy, combined with pathophysiologic processes unique to pregnancy, hormonally mediated damage to vascular tissue structure and a hypercoagulable state. The incidence of stroke during pregnancy and puerperium ranges from 4.3-69 per 100,000 deliveries. Stroke contributes to >12% of all maternal deaths. For intracerebral hemorrhage, the adjusted relative risk is 2.5 during pregnancy, and 28.3 in the postpartum period. Intracranial hemorrhages secondary to ruptured cerebral aneurysm or arteriovenous malformation (AVM) account for 5-12% of maternal mortality [1-3].

Ischemic stroke

Arterial hypertension, cardiovascular diseases, and thromboembolic complications are the most common non-obstetrical causes of maternal death. The increased risk of ischemic stroke is attributed to the physiologic hemodynamic changes occurring during pregnancy, change in cardiac output, volume overload, and peripheral arterial resistance. During pregnancy, there is a marked increase in intravascular volume which peaks in the third trimester, with a 30-40% increase in cardiac output, and a 15% increase in heart rate. Most pregnancy-related strokes are ischemic, often occurring in the third trimester, during delivery or puerperium. While most ischemic strokes are due to arterial occlusion, cardioembolic strokes are not uncommon, especially among patients with preexisting cardiomyopathy, valvulopathy, or cardiac arrhythmias. Specific changes contributing to stroke during pregnancy are related to arterial hypertension in patients with pre-eclampsia and eclampsia, paradoxical embolism, peripartum or postpartum cerebral angiopathy, peripartum cardiomyopathy (PPCM), cerebral dural venous sinus thrombosis (CDVST), and, rarely, choriocarcinoma (Table 1). In addition, the hypercoagulability state of pregnancy predisposes to both arterial and venous thromboembolism [1-5].

Table 1. Etiology of pregnancy-related stroke.

Ischemic	Hemorrhagic
Occlusive arterial disease	*Intraparenchymal hemorrhage*
Peripartum cardiomyopathy	Eclampsia
Atrial fibrillation	Arterial hypertension
Prosthetic heart valves	Choriocarcinoma
Infective and NBT endocarditis	Ruptured vascular malformation
Rheumatic heart disease	CDVST
Paradoxical embolism/PFO	*Subarachnoid hemorrhage*
Arterial hypotension	Aneurysm
Border zone infarction	AVM
Sheehan's syndrome	DIC
Others	
Amniotic fluid embolism	
Hematologic disorders (SCD, DIC, TTP, ITP)	

AVM = arteriovenous malformation; CDVST = cerebral dural venous sinus thrombosis; DIC = disseminated intravascular coagulation; ITP = idiopathic thrombocytopenic purpura; NBT = non-bacterial thrombotic; PFO = patent foramen ovale; SCD = sickle cell disease; TTP = thrombotic thrombocytopenic purpura

The occurrence of cardiac arrhythmias is increased during labor and delivery, mainly due to hemodynamic and electrophysiological changes of pregnancy [6-9]. Although most cardiac arrhythmias often do not require pharmacological treatment, high-risk arrhythmias such as atrial fibrillation, ventricular arrhythmias, and heart block pose a therapeutic challenge. Pharmacotherapy of cardiac arrhythmias in pregnant women is limited by fetal side effects. A multidisciplinary approach with collaboration between cardiologists and obstetricians is essential for good maternal and neonatal outcomes.

Patients with pre-existing cardiovascular abnormalities are at higher risk of stroke during pregnancy, with cardiovascular abnormalities being the first leading non-obstetric cause of morbidity and mortality during pregnancy. These include rheumatic heart disease, congenital cardiac anomalies, coronary artery disease, ischemic and dilated cardiomyopathies, pulmonary hypertension, and cardiac arrhythmias. Although pregnancy is well tolerated by most patients with cardiac conditions, the risk is greater in patients with severe cardiac dysfunction, pulmonary hypertension, cyanotic congenital heart disease, prosthetic valvular heart disease, and severe obstructive left-sided heart lesions.

Pregnant women with cardiac valvulopathies represent a unique patient group with increased risk for adverse fetal and maternal outcomes. Management of a pregnant woman with non-valvular heart disease presents a unique challenge to the anesthesiologist during labor and delivery. Intervention is of utmost importance in high-risk women, and percutaneous intervention or repair may be considered before a planned pregnancy. Mitral valve prolapse is present in 12-17% of young women of reproductive age [10-12]. The presence of a mechanical cardiac valve prosthesis is challenging to obstetrician and cardiologist, due to an increased risk of infective endocarditis, cardiac arrhythmias, valvular thrombosis and systemic embolization, in particular when anticoagulation is interrupted during pregnancy and delivery. The presence of valvular heart disease does not affect the course of pregnancy and is not a factor in the decision of mode of delivery [13-16]. Despite recent data showing that induction of labor after the 37th week of gestation in pregnant women with hypertension and mild pre-eclampsia is associated with improved maternal outcome, timing and mode of delivery should be decided upon jointly by the obstetrician, cardiologist, and anesthesiologist [17, 18].

There are no specific recommendations for the management of cardiac valvulopathy during labor and delivery. Most valvular heart diseases may be managed medically during pregnancy. In rare situations where patients become symptomatic, intervention with balloon-valvuloplasty or valve replacement may become a necessity. Valve replacement is best undertaken during the second trimester, with special care taken to maintain the blood pressure during cardiopulmonary bypass, and to avoid hypothermia due to substantial risk for the fetus [19].

Pregnancy carries no additional risk for infective endocarditis and prophylaxis is not routinely recommended in patients with valvular heart disease undergoing uncomplicated vaginal delivery or Caesarean section. Antibiotics should be considered in high-risk patients with prosthetic heart valves, a previous history of infective endocarditis, or in the setting of another systemic infection [19, 20] **(IIb/B)**.

Acute coronary syndrome (ACS) is a rare but potentially fatal cardiac complication in pregnant women. Risk factors include pre-eclampsia, older age, multiparity, pregnancy-associated coagulopathy, in addition to the pre-existing vascular risks. Management of ACS is similar to the therapeutic recommendations of non-pregnant women. While urgent reperfusion therapy remains the goal, limited data are available on therapeutic intervention in pregnant women. Beta-blockers may be used during pregnancy, with careful monitoring of fetal bradycardia and apnea at birth [21, 22] (IIa/B). Angiotensin-converting enzyme (ACE) inhibitors and angiotensin receptor antagonists are teratogenic and thus contraindicated in pregnancy [23, 24] (IV/C). There are insufficient data to determine the safety of statin use in pregnancy, although its use has been associated with an increased risk of birth defects [25, 26]. Limited data exist on the safety of thienopyridine derivatives during pregnancy and breastfeeding, thus they are better avoided during pregnancy (IV/C). Aspirin and heparin use is preferred [27]. Recommendations for the use of aspirin and heparin products are discussed later on in this chapter under primary and secondary stroke prevention.

A patent foramen ovale (PFO), especially when present in combination with an atrial septal aneurysm, confers an increased risk of paradoxical embolism and cryptogenic stroke, particularly in the setting of pregnancy-induced hypercoagulable state [28-31]. Management of stroke in the setting of PFO remains controversial. Percutaneous PFO closure has been safely performed in selected patients with recurrent strokes due to paradoxical embolism during pregnancy [32, 33] (IV/C). In the absence of recommendations or guidelines, options include medical therapy with antiplatelets or anticoagulants, or surgical intervention with percutaneous device closure or surgical repair. The American Heart Association/American Stroke Association strongly encourages referral of patients with PFO and cryptogenic strokes for enrollment in ongoing prospective randomized clinical trials [34].

Pregnancy-related conditions often complicated by stroke include CDVST, postpartum cerebral angiopathy (PPCA), ovarian hyperstimulation syndrome (OHS), and amniotic fluid embolism (AFE).

PPCM is a relatively uncommon life-threatening idiopathic pregnancy-related congestive cardiomyopathy, afflicting previously healthy women in the peripartum period. Patients develop symptoms of left ventricular heart failure in the last trimester of pregnancy or in the first 5 months following delivery. The incidence of PPCM is reported at 1 in 1000 to 1 in 15,000 pregnancies. PPCM is more common among women in the third decade of life, multiparous, with twin pregnancies, African-Americans, and in patients with pregnancy-associated hypertensive disorders such as pre-eclampsia or gestational hypertension [35-40]. The etiology of PPCM remains unclear; viral and autoimmune causes have been implicated. Previously healthy patients usually present with cardiac arrhythmias and heart failure secondary to dilated cardiomyopathy. Early diagnosis and treatment are essential to prevent irreversible cardiac injury. Management of PPCM is based on observational studies, and is directed at optimization of maternal hemodynamics and prevention of thromboembolism. It consists of the administration of loop diuretics, vasodilators, digoxin and β-blockers, sodium restriction, and treatment of symptomatic cardiac arrhythmias. PPCM carries a favorable prognosis, with 50% achieving full recovery. The mortality rate is often due to embolism and is estimated at 1-2%.

CDVST is more common during pregnancy and puerperium due to hemodynamic changes, anemia, and hypercoagulability associated with pregnancy [41]. The incidence of CDVST is 10-20 per 100,000 deliveries in western countries [42, 43]. Patients present with severe headaches, seizures, and focal neurological signs [42, 44, 45]. Diagnosis is often confirmed with cranial computed tomography (CCT) with contrast CT venography, or brain magnetic resonance imaging (MRI) with MR venography. Early administration of weight-adjusted subcutaneous low-molecular-weight heparin (LMWH) or dose-adjusted intravenous unfractionated heparin (UFH) may improve outcome **(IIb/B)**. Concomitant intracranial hemorrhage related to CDVST is not a contraindication for heparin therapy. Based upon limited evidence available, anticoagulant treatment for CDVST appears to be safe and is associated with a potentially important reduction in the risk of death or dependency which did not reach statistical significance [46-52].

Postpartum cerebral angiopathy (PPCA) is a rare cause of ischemic and hemorrhagic strokes in the puerperium. It is clinically characterized by thunderclap headache, seizures, altered consciousness, and focal neurologic deficits, and angiographically by reversible segmental cerebral vasoconstriction. PPCA is more common after use of vasoconstrictive agents, and has been reported in migraineurs following the use of triptans and ergot alkaloids [53-55]. Steroid therapy may improve symptoms. Calcium channel blockers, verapamil and nimodipine, may be used for symptomatic vasospasm **(IV/C)**.

Ovarian hyperstimulation syndrome (OHS) is a serious complication of fertility medications associated with thromboembolism, multiorgan failure, including renal insufficiency, liver dysfunction, adult respiratory distress syndrome, fluid overload, stroke, and death.

Amniotic fluid embolism (AFE) remains a common cause of maternal death. The incidence of AFE is estimated at 1:15,000 to 1:80,000 deliveries in the Western countries. Risk is increased with advanced maternal age, placental abnormalities, operative deliveries, eclampsia, poly-hydramnios, cervical lacerations, and uterine rupture. Patients may present with pulmonary hypertension and right ventricular failure, left ventricular failure, disseminated intravascular coagulation, or hemorrhage [38, 40, 56-60]. AFE is caused by embolization into the maternal circulation of amniotic fluid debris intrapartum or during the early postpartum [53-57]. Promising therapies include early recognition of the disorder, adequate oxygenation, selective pulmonary vasodilators, correction of coagulopathy, and recombinant activated Factor VIIa. Maternal and fetal mortality rates remain high.

Primary prevention of ischemic stroke during pregnancy

There are no randomized data regarding stroke prevention strategies in pregnant women. Management is largely similar to non-pregnant patients. Treatment of non-pregnancy-specific cardiac disorders during pregnancy is similar to that in non-pregnant patients. Patients with these conditions need counseling on the possible risks of pregnancy to both the fetus and the mother, and in advanced disease, avoidance or interruption of pregnancy should be advised. Management of cardiac arrhythmias during pregnancy is similar to that in non-pregnant patients. Choices of anti-arrhythmic agents need to be carefully discussed with obstetricians in order to avoid potential teratogenicity [7-9]. Routine endocarditis prophylaxis is not recommended at the time of delivery in patients with cardiac valvulopathies, except in selected cases [10, 12, 20, 61-65]. Hypertension is a common problem during pregnancy affecting 12% of women in the US. There are limited data on the effects of pregnancy on the pharmacokinetics of antihypertensive drugs. Pregnancy can cause a change in the elimination half-life of antihypertensive drugs, resulting in the need for modification of the dosing frequency [66].

Use of anticoagulants for primary stroke prevention is similar to that of non-pregnant women. Anticoagulation should be used with caution during pregnancy due to its potential teratogenic effect and bleeding complications during labor and delivery. Warfarin may lead to fetal loss, and should be avoided during pregnancy, especially in the first 12 weeks of gestation. In patients with high thromboembolic risk, such as those with known coagulopathies, symptomatic atrial fibrillation, venous thromboembolism, and mechanical heart valves, adjusted-dose UFH or LMWH is preferable. Alternatively, UFH or LMWH may be used up to the 13th week of gestation, followed by warfarin until the middle of the third trimester, when UFH or LMWH is then reinstituted until delivery. LMWH is preferred to UFH due to the risk of osteoporosis associated with long-term unfractionated therapy (IIb/B) [14-16, 65, 67].

Acute stroke management: the role of thrombolytic therapy

The use of intravenous thrombolytic therapy in the hyperacute phase of ischemic stroke has largely been limited to non-pregnant patients. There are no data from controlled randomized or non-randomized clinical trials to support the use of thrombolysis during pregnancy, as pregnant women have been excluded from acute ischemic stroke trials. Despite the evidence that recombinant tissue plasminogen activator (rt-PA) does not cross the placenta, and despite the lack of teratogenicity at least in animal models, the use of rt-PA remains a relative contraindication in pregnancy due to the potential risk of premature labor, abruption placenta, fetal loss or other fetal complications. Nevertheless, the use of intravenous and intra-arterial thrombolysis has been reported in over 15 patients at different stages of gestation, with good outcomes with a complication rate similar to non-pregnant women, and a fetal fatality rate of 8% (Table 2). In view of the devastating outcome and available data on its use in this selective patient population, thrombolytic therapy should not be withheld in pregnant women with ischemic stroke (IV/C) [68-77].

Secondary prevention of ischemic stroke during pregnancy

There are no direct randomized data for stroke prevention in pregnant women. Patients with non-cardioembolic ischemic strokes should receive antiplatelet therapy, preferably low-dose aspirin [78]. Caution should be taken due to the potential risk associated with the use of antiplatelets during pregnancy. While the use of aspirin often reduces the occurrence of perinatal deaths and pre-eclampsia in particular in women with historical risk factors for pre-eclampsia [79-81], aspirin is associated with decreased uterine contractility, delayed labor, antepartum and labor bleeding. For pregnant women with ischemic stroke or TIA, low-dose aspirin (<150mg/d) appears safe for both the mother and the fetus after the first trimester and for the remainder of the pregnancy, and puerperium (IV/C) [82].

Year	Author	Gestational week	Thrombolytic agent	Outcome mother	Outcome baby
2002	Elford [70]	1	IA rt-PA	Minor deficit; HT	Healthy
2002	Dapprich [71]	12	IV rt-PA	Improved; HT	Healthy
2005	Johnson [72]	37	IA rt-PA	Improved	Healthy
2006	Leonhardt [73]	23	IV	Improved	Unknown
2006	Wiese [74]	13	IV rt-PA	Improved	Healthy
2006	Murugappan [75]	12	IV rt-PA	Intrauterine hematoma	Termination of pregnancy
		4	IV rt-PA	Improved	Termination of pregnancy
		6	IV rt-PA	Died from arterial dissection	Dead
		37	IA rt-PA	Improved	Healthy
		6	IA UK	Improved	Healthy
		6	Local UK	Improved	Fetal demise
		8	Local UK	Improved, ICH	Termination of pregnancy
		2	Local UK	Improved, ICH	Spontaneous abortion
2008	Mendez [76]	Postpartum	IA UK	Full recovery	Healthy

Table 2. Thrombolysis in acute arterial ischemic stroke.

IA = intra-arterial; IV = intravenous; rt-PA = recombinant tissue plasminogen activator; UK = urokinase; ICH = intracerebral hemorrhage; HT = hemorrhagic transformation

In patients with underlying high-risk cardiac conditions defined as atrial fibrillation, or prosthetic heart valves, thrombosed heart valves, and in patients with CVDST and other conditions where anticoagulation is recommended, heparin may be administered. Although warfarin may be safe for the fetus after a certain early period (6-12 weeks), its use in pregnancy is not usually recommended by the ACCP in the United States due to concerns of fetal safety **(IV/C)** [14, 15, 19, 82-84].

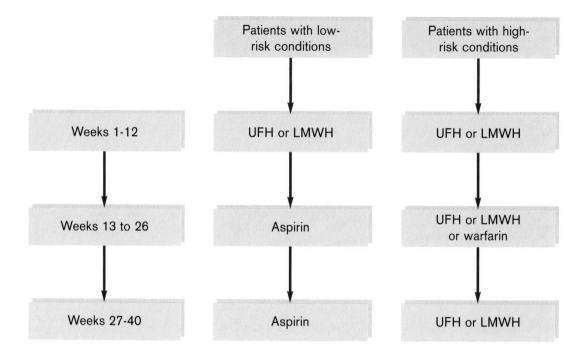

Figure 1. Antithrombotic drug use in TIA and stroke during pregnancy.

In summary, the followings are the recommendations by the ACCP for secondary stroke prevention during pregnancy (see Figure 1 above) [82, 83]:

♦ For pregnant women with ischemic stroke or TIA and a high risk of thromboembolism, e.g. coagulopathy or mechanical heart valves, options include:
  - adjusted-dose UFH throughout pregnancy;
  - adjusted-dose LMWH with Factor Xa monitoring throughout pregnancy;
  - UFH or LMWH until week 13, followed by warfarin until the middle of the third trimester, when UFH or LMWH is then reinstituted until delivery **(IV/C)**;
♦ For pregnant women with ischemic stroke or TIA and lower-risk conditions:
  - UFH or LMWH in the first trimester, followed by low-dose aspirin for the remainder of the pregnancy **(IV/C)**.

Hemorrhagic strokes

Intracerebral hemorrhage (ICH) may also occur during pregnancy, especially in the setting of pre-eclampsia and eclampsia, or due to, rupture of pre-existing cerebral vascular anomalies. The risk of ICH is increased during pregnancy and puerperium, in particular in women with arterial hypertension, eclampsia, advanced maternal age, tobacco use, and

African American ethnicity. Other causes of ICH include ruptured intracranial vascular anomalies, anticoagulant therapy, bleeding diatheses, CVDST, mycotic aneurysms, vasculitides, and metastatic choriocarcinoma.

Eclampsia is a common culprit of ICH during pregnancy mainly during the third trimester of pregnancy or puerperium. Patients often present with arterial hypertension, proteinuria, peripheral edema, seizure, focal neurological deficit, and coma. Aggressive blood pressure control and careful choice of antiepileptic agent are essential in the management of eclampsia.

The treatment of central nervous system (CNS) vasculitides remains problematic in the general population, and is often based on observational studies. Specifically, treatment of symptomatic CNS vasculitis with ICH during pregnancy remains a challenge, due to an increased risk of fetal and maternal complications associated with the use of corticosteroids and immunosuppressant agents, the latter to be avoided during pregnancy due to embryopathy [85] **(IV/C)**.

Gestational choriocarcinoma is a potentially curable, rapidly growing malignant tumor of gestational trophoblastic neoplasia, affecting 300 to 500 women a year in the United States. It may occur following a normal pregnancy or following a hydatidiform mole, miscarriage, or ectopic pregnancy [86-88]. Intracranial metastatic choriocarcinoma may present as ICH, subarachnoid hemorrhage, subdural hematoma, multiple arterial occlusions, and seldom as a neoplastic intracranial aneurysm or neoplastic carotid-cavernous fistula. Treatment of choriocarcinoma metastatic to the brain combines craniotomy or stereotactic radiosurgery combined with chemotherapy. Radiation therapy should be avoided during pregnancy.

Management of cerebrovascular malformations during pregnancy

Ruptured arteriovenous malformations (AVM) and cerebral aneurysms are a rare but not uncommon cause of lobar intracerebral hemorrhages or subarachnoid hemorrhage (SAH) during pregnancy and puerperium, responsible for 5-12% of all maternal deaths [89-93]. Intracranial cerebral aneurysmal rupture accounts for more than three quarters of causes of SAH in pregnancy, with a significant mortality rate of 40%. The estimated incidence of ruptured intracranial aneurysm is 1-5 in 10,000 pregnancies, occurring mainly in the third trimester of pregnancy and during labor and delivery, or in early puerperium. Predisposing factors to aneurysmal rupture include earlier age at menarche, advanced gestational age and primi-parity [94]. The presence of an unruptured cerebral aneurysm does not confer a contraindication for pregnancy and should not affect the obstetrical decision for the method of delivery. Management of aneurysmal SAH during pregnancy should be similar to non-pregnant patients [95-98]. Unruptured intracranial aneurysms are better left alone **(IIa/B)**. Nimodipine is teratogenic in animals, but there are no data on its teratogenicity in humans. Nimodipine should be used with caution in pregnancy due to the potential risk of hypotension and its deleterious effect on the fetus. Ruptured aneurysms may be treated with endovascular coiling or clipping based on neurosurgical indications **(Ia/A)**. Digital substraction angiography (DSA) and coil embolization may confer radiation risks to the fetus, thus special considerations with abdominal shielding should be taken to decrease the risk of radiation.

Surgical clipping may be preferred to coiling in pregnant patients with a ruptured cerebral aneurysm during pregnancy to eliminate the radiation risk to fetus, and to avoid the potential risk of rebleeding in partially coiled aneurysm during labor and delivery. Caesarean section may be an option in pregnant women with complications of SAH [95, 99, 100].

Intracranial AVMs are relatively uncommon, but are an increasingly recognized cause of serious neurological symptoms and signs, ICH, and death in pregnant women. While the risk of hemorrhage of an AVM is inconclusive, it is estimated that the incidence of ICH due to a ruptured AVM is 3.5% during pregnancy compared to 1-2% in non-pregnant women, with a much higher rebleeding rate of 26-31% in the first year, which decreases to 5.5% for each consecutive year [101, 102]. It remains, however, unclear whether pregnancy alters the natural tendency of existing AVMs to rupture [91, 103-105]. Data from the New York islands did not show a greater risk of AVM rupture during pregnancy compared to non-pregnant women (0.50 vs. 0.33 per 100,000 person-years) or an increase in the rate of first cerebral hemorrhage from a ruptured AVM [106].

In the absence of randomized clinical trials, guidelines for the management of AVMs are not available. While awaiting the results of the ARUBA trial, management of unruptured AVMs remains controversial and the recommendations for surgical intervention are generally elective. Specifically, management of symptomatic AVM during pregnancy remains a dilemma. Pregnant women with asymptomatic and symptomatic AVM should be treated similar to non-pregnant women, irrespective of gestational age. Patients with unruptured AVM should be cautiously monitored. Counseling on pregnancy is necessary, specifically in patients with a prior history of bleeding, and patients should be advised to postpone pregnancy beyond 1 year of the initial bleeding. The presence of an AVM should not affect the decision on delivery method which should be left to the discretion of the obstetrician based on obstetrical indications. In patients with hemorrhage secondary to an AVM, surgical intervention may be considered **(IV/C)**. In cases of a ruptured AVM, caution is advocated when considering radiation therapy in the first 12 weeks of gestation due to potential fetal injury [107, 108]. The choice of anesthetic technique during pregnancy in a patient with an AVM is a challenge for anesthesiologists and obstetricians, and is aimed at maintaining good oxygenation, avoiding increased intracranial pressure, and stable hemodynamics. Regional anesthetic techniques are preferred to avoid hemodyamic stress.

As for AVMs and aneurysms, management of dural AV or carotid cavernous fistulae in pregnancy remains unclear. It is postulated that pregnancy may increase the risk of spontaneous carotid cavernous fistulae, mainly in the third trimester or during labor and delivery. Treatment should be considered in symptomatic patients on a case by case basis. Endovascular intervention could be curative, and may be considered alone or in combination with surgery to prevent stroke or hemorrhage [109, 110] **(IV/C)**.

Conclusions

Stroke, ischemic and hemorrhagic, is a relatively rare complication of pregnancy and puerperium, and its incidence compared to non-pregnant women of matched age remains unknown. There are no adequate trials demonstrating that prophylactic regimens are effective, and data from randomized clinical trials are lacking. In the absence of prospective studies, the management of stroke in pregnancy is driven by observational studies. The choice of platelet anti-aggregants for primary and secondary prevention should be based on individual clinical scenarios. When anticoagulation is indicated in high-risk patients, LMWH or UFH is the anticoagulant of choice in pregnancy. Expert consensus panels disagree over the optimal management of pregnant women with primary and secondary stroke prevention. Randomized controlled trials during pregnancy are needed.

Key points	Evidence level
◆ Thrombolysis for acute ischemic stroke should not be withheld due to pregnancy, but should be used with caution.	IV/C
◆ Aspirin may be used for secondary stroke prevention during pregnancy after the first trimester.	IV/C
◆ There are limited data on the safety of thienopyridine derivatives during pregnancy and breastfeeding; therefore, they should be avoided whenever possible.	IV/C
◆ Warfarin is better avoided during pregnancy, but may be used after the 13th week of gestation.	IV/C
◆ UFH or LMWH may be used throughout pregnancy in patients with mechanical valve prosthesis, atrial fibrillation, CDVST, and venous-thrombotic events.	IV/C
◆ In patients with ACS, β-blockers may be used during pregnancy.	IIa/B
◆ Based on teratogenicity ACE-Is and ARBs should be avoided during pregnancy.	IV/C
◆ Antibiotic prophylaxis of infective endocarditis in valvular heart disease is not routinely recommended, and should only be considered in high-risk patients with systemic infection or with prior history of endocarditis.	IIb/B
◆ There is no justification for percutaneous PFO closure in pregnancy.	IV/C
◆ There is no justification for treatment of unruptured cerebral aneurysms or unruptured AVMs during pregnancy.	IIa/B
◆ Ruptured cerebral aneurysms may be treated with endovascular coiling or clipping based on neurosurgical indications.	Ia/A
◆ In symptomatic AVM or AV fistulae, surgical or endovascular interventions may be considered.	IV/C
◆ Management of pregnancy-specific conditions such as PPCA, PPCM, and OHS is based on case reports and expert opinions.	IV/C

References

1. Wiebers DO. Ischemic cerebrovascular complications of pregnancy. *Arch Neurol* 1985; 42(11):1106-13.
2. Sharshar T, Lamy C, Mas JL. Incidence and causes of strokes associated with pregnancy and puerperium. A study in public hospitals of Ile de France. Stroke in Pregnancy Study Group. *Stroke* 1995; 26(6): 930-6.
3. Kittner SJ, Stern BJ, Feeser BR, *et al*. Pregnancy and the risk of stroke. *N Engl J Med* 1996; 335(11): 768-74.
4. Pruitt AB, Mole HW. Middle cerebral artery occlusion in pregnancy. Review of the literature and report of a case. *Obstet Gynecol* 1967; 29(4): 545-50.
5. Maitra G, Sengupta S, Rudra A, Debnath S. Pregnancy and non-valvular heart disease - anesthetic considerations. *Ann Card Anaesth* 2010; 13(2): 102-9.
6. Wilson MR, Hughes SJ. The effect of maternal protein deficiency during pregnancy and lactation on glucose tolerance and pancreatic islet function in adult rat offspring. *J Endocrinol* 1997; 154(1): 177-85.
7. Ferrero S, Colombo BM, Ragni N. Maternal arrhythmias during pregnancy. *Arch Gynecol Obstet* 2004; 269(4): 244-53.
8. Gowda RM, Khan IA, Mehta NJ, Vasavada BC, Sacchi TJ. Cardiac arrhythmias in pregnancy: clinical and therapeutic considerations. *Int J Cardiol* 2003; 88(2-3): 129-33.
9. Wolbrette D. Treatment of arrhythmias during pregnancy. *Curr Womens Health Rep* 2003; 3(2): 135-9.
10. Degani S, Abinader EG, Scharf M. Mitral valve prolapse and pregnancy: a review. *Obstet Gynecol Surv* 1989; 44(9): 642-9.
11. Jeng JS, Tang SC, Yip PK. Incidence and etiologies of stroke during pregnancy and puerperium as evidenced in Taiwanese women. *Cerebrovasc Dis* 2004; 18(4): 290-5.
12. Tang LC, Chan SY, Wong VC, Ma HK. Pregnancy in patients with mitral valve prolapse. *Int J Gynaecol Obstet* 1985; 23(3): 217-21.
13. Martinez-Diaz JL. Valvular heart disease in pregnancy: a review of the literature. *Bol Asoc Med P R* 2008; 100(4): 55-9.
14. Geelani MA, Singh S, Verma A, Nagesh A, Betigeri V, Nigam M. Anticoagulation in patients with mechanical valves during pregnancy. *Asian Cardiovasc Thorac Ann* 2005; 13(1): 30-3.
15. Akhtar RP, Abid AR, Zafar H, Cheema MA, Khan JS. Anticoagulation in pregnancy with mechanical heart valves: 10-year experience. *Asian Cardiovasc Thorac Ann* 2007; 15(6): 497-501.
16. Pavankumar P, Venugopal P, Kaul U, *et al*. Pregnancy in patients with prosthetic cardiac valve. A 10-year experience. *Scand J Thorac Cardiovasc Surg* 1988; 22(1): 19-22.
17. Lavy S, Kahana E. Cerebral arterial occlusion during pregnancy and puerperium. Report of 3 cases. *Obstet Gynecol* 1970; 35(6): 916-23.
18. Koopmans CM, Bijlenga D, Groen H, *et al*. Induction of labour versus expectant monitoring for gestational hypertension or mild pre-eclampsia after 36 weeks' gestation (HYPITAT): a multicentre, open-label randomised controlled trial. *Lancet* 2009; 374(9694): 979-88.
19. Bonow RO, Carabello B, de Leon AC, Jr., *et al*. Guidelines for the Management of Patients with Valvular Heart Disease: Executive Summary. A report of the American College of Cardiology/American Heart Association Task Force on Practice Guidelines (Committee on Management of Patients with Valvular Heart Disease). *Circulation* 1998; 98(18): 1949-84.
20. Wilson W, Taubert KA, Gewitz M, *et al*. Prevention of Infective Endocarditis: Guidelines from the American Heart Association: a Guideline from the American Heart Association Rheumatic Fever, Endocarditis, and Kawasaki Disease Committee, Council on Cardiovascular Disease in the Young, and the Council on Clinical Cardiology, Council on Cardiovascular Surgery and Anesthesia, and the Quality of Care and Outcomes Research Interdisciplinary Working Group. *Circulation* 2007; 116(15): 1736-54.
21. Roth A, Elkayam U. Acute myocardial infarction associated with pregnancy. *J Am Coll Cardiol* 2008; 52(3): 171-80.
22. Hunt SA, Abraham WT, Chin MH, *et al*. 2009 focused update incorporated into the ACC/AHA 2005 Guidelines for the Diagnosis and Management of Heart Failure in Adults: a report of the American College of Cardiology Foundation/American Heart Association Task Force on Practice Guidelines: developed in collaboration with the International Society for Heart and Lung Transplantation. *Circulation* 2009; 119(14): e391-479.

23. Qasqas SA, McPherson C, Frishman WH, Elkayam U. Cardiovascular pharmacotherapeutic considerations during pregnancy and lactation. *Cardiol Rev* 2004; 12(5): 240-61.

24. Shotan A, Widerhorn J, Hurst AK, Elkayam U. Angiotensin-converting enzyme inhibitors and pregnancy. In: *Cardiac Problems in Pregnancy: Diagnosis and Management of Maternal and Fetal Disease*, 3rd ed. Elkayam U, Gleicher N, Eds. New York, USA: Wiley-Liss, 1998: 399-406.

25. Becerra JE, Khoury MJ, Cordero JF, Erickson JD. Diabetes mellitus during pregnancy and the risks for specific birth defects: a population-based case-control study. *Pediatrics* 1990; 85(1): 1-9.

26. Waller DK, Shaw GM, Rasmussen SA, *et al*. Prepregnancy obesity as a risk factor for structural birth defects. *Arch Pediatr Adolesc Med* 2007; 161(8): 745-50.

27. Bates SM, Greer IA, Hirsh J, Ginsberg JS. Use of antithrombotic agents during pregnancy: the Seventh ACCP Conference on Antithrombotic and Thrombolytic Therapy. *Chest* 2004; 126(3 Suppl): 627S-44.

28. Webster MW, Chancellor AM, Smith HJ, *et al*. Patent foramen ovale in young stroke patients. *Lancet* 1988; 2(8601): 11-2.

29. Lechat P, Mas JL, Lascault G, *et al*. Prevalence of patent foramen ovale in patients with stroke. *N Engl J Med* 1988; 318(18): 1148-52.

30. Hagen PT, Scholz DG, Edwards WD. Incidence and size of patent foramen ovale during the first 10 decades of life: an autopsy study of 965 normal hearts. *Mayo Clin Proc* 1984; 59(1): 17-20.

31. Messe SR, Silverman IE, Kizer JR, *et al*. Practice parameter: recurrent stroke with patent foramen ovale and atrial septal aneurysm: report of the Quality Standards Subcommittee of the American Academy of Neurology. *Neurology* 2004; 62(7): 1042-50.

32. Schrale RG, Ormerod J, Ormerod OJ. Percutaneous device closure of the patent foramen ovale during pregnancy. *Catheter Cardiovasc Interv* 2007; 69(4): 579-83.

33. Daehnert I, Ewert P, Berger F, Lange PE. Echocardiographically guided closure of a patent foramen ovale during pregnancy after recurrent strokes. *J Interv Cardiol* 2001; 14(2): 191-2.

34. O'Gara PT, Messe SR, Tuzcu EM, Catha G, Ring JC. Percutaneous device closure of patent foramen ovale for secondary stroke prevention: a call for completion of randomized clinical trials: a science advisory from the American Heart Association/American Stroke Association and the American College of Cardiology Foundation. *Circulation* 2009; 119(20): 2743-7.

35. Elkayam U, Akhter MW, Singh H, *et al*. Pregnancy-associated cardiomyopathy: clinical characteristics and a comparison between early and late presentation. *Circulation* 2005 ;111(16): 2050-5.

36. Sliwa K, Tibazarwa K, Hilfiker-Kleiner D. Management of peripartum cardiomyopathy. *Curr Heart Fail Rep* 2008; 5(4): 238-44.

37. Brar SS, Khan SS, Sandhu GK, *et al*. Incidence, mortality, and racial differences in peripartum cardiomyopathy. *Am J Cardiol* 2007; 100(2): 302-4.

38. Mielniczuk LM, Williams K, Davis DR, *et al*. Frequency of peripartum cardiomyopathy. *Am J Cardiol* 2006; 97(12): 1765-8.

39. Kawano H, Tsuneto A, Koide Y, *et al*. Magnetic resonance imaging in a patient with peripartum cardiomyopathy. *Intern Med* 2008; 47(2): 97-102.

40. Fett JD, Christie LG, Carraway RD, Murphy JG. Five-year prospective study of the incidence and prognosis of peripartum cardiomyopathy at a single institution. *Mayo Clin Proc* 2005; 80(12): 1602-6.

41. Coutinho JM, Ferro JM, Canhao P, *et al*. Cerebral venous and sinus thrombosis in women. *Stroke* 2009; 40(7): 2356-61.

42. Preter M, Tzourio C, Ameri A, Bousser MG. Long-term prognosis in cerebral venous thrombosis. Follow-up of 77 patients. *Stroke* 1996; 27(2): 243-6.

43. Canhao P, Ferro JM, Lindgren AG, Bousser MG, Stam J, Barinagarrementeria F. Causes and predictors of death in cerebral venous thrombosis. *Stroke* 2005; 36(8): 1720-5.

44. Daif A, Awada A, al-Rajeh S, *et al*. Cerebral venous thrombosis in adults. A study of 40 cases from Saudi Arabia. *Stroke* 1995; 26(7): 1193-5.

45. Krayenbuhl HA. Cerebral venous and sinus thrombosis. *Clin Neurosurg* 1966; 14: 1-24.

46. Stam J, De Bruijn SF, DeVeber G. Anticoagulation for cerebral sinus thrombosis. *Cochrane Database Syst Rev* 2002(4): CD002005.

47. Einhaupl K, Stam J, Bousser MG, *et al*. EFNS guideline on the treatment of cerebral venous and sinus thrombosis in adult patients. *Eur J Neurol* 2010; 17(10): 1229-35.

48. Ferro JM, Canhao P, Stam J, *et al.* Delay in the diagnosis of cerebral vein and dural sinus thrombosis: influence on outcome. *Stroke* 2009; 40(9): 3133-8.

49. Ferro JM, Canhao P, Bousser MG, Stam J, Barinagarrementeria F, Stolz E. Cerebral venous thrombosis with nonhemorrhagic lesions: clinical correlates and prognosis. *Cerebrovasc Dis* 2010; 29(5): 440-5.

50. Einhaupl KM, Villringer A, Meister W, *et al.* Heparin treatment in sinus venous thrombosis. *Lancet* 1991; 338(8767): 597-600.

51. de Bruijn SF, Stam J. Randomized, placebo-controlled trial of anticoagulant treatment with low-molecular-weight heparin for cerebral sinus thrombosis. *Stroke* 1999; 30(3): 484-8.

52. Nagaraja D, Haridas T, Taly AB, Veerendrakumar M, SubbuKrishna DK. Puerperal cerebral venous thrombosis: therapeutic benefit of low-dose heparin. *Neurol India* 1999; 47(1): 43-6.

53. Crippa G, Sverzellati E, Pancotti D, Carrara GC. Severe postpartum hypertension and reversible cerebral angiopathy associated with ergot derivative (methergoline) administration. *Ann Ital Med Int* 2000; 15(4): 303-5.

54. Konstantinopoulos PA, Mousa S, Khairallah R, Mtanos G. Postpartum cerebral angiopathy: an important diagnostic consideration in the postpartum period. *Am J Obstet Gynecol* 2004; 191(1): 375-7.

55. Granier I, Garcia E, Geissler A, Boespflug MD, Durand-Gasselin J. Postpartum cerebral angiopathy associated with the administration of sumatriptan and dihydroergotamine - a case report. *Intensive Care Med* 1999; 25(5): 532-4.

56. Conde-Agudelo A, Romero R. Amniotic fluid embolism: an evidence-based review. *Am J Obstet Gynecol* 2009; 201(5): 445: e1-13.

57. Fett JD. Peripartum cardiomyopathy (PPCM) in both surrogate and biological mother. *Hum Reprod* 2005; 20(9): 2666-8.

58. Murali S, Baldisseri MR. Peripartum cardiomyopathy. *Crit Care Med* 2005; 33(10 Suppl): S340-6.

59. Abboud J, Murad Y, Chen-Scarabelli C, Saravolatz L, Scarabelli TM. Peripartum cardiomyopathy: a comprehensive review. *Int J Cardiol* 2007; 118(3): 295-303.

60. Lamparter S, Pankuweit S, Maisch B. Clinical and immunologic characteristics in peripartum cardiomyopathy. *Int J Cardiol* 2007; 118(1): 14-20.

61. Wong MC, Giuliani MJ, Haley EC, Jr. Cerebrovascular disease and stroke in women. *Cardiology* 1990; 77 Suppl 2: 80-90.

62. Chia YT, Yeoh SC, Lim MC, Viegas OA, Ratnam SS. Pregnancy outcome and mitral valve prolapse. *Asia Oceania J Obstet Gynaecol* 1994; 20(4): 383-8.

63. Cowles T, Gonik B. Mitral valve prolapse in pregnancy. *Semin Perinatol* 1990; 14(1): 34-41.

64. Jana N, Vasishta K, Khunnu B, Dhall GI, Grover A. Pregnancy in association with mitral valve prolapse. *Asia Oceania J Obstet Gynaecol* 1993; 19(1): 61-5.

65. Bonow RO, Carabello BA, Kanu C, *et al.* ACC/AHA 2006 Guidelines for the Management of Patients with Valvular Heart Disease: a report of the American College of Cardiology/American Heart Association Task Force on Practice Guidelines (Writing Committee to revise the 1998 Guidelines for the Management of Patients With Valvular Heart Disease): developed in collaboration with the Society of Cardiovascular Anesthesiologists: endorsed by the Society for Cardiovascular Angiography and Interventions and the Society of Thoracic Surgeons. *Circulation* 2006; 114(5): e84-231.

66. Anderson GD, Carr DB. Effect of pregnancy on the pharmacokinetics of antihypertensive drugs. *Clin Pharmacokinet* 2009; 48(3): 159-68.

67. Suri V, Sawhney H, Vasishta K, Renuka T, Grover A. Pregnancy following cardiac valve replacement surgery. *Int J Gynaecol Obstet* 1999; 64(3): 239-46.

68. Young SK, Al-Mondhiry HA, Vaida SJ, Ambrose A, Botti JJ. Successful use of argatroban during the third trimester of pregnancy: case report and review of the literature. *Pharmacotherapy* 2008; 28(12): 1531-6.

69. Tang SC, Jeng JS. Management of stroke in pregnancy and the puerperium. *Expert Rev Neurother* 2010; 10(2): 205-15.

70. Elford K, Leader A, Wee R, Stys PK. Stroke in ovarian hyperstimulation syndrome in early pregnancy treated with intra-arterial rt-PA. *Neurology* 2002; 59(8): 1270-2.

71. Dapprich M, Boessenecker W. Fibrinolysis with alteplase in a pregnant woman with stroke. *Cerebrovasc Dis* 2002; 13(4): 290.

72. Johnson DM, Kramer DC, Cohen E, Rochon M, Rosner M, Weinberger J. Thrombolytic therapy for acute stroke in late pregnancy with intra-arterial recombinant tissue plasminogen activator. *Stroke* 2005; 36(6): e53-5.

73. Leonhardt G, Gaul C, Nietsch HH, Buerke M, Schleussner E. Thrombolytic therapy in pregnancy. *J Thromb Thrombolysis* 2006; 21(3): 271-6.

74. Wiese KM, Talkad A, Mathews M, Wang D. Intravenous recombinant tissue plasminogen activator in a pregnant woman with cardioembolic stroke. *Stroke* 2006; 37(8): 2168-9.

75. Murugappan A, Coplin WM, Al-Sadat AN, *et al*. Thrombolytic therapy of acute ischemic stroke during pregnancy. *Neurology* 2006; 66(5): 768-70.

76. Mendez JC, Masjuan J, Garcia N, de Lecinana M. Successful intra-arterial thrombolysis for acute ischemic stroke in the immediate postpartum period: case report. *Cardiovasc Intervent Radiol* 2008; 31(1): 193-5.

77. Weatherby SJ, Edwards NC, West R, Heafield MT. Good outcome in early pregnancy following direct thrombolysis for cerebral venous sinus thrombosis. *J Neurol* 2003; 250(11): 1372-3.

78. Helms AK, Drogan O, Kittner SJ. First trimester stroke prophylaxis in pregnant women with a history of stroke. *Stroke* 2009; 40(4): 1158-61.

79. Louden KA, Broughton Pipkin F, Symonds EM, *et al*. A randomized placebo-controlled study of the effect of low-dose aspirin on platelet reactivity and serum thromboxane B2 production in non-pregnant women, in normal pregnancy, and in gestational hypertension. *Br J Obstet Gynaecol* 1992; 99(5): 371-6.

80. Benigni A, Gregorini G, Frusca T, *et al*. Effect of low-dose aspirin on fetal and maternal generation of thromboxane by platelets in women at risk for pregnancy-induced hypertension. *N Engl J Med* 1989; 321(6): 357-62.

81. Walsh SW. Low-dose aspirin: treatment for the imbalance of increased thromboxane and decreased prostacyclin in pre-eclampsia. *Am J Perinatol* 1989; 6(2): 124-32.

82. Sacco RL, Adams R, Albers G, *et al*. Guidelines for Prevention of Stroke in Patients with Ischemic Stroke or Transient Ischemic Attack: a Statement for Healthcare Professionals from the American Heart Association/American Stroke Association Council on Stroke: co-sponsored by the Council on Cardiovascular Radiology and Intervention: the American Academy of Neurology affirms the value of this guideline. *Stroke* 2006; 37(2): 577-617.

83. Bates SM, Greer IA, Pabinger I, Sofaer S, Hirsh J. Venous Thromboembolism, Thrombophilia, Antithrombotic Therapy, and Pregnancy: American College of Chest Physicians Evidence-Based Clinical Practice Guidelines (8th Edition). *Chest* 2008; 133(6 Suppl): 844S-86.

84. Yinon Y, Siu SC, Warshafsky C, *et al*. Use of low-molecular-weight heparin in pregnant women with mechanical heart valves. *Am J Cardiol* 2009; 104(9): 1259-63.

85. Mukhtyar C, Guillevin L, Cid MC, *et al*. EULAR recommendations for the management of large vessel vasculitis. *Ann Rheum Dis* 2009; 68(3): 318-23.

86. Verzar Z, Kover E, Doczi T, Kalman E, Koppan M, Bodis J. Successful treatment of FIGO stage IV gestational choriocarcinoma occurring 2 months after delivery. *Eur J Obstet Gynecol Reprod Biol* 2008; 140(2): 275-6.

87. Huang CY, Chen CA, Hsieh CY, Cheng WF. Intracerebral hemorrhage as initial presentation of gestational choriocarcinoma: a case report and literature review. *Int J Gynecol Cancer* 2007; 17(5): 1166-71.

88. Nugent D, Hassadia A, Everard J, Hancock BW, Tidy JA. Postpartum choriocarcinoma presentation, management and survival. *J Reprod Med* 2006; 51(10): 819-24.

89. Dias MS, Sekhar LN. Intracranial hemorrhage from aneurysms and arteriovenous malformations during pregnancy and the puerperium. *Neurosurgery* 1990; 27(6): 855-65; discussion 65-6.

90. Horton JC, Chambers WA, Lyons SL, Adams RD, Kjellberg RN. Pregnancy and the risk of hemorrhage from cerebral arteriovenous malformations. *Neurosurgery* 1990; 27(6): 867-71; discussion 71-2.

91. Mast H, Young WL, Koennecke HC, *et al*. Risk of spontaneous haemorrhage after diagnosis of cerebral arteriovenous malformation. *Lancet* 1997; 350(9084): 1065-8.

92. Barno A, Freeman DW. Maternal deaths due to spontaneous subarachnoid hemorrhage. *Am J Obstet Gynecol* 1976; 125(3): 384-92.

93. Yang CY, Chang CC, Kuo HW, Chiu HF. Parity and risk of death from subarachnoid hemorrhage in women: evidence from a cohort in Taiwan. *Neurology* 2006; 67(3): 514-5.

94. Mhurchu CN, Anderson C, Jamrozik K, Hankey G, Dunbabin D. Hormonal factors and risk of aneurysmal subarachnoid hemorrhage: an international population-based, case-control study. *Stroke* 2001; 32(3): 606-12.

95. Molyneux A, Kerr R, Stratton I, *et al*. International Subarachnoid Aneurysm Trial (ISAT) of neurosurgical clipping versus endovascular coiling in 2143 patients with ruptured intracranial aneurysms: a randomised trial. *Lancet* 2002; 360(9342): 1267-74.

96. Molyneux AJ, Kerr RS, Yu LM, *et al.* International subarachnoid aneurysm trial (ISAT) of neurosurgical clipping versus endovascular coiling in 2143 patients with ruptured intracranial aneurysms: a randomised comparison of effects on survival, dependency, seizures, rebleeding, subgroups, and aneurysm occlusion. *Lancet* 2005; 366(9488): 809-17.

97. Marshman LA, Aspoas AR, Rai MS, Chawda SJ. The implications of ISAT and ISUIA for the management of cerebral aneurysms during pregnancy. *Neurosurg Rev* 2007; 30(3): 177-80; discussion 80.

98. Selo-Ojeme DO, Marshman LA, Ikomi A, *et al.* Aneurysmal subarachnoid haemorrhage in pregnancy. *Eur J Obstet Gynecol Reprod Biol* 2004; 116(2): 131-43.

99. Wiebers DO, Whisnant JP, Huston J, 3rd, *et al.* Unruptured intracranial aneurysms: natural history, clinical outcome, and risks of surgical and endovascular treatment. *Lancet* 2003; 362(9378): 103-10.

100. Piotin M, de Souza Filho CB, Kothimbakam R, Moret J. Endovascular treatment of acutely ruptured intracranial aneurysms in pregnancy. *Am J Obstet Gynecol* 2001; 185(5): 1261-2.

101. Robinson JL, Hall CS, Sedzimir CB. Arteriovenous malformations, aneurysms, and pregnancy. *J Neurosurg* 1974; 41(1): 63-70.

102. Bateman BT, Schumacher HC, Bushnell CD, *et al.* Intracerebral hemorrhage in pregnancy: frequency, risk factors, and outcome. *Neurology* 2006; 67(3): 424-9.

103. Finnerty JJ, Chisholm CA, Chapple H, Login IS, Pinkerton JV. Cerebral arteriovenous malformation in pregnancy: presentation and neurologic, obstetric, and ethical significance. *Am J Obstet Gynecol* 1999; 181(2): 296-303.

104. Sadasivan B, Malik GM, Lee C, Ausman JI. Vascular malformations and pregnancy. *Surg Neurol* 1990; 33(5): 305-13.

105. Velut S, Vinikoff L, Destrieux C, Kakou M. [Cerebro-meningeal hemorrhage secondary to ruptured vascular malformation during pregnancy and post-partum]. *Neurochirurgie* 2000; 46(2): 95-104.

106. Stapf C, Mast H, Sciacca RR, *et al.* The New York Islands AVM Study: design, study progress, and initial results. *Stroke* 2003; 34(5): e29-33.

107. Piotin M, Mounayer C, Spelle L, Moret J. [Cerebral arteriovenous malformations and pregnancy: management of a dilemma]. *J Neuroradiol* 2004; 31(5): 376-8.

108. Ogilvy CS, Stieg PE, Awad I, *et al.* AHA Scientific Statement: Recommendations for the Management of Intracranial Arteriovenous Malformations: a Statement for Healthcare Professionals from a Special Writing Group of the Stroke Council, American Stroke Association. *Stroke* 2001; 32(6): 1458-71.

109. Lin TK, Chang CN, Wai YY. Spontaneous intracerebral hematoma from occult carotid-cavernous fistula during pregnancy and puerperium. Case report. *J Neurosurg* 1992; 76(4): 714-7.

110. Toya S, Shiobara R, Izumi J, Shinomiya Y, Shiga H, Kimura C. Spontaneous carotid-cavernous fistula during pregnancy or in the postpartum stage. Report of two cases. *J Neurosurg* 1981; 54(2): 252-6.

Chapter 13

Oral contraceptives, hormonal therapy and stroke

Kerstin Bettermann MD PhD, Assistant Professor of Neurology
Department of Neurology, Penn State College of Medicine
Hershey, Pennsylvania, USA

Introduction

Oral contraceptives (OCs) and hormone replacement therapy (HRT) are widely used in Western industrialized nations [1]. While the use of HRT for treatment of menopause-related symptoms in women has declined following publication of the results from the Women's Health Initiative study (WHI), there is growing interest in the use of androgens for treatment of male hypogonadism and, more recently, treatment of postmenopausal symptoms in women [2]. OCs are frequently and widely used, and there is continuing debate regarding the stroke risk associated with these drugs. Current evidence suggests that HRT is associated with an increased risk of cardiovascular disease and ischemic stroke, while the stroke risk associated with testosterone replacement therapy has not been well examined. The literature surrounding hormonal therapy remains controversial. This chapter will focus on the current evidence of sex hormone therapy and associated stroke risk.

Hormone replacement therapy and stroke risk in women

Types of hormonal regimens used for replacement therapy

Hormonal regimens used for replacement therapy in women include estrogen-progestin combination therapy, estrogen monotherapy and, increasingly, androgen supplementation. Estrogen and estrogen-progestin combination regimens are routinely used in clinical practice to alleviate menopausal symptoms in women. Medroxyprogesterone acetate (MPA), a synthetic progestagen that emulates the bioeffects of naturally occurring progesterone on the uterus in premenopausal women, has been widely prescribed in combination with estrogen and has been used for combination therapy in recent randomized clinical trials which studied the effect of HRT on risk of coronary artery disease and stroke [3, 4].

The Women's Health Initiative (WHI) study compared continuous hormonal combination therapy of 0.625mg conjugated equine estrogen plus 2.5mg MPA daily to placebo. The Heart and Estrogen/Progestin Replacement studies (HERS-I and HERS-II) used the same combination of MPA (2.5mg per day) and estrogen (0.625mg per day). The choice of MPA as progestin in these trials has been subsequently critiqued as it has adverse metabolic and thrombogenic properties [5], but MPA was a routinely prescribed component of combination regimens at the time these studies were conducted.

Estrogen monotherapy is often given for a short period of time to postmenopausal women following hysterectomy. Orally administered estrogen decreases LDL cholesterol, increases HDL cholesterol levels [6, 7], and may improve insulin sensitivity and endothelial function in younger women [8, 9]. On the other hand it increases triglycerides and C-reactive protein levels and has prothrombotic properties [10, 11]. The association of estrogen monotherapy and stroke risk has been recently studied in the large randomized unopposed estrogen versus placebo WHI trial [12].

Recently, androgens are increasingly being considered for the treatment of postmenopausal symptoms in women. Androgens are produced in the ovaries and adrenal glands and are converted to estrogen in peripheral tissues until menopause. After menopause, ovarian production of estrogen and androgens ceases and therefore androgen supplementation is thought to be helpful to ameliorate postmenopausal symptoms. However, this practice is controversial as it has been shown that an androgen-dominant stage may have adverse effects on lipid metabolism and insulin function. LDL cholesterol concentrations and insulin resistance increase, while HDL concentrations decrease, which may promote obesity and atherosclerosis [12]. Similarly, supplemental androgens can impair endothelium-dependent vasodilation in the forearm, and can decrease cerebral blood flow in the middle cerebral artery in postmenopausal women [13]. However, the effects of androgens on the cerebral vasculature are poorly understood.

The question of cardiovascular and cerebrovascular safety of androgen therapy in women remains currently unanswered, and there are no USA Food and Drug Administration (FDA)-approved androgen preparations on the market for treating androgen insufficiency in women [14]. The current lack of knowledge about the effects of androgens on vascular function, atherosclerotic plaque formation and stroke risk does not allow translation of results from preliminary studies into clinical practice guidelines. Future randomized controlled trials of androgenic agents are required to address these questions.

Observational studies of estrogen and estrogen-progestin combination therapy and associated stroke risk

Observational and clinical data show that women rarely have cardiovascular disease and stroke during their reproductive years. In the past, this had been attributed to the protective effects of ovarian sex hormones, including estrogen and progesterone [15, 16]. Based on these observations, it had been clinical practice to use HRT for prevention of coronary artery disease and stroke.

Epidemiological studies of HRT and stroke risk have yielded conflicting results. More recent case-control and observational studies have not found an increased stroke risk for menopausal women using unopposed estrogen or estrogen/progestin combination therapy [17-21], or have even reported a decreased stroke risk associated with HRT [22].

In contrast to these reports, data from the observational Nurses' Health Study demonstrated an increased stroke risk with estrogen monotherapy (HR 1.39; 95% CI, 1.18-1.63), as well as with estrogen/progestin combination treatment (HR 1.27; 95% CI, 1.04-1.56) [23]. The increased risk was independent of timing of HRT or type of hormonal replacement regimen used. The stroke risk in younger women in this trial was modestly elevated which is probably due to the overall very low stroke rate in this population [24]. However, data from observational studies are influenced by confounding and multiple biases inherent to these analyses and may not capture all clinical events.

Clinical studies of estrogen and estrogen-progestin combination therapy and associated stroke risk

Recent randomized clinical trials have failed to prove any benefit of HRT for the prevention of coronary heart disease or stroke (WHIMS studies, HERS trials). Additionally, epidemiological studies indicate that independent of HRT use, female gender is associated with a reduced stroke risk that persists throughout life, starting at birth and lasting beyond menopause [25-27], that further questions the role of HRT for stroke prevention.

In contrast to epidemiological studies which indicate a benefit or no effect of HRT on stroke risk [22], data from large randomized clinical trials and subsequent meta-analyses of these studies suggest that the use of HRT in women is associated with an increased risk of ischemic stroke [3, 4, 12, 28-30]. Data from the most relevant clinical trials and meta-analyses exploring the stroke risk associated with HRT are summarized in Table 1.

The WHI trials included two hormonal studies of healthy postmenopausal women ages 50-79:

- ❖ the combination trial of estrogen-progestin versus placebo in more than 16,000 women; and
- ❖ the unopposed estrogen versus placebo trial conducted in about 11,000 participants.

Table 1. Hormone replacement therapy in postmenopausal women and risk of ischemic stroke. Results from randomized controlled studies.

Study	Average follow-up	Number of participants/ age	Ischemic stroke risk, HR (95% CI)	Hemorrhagic stroke risk, HR (95% CI)
WHIMS unopposed estrogen trial	7.1 years	10,739/ 50-79 years	1.55 (1.19-2.01)	0.64 (0.35-1.18)
WHIMS combination trial	5.6 years	16, 608/ 50-79 years	1.44 (1.09-1.9)	0.82 (0.43-1.56)
HERS	6.8 years	2763/ ≤79 years	1.18 (0.83-1.67)	1.65 (0.47-5.72)
WEST	2.8 years	664/ >44 years	1.0 (0.6-1.4)	1.3 (0.3-6.0)
Meta-analysis of the studies above	5.6 years	30,774/ >44 years	1.29 (1.06 to 1.56)	1.07 (0.65 to 1.75)

Both studies were designed as clinical primary prevention trials of cardiovascular disease with stroke being a secondary outcome measure. The combination trial was terminated early after 5.2 years due to an observed increased risk in breast cancer, venous thromboembolism, coronary heart disease and stroke in women using HRT. The risk for colon cancer and bone fractures in women on HRT was reduced.

The estrogen monotherapy trial was also terminated early due to an observed increased risk for ischemic stroke showing a hazard ratio (HR) of 1.55 (95% CI, 1.19-2.01) in the intention-to-treat analysis of conjugated equine estrogen versus placebo. The risk of venous thromboembolism also was significantly increased [3]. The stroke risk did not vary by age, race, years since menopause or presence of traditional vascular risk factors. The increased stroke risk was similar in women with and without history of previous stroke. The event rate on estrogen monotherapy was slightly higher than that observed on combination therapy. The overall stroke risk due to estrogen monotherapy use in the WHI study was increased by 39% (HR 1.39; 95% CI, 1.1-1.77), but was not increased for hemorrhagic stroke (HR 0.64; 95% CI, 0.35-1.18) [12].

In the intention-to-treat analysis of the WHI estrogen-progestin combination trial, the risk for ischemic stroke was increased by 44% (HR 1.44; 95% CI, 1.09-1.90), while HRT use did not increase the risk for hemorrhagic stroke (HR 0.82; 95% CI, 0.43-1.56). The observed stroke risk was not influenced by age, presence of traditional vascular risk factors or use of statin drugs or aspirin. As observed in the monotherapy trial, the increased stroke risk was similar in women with and without history of previous stroke.

In a pooled data analysis, which combined results from both WHI hormonal studies, the observed increased stroke risk was not associated with age or time since menopause [31]. The overall stroke rate, including ischemic and hemorrhagic strokes, was relatively low in these trials. No absolute excess risk in stroke was observed due to the small number of strokes at baseline and an only modest number of events occurring in this study population of relatively young women, 50-59 years of age. Combination of both trials did not show any increase of hemorrhagic stroke risk associated with HRT.

The Heart and Estrogen-Progestin Replacement Studies (HERS-I and HERS-II) were secondary prevention studies of combined estrogen-progestin replacement therapy versus placebo in postmenopausal women with a history of coronary heart disease [32, 33]. HERS-I included 2763 postmenopausal women up to 80 years of age with an average 4 years of follow-up. HERS-II was a continuation of the HERS-I trial with additional follow-up of 93% of all participants for an additional 2.7 years. HRT did not significantly change the primary outcome measure (myocardial infarct or death from cardiovascular disease), but showed a trend towards increased stroke risk associated with HRT (HR 1.23; 95% CI, 0.89-1.7).

The Women's International Study of Long Duration Oestrogen after Menopause (WISDOM) trial aimed to study the effects of long-term HRT (monotherapy with 0.625mg estrogen daily or combined hormone therapy with MPA plus estrogen, 5.0mg/0.625mg orally daily versus placebo) on cardiovascular disease in women ages 50-69 years with a planned study follow-up of 10 years [34]. Cerebrovascular disease was a secondary outcome measure. However, the trial was terminated early, after about 1 year, when the results of the WHI studies became available. During the relatively short duration of the trial neither HRT combination therapy, nor estrogen monotherapy increased the risk of stroke (HR 0.73, and 0.99, respectively). However, the overall stroke risk in this cohort of relatively young women was, as anticipated, relatively low (37 events/5692 participants).

The randomized clinical Women's Estrogen for Stroke Trial (WEST) of estrogen monotherapy versus placebo in postmenopausal women with previous history of cerebrovascular disease showed an increased risk of fatal stroke (RR 2.9), and had no effect on stroke recurrence or death rate [28]. In contrast to the WHI estrogen trial, WEST did not show an increase in the risk for ischemic stroke in women with established cerebrovascular disease associated with estrogen monotherapy.

A large meta-analysis of randomized trials of HRT, including mono- and combination therapy trials (WEST, HERS and WHI trials) showed that both hormonal replacement regimens are associated with a higher risk of ischemic stroke (HR 1.29; 95% CI, 1.06-1.56), but not for hemorrhagic stroke or transient ischemic attacks [30].

The Kronos Early Estrogen Prevention Study (KEEPS) is a primary prevention trial of transdermal HRT to prevent progression of carotid and coronary atherosclerosis measured by surrogate outcome measures over 5 years [35]. Results from this study are currently pending.

A meta-analysis [36] of 21 randomized controlled trials analyzing estrogen/progestin combination therapy, estrogen monotherapy and including four trials of raloxifene, in more than 44,000 women is presented in Figure 1. In this analysis, HRT increased the overall risk of ischemic stroke by 32% (OR 1.32; 95% CI, 1.14-1.53) and HRT use was associated with worse stroke severity (HR 1.31; 95% CI, 1.12-1.54).

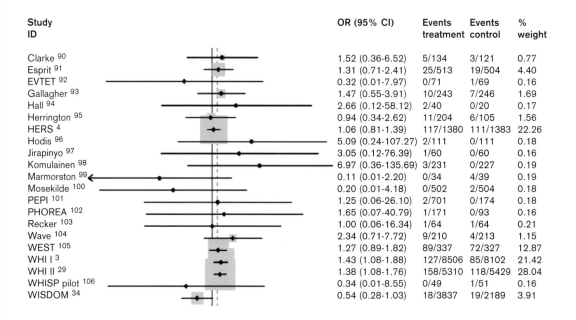

Study ID	OR (95% CI)	Events treatment	Events control	% weight
Clarke [90]	1.52 (0.36-6.52)	5/134	3/121	0.77
Esprit [91]	1.31 (0.71-2.41)	25/513	19/504	4.40
EVTET [92]	0.32 (0.01-7.97)	0/71	1/69	0.16
Gallagher [93]	1.47 (0.55-3.91)	10/243	7/246	1.69
Hall [94]	2.66 (0.12-58.12)	2/40	0/20	0.17
Herrington [95]	0.94 (0.34-2.62)	11/204	6/105	1.56
HERS [4]	1.06 (0.81-1.39)	117/1380	111/1383	22.26
Hodis [96]	5.09 (0.24-107.27)	2/111	0/111	0.18
Jirapinyo [97]	3.05 (0.12-76.39)	1/60	0/60	0.16
Komulainen [98]	6.97 (0.36-135.69)	3/231	0/227	0.19
Marmorston [99]	0.11 (0.01-2.20)	0/34	4/39	0.19
Mosekilde [100]	0.20 (0.01-4.18)	0/502	2/504	0.18
PEPI [101]	1.25 (0.06-26.10)	2/701	0/174	0.18
PHOREA [102]	1.65 (0.07-40.79)	1/171	0/93	0.16
Recker [103]	1.00 (0.06-16.34)	1/64	1/64	0.21
Wave [104]	2.34 (0.71-7.72)	9/210	4/213	1.15
WEST [105]	1.27 (0.89-1.82)	89/337	72/327	12.87
WHI I [3]	1.43 (1.08-1.88)	127/8506	85/8102	21.42
WHI II [29]	1.38 (1.08-1.76)	158/5310	118/5429	28.04
WHISP pilot [106]	0.34 (0.01-8.55)	0/49	1/51	0.16
WISDOM [34]	0.54 (0.28-1.03)	18/3837	19/2189	3.91

Figure 1. Summary of observational studies and randomized clinical trials analyzing the relation between hormonal replacement therapy and stroke risk. *Modified, with permission, from Oxford University Press and the European Society of Cardiology. Sare GM, et al* [36].

Androgens, hormone therapy and stroke risk in men

The association of stroke risk and androgen (testosterone, dehydroepiandrosterone [DHEA] and dehydroepiandrosterone-sulfate [DHEA-S]) use in men is receiving increasing research interest. Observational studies report a relation between increased stroke risk and cardiovascular risk in older men who have reduced circulating testosterone levels. Several studies suggest that testosterone supplementation may improve arterial vasoreactivity and may reduce levels of pro-inflammatory cytokines, total cholesterol and triglycerides [14]. However, it remains unclear whether these surrogate measures of vascular risk will translate into protection from ischemic stroke by testosterone supplementation in the clinical setting. Furthermore, adverse cardiovascular and cerebrovascular events, including myocardial infarct, pulmonary embolism and stroke have been reported following androgen use [14].

The current literature on stroke risk associated with androgen use is limited as results are predominantly based on single case reports. Single case reports suggest that ischemic stroke may be associated with high-dose use or abuse of synthetic androgens [37-41]. In some of the reported cases, individuals who used androgens and suffered from an ischemic stroke also had contributing vascular risk factors, making it difficult to interpret the findings of increased stroke risk [42].

A meta-analysis of 30 clinical trials in 1642 men including 808 men who were treated with testosterone, showed a weak trend indicating that testosterone is not associated with any important adverse cardiovascular effects [43]. However, this analysis was based on pooled data and included studies which had methodological limitations and used different study approaches.

The stroke risk is higher in men than in women. There is a well established association between stroke risk and advanced age in men, but based on the limited data available it is difficult to comment on an increased stroke risk associated with menopause-related decreased androgen levels. Case-control studies reported that men with stroke have lower testosterone concentrations in their blood and cerebrospinal fluid than those without stroke [44-46]. However, it remains unclear whether lowered blood testosterone levels are the cause, or a reaction following acute ischemic stroke in men, or if there is any relation at all.

Cross-sectional studies indicate that endogenous testosterone concentrations are inversely related with carotid artery intima media thickness, which is an independent marker of stroke risk and other atherosclerosis-related events [47]. In an observational study of 3443 men, age 17 years and older with a mean follow-up of 3.5 years, the incidence of first ischemic stroke and TIA was rather small at 3.7% [48]. Low testosterone levels were associated with an increased risk for ischemic stroke or TIA (HR 1.99; 95% CI, 1.33-2.99). The increased risk of cerebrovascular events persisted after adjustment for traditional vascular risk factors.

The Health in Men Study (HIMS) followed 3638 men. Fatal ischemic stroke occurred in five men in this study, and 140 men had a non-fatal ischemic stroke or TIA, resulting in a stroke incidence rate of 3.5% [49]. Baseline total and free testosterone levels were lower in men who experienced a first stroke or TIA compared to those without cerebrovascular events. Only free testosterone levels were significantly different between the groups (p=0.03). Men with a total testosterone level below 8nmol/L had a HR of 1.39 for incidence stroke or TIA (95% CI, 0.64-3.02). Men with low to normal low total testosterone levels had a HR of 2.08 (95% CI, 1.35-3.2) for cerebrovascular events. Results from this study suggest that free testosterone levels are associated with an increased risk for ischemic stroke and TIA. However, the study is limited by biases inherent to observational study designs and will require confirmation by future randomized controlled clinical trials.

In animal studies of acute stroke, administration of testosterone was associated with increased infarct volume and worse clinical outcome [50] suggesting an adverse effect. These data remain controversial as other groups have either reported no change or improved cell survival outcome following testosterone treatment in animal models of ischemic stroke [51]. The discrepancies between these studies may suggest that dose and duration of testosterone administration are important factors in acute ischemic stroke. The role of androgens for outcome in acute stroke, if any, remains currently unclear.

Oral contraceptives and associated stroke risk

Most oral contraceptives (OCs) today contain combinations of low-dose estrogen (most regimens now contain ≤50μg ethinyl estradiol) and progestin components. Reduction in both hormone concentrations has decreased the risk of adverse events including that of ischemic stroke [52]. The risk of deep venous thrombosis has remained unchanged despite introduction of low-dose combination formulations. Overall, the attributable absolute risk of stroke and sinus venous thrombosis in healthy young women who do not smoke is rare [53].

Evidence of stroke risk associated with the use of OCs is based on epidemiological studies which clearly have limitations due to multiple biases and methodological limitations. A summary of a meta-analysis of 16 epidemiological studies on the stroke risk associated with OC use is shown in Figure 2 [54]. In this analysis, the stroke risk associated with the use of low-dose estrogen-containing combination regimens was increased by 93% compared to non-users (HR 1.93, 95% CI 1.35-2.74), which persisted after adjustment for tobacco use and hypertension. The stroke risk associated with OCs containing higher doses of estrogen (>50μg estrogen) was slightly higher in this meta-analysis (see Figure 2). Most, but not all studies show a relatively small, but significant increase in ischemic stroke risk associated with OC use [55], whereas the risk of hemorrhagic stroke does not seem to be influenced by OC use.

A multicenter case-control study of stroke risk associated with OC use containing an estrogen/progestin combination studied women in Europe and in developing countries of Africa, Asia and Latin America. The observed stroke risk associated with OC use was increased in Europe (HR 2.99; 95% CI, 1.65-5.4), as well as in developing countries (HR 2.93; 95% CI, 2.15-4.0) [56]. In this study, the HR associated with the use of OCs containing low-dose estrogen was lower (HR1.53; 95% CI, 0.71-3.31) than in women using OCs which contained higher doses of estrogen (>50μg ethinyl estradiol) in Europe (HR 5.3; 95% CI

2.56-11). In developing countries both high- and low-dose estrogen was associated with a significantly increased stroke risk and did not differ significantly between groups (HR 3.26; 95% CI, 2.19-4.86 on low-dose estrogen versus HR 2.71; 95% CI, 1.75-4.19 on higher-dose estrogen). However, confidence intervals were relatively large and the study had methodological limitations so the translation of these data to clinical practice remains somewhat problematic. Similar to other studies stroke risk was higher in older women, in smokers and in those with a history of hypertension.

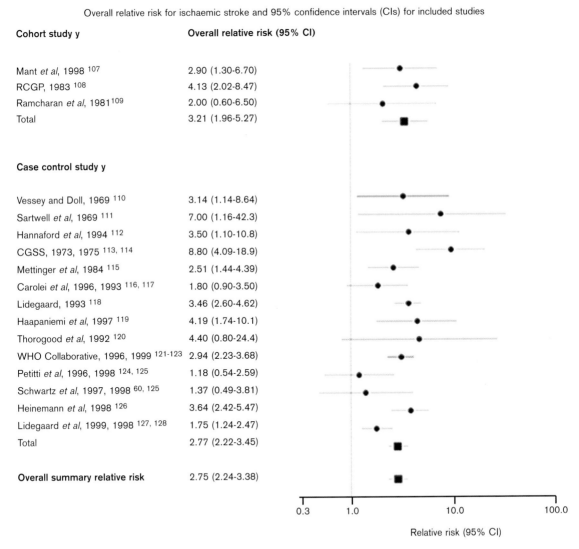

Figure 2. Stroke risk and use of oral contraceptives. Results of a meta-analysis of epidemiological studies. *Reproduced with permission from Gillum LA, et al* [54]. *Copyright © 2000 American Medical Association. All rights reserved.*

An increased ischemic stroke risk associated with OC use was reported in several case-control studies [57, 58], but could not be confirmed by other similar studies [52, 59-61]. In a multicenter case-control study [62] that examined the effect of different types of contraceptives on stroke risk (first generation OC containing lynestrenol or norethindrone, versus second generation OC containing levonorgestrel, versus third generation OC containing desogestrel or gestodene), the risk for ischemic stroke was increased in all OC users compared to non-users (HR 2.3; 95% CI, 0.7-4.4). Third generation OCs carried a similar increase in risk as second generation regimens (HR 1.0; 95%, CI 0.6-1.8).

The association of stroke risk and use of OCs which only contain progestogen was studied in a meta-analysis of six case-control studies [63]. Although only limited data are available regarding the use of progestogen monotherapy, these studies seem to indicate that progestogen is not associated with an increased risk for ischemic stroke (pooled HR 0.96; 95% CI, 0.70-1.31).

A pooled meta-analysis of four cohort and 16 case-control studies reported no increase in stroke risk associated with OC use (OR 0.95; 95% CI, 0.51-1.78) [55], whereas the pooled HR from all the case-control studies showed a significant association between risk of ischemic stroke and OC use (HR 2.74; 95% CI, 2.24-3.35) [55]. Women older than 35 years of age, those who use tobacco and hypertensive women had a higher risk of ischemic stroke. Risk of hemorrhagic stroke and stroke mortality was not increased in users of OCs.

Migraine, use of oral contraceptives and stroke risk

Migraine headaches are associated with a somewhat higher risk of stroke in women [64, 65]. The risk is especially high in women who have migraine with auras. Current evidence regarding stroke risk associated with the use of OCs in women with migraine is based on a limited number of studies. Best evidence currently comes from a meta-analysis of 11 case-control studies and three cohorts studies [66]. Based on this meta-analysis, the pooled relative risk (RR) for ischemic stroke among women with any type of migraine, with or without aura, was 2.16. This risk increased significantly in women who took oral contraceptives (RR 8.72) [66]. In women with migraines who have auras, but no other vascular risk factors, the frequency and severity of the auras is likely to be important [67]. Women with frequent auras should not receive OCs as there is a higher risk for ischemic stroke. However, the risk: benefit ratio of OC use needs to be thoroughly evaluated on an individual case basis [67, 68].

Hormonal therapy in women and risk of venous thrombosis

Deep vein thrombosis, pulmonary embolism and cerebral venous thrombosis are serious side effects of OCs and hormonal replacement therapy. Most data available are based on observational and case-control studies [69]. Results from observational and case-control studies are summarized in Table 2. Use of OCs, independent of estrogen dose, modestly, but significantly, increases the risk of venous thromboembolic events, including that of cerebral venous thrombosis [70-72]. Overall, the risk for venous thromboembolic events in women using HRT or OCs are increased by about 2 to 6-fold compared to non-users [53].

Table 2. Relative risk for thromboembolism (pulmonary embolism and deep venous thrombosis) in current users of oral contraceptives containing low doses of estrogen. *Reproduced with permission from Chasan-Taber L, et al* [69].

Study, year (reference)	Study period	Dose µg	Women using oral contraceptives n	Relative risk (95% CI)
Case control studies				
Helmrich *et al*, 1987 [81]	1976-1983	<50	5	11 (3.7-32)
World Health Organisation, 1989 [129]	1979-1984	NA†	41	2.9 (1.4-6.1)
Thorogood *et al*, 1992 [82]	1986-1988	≤50	29‡	1.6 (0.7-3.4)
Vandenbroucke *et al*, 1994 [85]	1988-1993	≤50 (inferred)	109	3.8 (2.4-6.0)
Beaumont *et al*, 1992 [130]	1992	50	21	1.00
		30	79	0.61 (0.29-1.28)
Cohort studies				
Hirvonen and Idänpään-Heikkilä, 1990 [131]	1975-1984	≤50	4‡	1.2 (0.4-3.7)
Porter *et al*, 1987 [132]	1977-1981	NA†	0	-
Porter *et al*, 1985 [70]	1980-1982	≤50	3	2.8 (0.9-8.2)
Gerstman *et al*, 1991 [133]	1980-1986	<50	53	1.0
		50	69	1.5 (1.0-2.1)
		>50	20	1.7 (0.9-3.0)

NA = not available
† = no information on estrogen dose, results given for entire sample
‡ = fatal cases only

Progesterone type

Case-control studies suggest that the risk of venous thromboembolism (VTE) is higher with use of third generation progestins, desogestrel and gestodene [73-75] compared to second generation regimens [73]. In a large case-control study, hazard ratios for second generation OCs containing low-dose ethinyl estradiol (no gestodene or desogestrel) were 3.2 and for third generation OCs (low-dose ethinyl estradiol with gestodene or desogestrel) 4.8, respectively [73]. The HR associated risk for venous thromboembolism with use of third versus second generation was 1.5. Similarly, the UK General Practice Research Database showed a RR of 1.9 for desogestrel and a RR of 1.8 for gestodene compared to levonorgestrel [75].

A case-control study demonstrated a higher risk of VTE associated with desogestrel compared to levonorgestrel (HR 1.7) [76]. Women receiving third generation OCs were often more obese and older which could have led to confounding of these study results.

There seems to be an increased risk associated with thromboembolism in women using newer generation progesterone compared to women using older oral contraceptives. The increase in risk was similar for users on desogestrel and uses of gestodene. This risk increase seems to persist despite adjustment for the other risk factors of venous thromboembolic events. Overall data from current studies between 1989 and 1995 suggest that there is an increased risk associated with OC use, but that there is a significant amount of confounding and biases associated with these studies. Further randomized trials are necessary to comment on the use of third versus older generation progestins.

Estrogen dose

The risk of venous thrombosis and pulmonary embolism is increased in women taking high-dose estrogen of 50μg or more. The risk with low-level estrogen, containing 50μg or less, may be somewhat lower. Gerstman and coworkers have found a direct dose-response relationship between estrogen dose and occurrence of venous thromboembolism [77].

Lowering the estrogen component from 100 to 50μg has been associated with a significant decrease in risk of thromboembolism. Overall, currently available OCs increase the risk of venous thrombosis by about five-fold compared to non-use (OR 5; 95% CI, 4.2-5.8). The risk of venous thrombosis seems to be highest during the first few months of OC administration irrespective of OC type [78]. Levonorgestrel is associated with an almost four-fold increased risk of DVT or cerebral venous thrombosis (OR 3.6; 95% CI, 2.9-4.6), and gestodene has an OR of 5.6 (95% CI, 3.7-8.4). VTE risk is also increased for desogestrel, (OR 7.5; 95% CI, 5.3-10), for cyproterone acetate (OR 6.8, 95% CI, 4.7-10), and for drospirenone (OR 6.3; 95% CI, 2.9-13.7). Overall, the risk for venous thrombosis is clearly associated with the type of progestogen, and estrogen dose.

The safest combination with regards to risk of venous thrombosis in OCs was observed with levonorgestrel combined with low-dose estrogen. The use of OCs is associated with a 2-6-fold increase of venous thromboembolic risk. The information regarding the new type of OCs containing drospirenone is currently limited.

A randomized controlled trial showed no difference in almost 5000 users of mestranol, 75µg versus controls using an alternative method of contraception, but the study had several methodological limitations [79]. Böttiger and colleagues noted a marked decline in VTE events in women who used low-dose estrogen OCs compared to those using high-dose preparations [80]. A case-control study reported a relative risk of venous thromboembolism of 11 (95% CI, 3.7-32) based on five cases in women using high-dose compared to women using low-dose estrogen contraceptives [81]. However, due to the overall small number of participants, the confidence intervals in this study were rather large. The WHO hospital-based case-control study reported a relative risk of 2.5 (95% CI, 1.42-6.1) among users of OCs. There was no sub-analysis adjusting for estrogen type or dose [82].

Comparing the association of risk of VTE and hormonal therapy suggests that progestin only contraceptives and transdermal HRT may be associated with a somewhat smaller risk of thrombembolism than other modes of hormonal treatment, such as oral OCs or oral HRT in women in whom use of oral hormonal administration is contraindicated [83, 84]. However, data on these regimens are very limited (III/B).

Hypercoaguable state and vascular risk factors

Women using OCs who have a hypercoaguable state or history of cardiovascular disease have a higher risk for VTE than non-users [85, 86]. For instance, in one study, women with a Factor V Leiden gene mutation had a 30-fold increased risk of venous thromboembolism compared to women without thrombophilia or to women who did not use OCs [85]. Women with a hypercoaguable state taking OCs are also at higher risk to develop cerebral sinus venous thrombosis, a potential devastating adverse event associated with the use of OCs (see Figure 3).

Women with a history of Factor V Leiden gene mutation, prothrombin gene mutation, protein S, protein C or antithrombin efficiency are at higher risk of cerebral thrombosis and should therefore not receive OCs. The risk is also somewhat increased in women with vascular risk factors, such as obesity, arterial hypertension, hyperhomocysteinemia, and nephrotic syndrome. Carriers of Factor V Leiden mutation that represent about 3% of the overall population have a seven-fold increase in thrombosis compared to non-carriers. Users of new generation progestogen have an about six-fold increased risk for VTE if they have a Factor V Leiden gene mutation [87]. It has been suggested that third generation progestogens could potentially induce a prothrombotic state via acquired resistance to activated protein C which is similar to that associated with Factor V Leiden mutations [88].

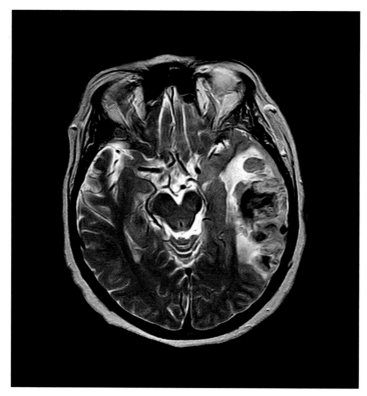

Figure 3. Magnetic resonance image of a 34-year-old woman with left sigmoid and transverse sinus thrombosis, resulting in a large left temporal-parietal hemorrhagic stroke with surrounding edema. The patient used oral contraceptives and had no other vascular risk factors.

Current practice guidelines for use of oral contraceptives

There is some controversy as well as overlap between current American College of Obstetricians and Gynecologists (ACOG) and WHO guidelines [89]. In general, women who are older than 35 years of age and who smoke more than 15 cigarettes daily should not receive estrogen/progestin oral contraceptives or hormonal replacement treatment [52]. Uncontrolled blood pressure also is associated with unacceptable risk and, as per guidelines of both societies, should not receive OCs. Women who have a history of stroke, ischemic heart disease, or a history of venous thromboembolism should not receive oral contraceptives. Also, women with migraine headache who are older than 35 years typically should not receive OCs, as the risk was found to typically outweigh the benefits. The risk is felt to be unacceptable if there is a history of focal neurological symptoms associated with migraine headaches. In women with hypercholesterolemia, ACOG guidelines state that the risk is acceptable if the LDL-cholesterol can be lowered to less than 160mg/dL, and if there are no other vascular risk factors present. Per WHO guidelines the benefit: risk ratio depends on the presence or absence of other cardiovascular risk factors. Both societies state that the risk of OC use is acceptable in women with controlled blood pressure. There is some controversy in women older than 35 years of age who smoke less than 15 cigarettes daily. ACOG guidelines state that the risk is unacceptable, while WHO guidelines state that the risk typically outweighs the benefit, but that there are no clear contraindications for use of OCs in this population.

Conclusions

HRT (estrogen monotherapy or combination therapy) should not be used for primary or secondary prevention of stroke in postmenopausal women **(Ia/A)**. In women who experienced a stroke while on HRT, the medication should be stopped. Short-term use, i.e. <5 years, of HRT in peri-or postmenopausal women with moderate to severe menopause-related symptoms is safe but risk: benefit ratios need to be weighted on a case by case basis **(Ia/A)**. The lowest effective estrogen concentration should be prescribed. Based on current evidence the risk of hemorrhagic stroke is not increased in users of HRT **(Ia/A)**.

There are no existing randomized trials of testosterone therapy or sufficiently statistically powered studies to comment on the potential benefits of androgens for stroke prevention in men. The stroke risk associated with androgen replacement remains currently unclear, although observational studies and meta-analyses of randomized clinical trials seem to suggest that they are safe and not associated with any increased risk of stroke. However, unexplained inconsistent results across trials, wide confidence intervals, and possible reporting bias among other limitations weaken the evidence **(IIa/B)**. The potential role of androgens in acute ischemic stroke is currently investigational. The safety and, if any, benefit of androgen use in men and women for primary and secondary stroke prevention remains uncertain until data from clinical randomized trials become available.

Due to limitations of observational studies by confounding and various biases, the association between OC and stroke risk remains currently uncertain **(IIa/B)**. Use of modern OC regimens with low-dose estrogen may be associated with a small increased risk of ischemic stroke. However, the absolute risk attributable to OC use in young women without hypertension who do not smoke, seems to be extremely low **(IIa/B)**. The baseline incidence of stroke in young women has been estimated to be less than 10/100,000 [52]. Older women, smokers, those with hypertension and women who have migraine with aura seem to have a higher ischemic stroke risk using OCs. The risk for stroke seems to be comparable for second and third generation progestins. The risk of hemorrhagic stroke associated with OCs is probably not increased. In women who have a stroke while they are on an OC, the medication should be discontinued.

Based on the currently available data **(IIb/B)**, the WHO and the American College of Obstetricians and Gynecologists (ACOG) conclude that women who have a history of migraine and who take OCs are at increased risk for thromboembolic events. The risks of OC use generally outweighs any benefits in this population, especially in women age 35 and above. Both societies therefore suggest that women who have migraines with aura or any focal neurological deficits associated with headaches that may indicate complicated migraine are at increased risk for stroke and should therefore not use any oral contraceptives or HRT. In women who have migraines without aura, other modifiable risk factors should be addressed and treated appropriately before considering OC use or HRT. In women with migraines who have auras, but no other vascular risk factors, the frequency and severity of the auras is likely to be important [67]. Women with frequent auras should not receive OCs considering that they are at higher risk for ischemic stroke. However, risks and benefits of OC use need to thoroughly evaluated on a case by case basis [67, 68].

The risk for VTE associated with third generation progestins seems to be the highest (IIa/B). However, in healthy women who are taking an OC containing third generation progestin and who do not have any history of thromboembolic event or any predisposing factors, change to an older preparation of progestin drug is probably not necessary. In general, if an OC is initiated, a second generation progestin is now the preferred combination regimen.

Data from prospective randomized trials are sparse due to the overall low risk of venous thromboembolism in otherwise healthy young women. Current evidence suggests that OCs containing more than 50µg of estrogen are associated with the highest risk of thromboembolic events and therefore low-dose estrogen combination regimens should be used (IIa/B).

Women who have hyperhomocysteinemia, nephrotic syndrome or those with a personal or family history of VTE or antiphospholipid antibodies should not receive OCs (IIb/B). Also, other hormonal contraceptives or HRT should not be used in this population. Routine screening for a hypercoaguable state in women of childbearing age is currently not recommended. Vascular risk factors should be treated whenever possible before considering use of an OC or HRT.

In summary, the current evidence suggests that the use of oral contraceptives and HRT in women is associated with an overall relatively small but significantly increased risk of ischemic stroke, while the stroke risk associated with testosterone replacement therapy has not been well examined. There seems to be no associated increased risk of intracranial hemorrhage with use of hormonal therapy. Risks and benefits of hormonal therapy need to weighted on an individual basis considering the patient's age, presence of comorbidities, history of cerebral ischemia, and associated stroke risk factors. The lowest effective hormone dose should be used. The literature surrounding hormonal therapy remains controversial, which is partly due to the small number of randomized controlled trials conducted. Recommendations based on currently available evidence and the level of evidence is shown in the key points.

Key points	Evidence level
♦ Estrogen monotherapy or estrogen-progestin combination therapy should not be used for primary or secondary prevention of stroke in postmenopausal women.	Ia/A
♦ The risk of hemorrhagic stroke is not increased in users of HRT.	Ia/A
♦ Short-term use, i.e. <5 years, of HRT in peri-or postmenopausal women with moderate to severe menopause-related symptoms is safe, but risk/benefit ratios need to be weighted on a case by case basis.	Ia/A
♦ The stroke risk associated with androgen replacement remains currently unclear, although observational studies seem to suggest that they are not associated with an increased risk for stroke.	IIa/B
♦ Use of modern OC regimens with low-dose estrogen may be associated with a small increased risk of ischemic stroke. However, the absolute risk attributable to OC use in young women without hypertension who do not smoke, seems to be low.	IIa/B
♦ The risk for venous thromboembolic events associated with third generation progestins seems to be higher than with older generation progestins.	IIa/B
♦ OCs containing more than 50µg of estrogen are associated with the highest risk of thromboembolic events and therefore low-dose estrogen combination regimens should be used	IIa/B

References

1. Lundberg V, Tolonen H, Stegmayr B, Kuulasmaa K, Asplund K; WHO MONICA Project. Use of oral contraceptives and hormone replacement therapy in the WHO MONICA project. *Maturitas* 2004; 48: 39-49.
2. Cameron DR, Braunstein GD. Androgen replacement therapy in women. *Fertil Steril* 2004; 82: 273-89.
3. Wassertheil-Smoller S, Hendrix SL, Limacher M, *et al.* WHI Investigators. Effect of estrogen plus progestin on stroke in postmenopausal women: the Women's Health Initiative: a randomized trial. *JAMA* 2003; 289: 2673-84.
4. Simon JA, Hsia J, Cauley JA, *et al.* Postmenopausal hormone therapy and risk of stroke: The Heart and Estrogen-progestin Replacement Study (HERS). *Circulation* 2001; 103: 638-42.
5. Herkert O, Kuhl H, Sandow J, Busse R, Schini-Kerth VB. Sex steroids used in hormonal treatment increase vascular procoagulant activity by inducing thrombin receptor (PAR-1) expression: role of the glucocorticoid receptor. *Circulation* 2001; 104: 2826-31.
6. Walsh BW, Schiff I, Rosner B, *et al.* Effects of postmenopausal estrogen replacement on the concentrations and metabolism of plasma lipoproteins. *N Engl J Med* 1991; 325: 1196-204.
7. Binder EF, Williams DB, Schechtman KB, Jeffe DB, Kohrt WM. Effects of hormone replacement therapy on serum lipids in elderly women. a randomized, placebo-controlled trial. *Ann Intern Med* 2001; 134: 754-60.
8. Yeboah J, Reboussin DM, Waters D, Kowalchuk G, Herrington DM. Effects of estrogen replacement with and without medroxyprogesterone acetate on brachial flow-mediated vasodilator responses in postmenopausal women with coronary artery disease. *Am Heart J* 2007; 153: 439-44.

9.   Rosano GM, Vitale C, Fini M. Hormone replacement therapy and cardioprotection: what is good and what is bad for the cardiovascular system? *Ann N Y Acad Sci* 2006; 1092: 341-8.

10. Brosnan JF, Sheppard BL, Norris LA. Haemostatic activation in post-menopausal women taking low-dose hormone therapy: less effect with transdermal administration? *Thromb Haemost* 2007; 97(4): 558-65.

11. Sumino H, Ichikawa S, Kasama S, *et al*. Different effects of oral conjugated estrogen and transdermal estradiol on arterial stiffness and vascular inflammatory markers in postmenopausal women. *Atherosclerosis* 2006; 189: 436-42.

12. Hendrix SL, Wassertheil-Smoller S, Johnson KC, *et al*. WHI Investigators. Effects of conjugated equine estrogen on stroke in the Women's Health Initiative. *Circulation* 2006; 113: 2425-34.

13. Schneider HPG. Androgenes and antiandrogenes. *Ann NY Acad Sci* 2003; 997: 292-306.

14. Liu PY, Death AK, Handelsman DG. Androgens and cardiovascular disease. *Endocrine Reviews* 2003; 24: 313-40.

15. Liu M, Dziennis S, Hurn PD, Alkayed NJ. Mechanisms of gender-linked ischemic brain injury. *Restor Neurol Neurosci* 2009; 27: 163-79.

16. Hurn PD, Macrae IM. Estrogen as a neuroprotectant in stroke. *J Cereb Blood Flow Metab* 2000; 20: 631-52.

17. Lemaitre RN, Weiss NS, Smith NL, *et al*. Esterified estrogen and conjugated equine estrogen and the risk of incident myocardial infarction and stroke. *Arch Intern Med* 2006; 166: 399-404

18. Arana A, Varas C, Gonzalez-Perez A, *et al*. Hormone therapy and cerebrovascular events: a populated based nested cohort study. *Menopause* 2006; 13: 1-7.

19. Li C, Engstrom G, Hedblad B, *et al*. Risk of stroke and hormone replacement therapy - a prospective cohort study. *Maturitas* 2006; 54: 11-18.

20. Lokkegaard E, Jovanovic Z, Heitmann BL, *et al*. Increased risk of stroke in hypertensive women using hormone therapy: analyses based on the Danish nurse study. *Arch Neurol* 2003; 60: 1379-84.

21. Heikkinen J, Vaheri R, Timonen U. A 10-year follow-up of postmenopausal women on long-term combined hormonal replacement therapy: update of safety and quality-of-life findings. *J Br Menopause Soc* 2006; 12: 115-25.

22. Finucane FF, Madans JH, Bush TL, Wolf PH, Kleinman JC. Decreased risk of stroke among postmenopausal hormone users. Results from a national cohort. *Arch Intern Med* 1993; 153: 73-9.

23. Stampfer MJ, Colditz GA, Willett WC, *et al*. Postmenopausal estrogen therapy and cardiovascular disease. Ten-year follow-up from the Nurses' Health Study. *N Engl J Med* 1991; 325: 756-62.

24. Grodstein F, Manson JE, Stampfer MJ, Rexrode K. Postmenopausal hormone therapy and stroke: role of time since menopause and age at initiation of hormone therapy. *Arch Intern Med* 2008; 168: 861-6.

25. Giroud M, Milan C, Beuriat P, *et al*. Incidence and survival rates during a two-year period of intracerebral and subarachnoid haemorrhages, cortical infarcts, lacunes and transient ischaemic attacks. The Stroke Registry of Dijon: 1985-1989. *Int J Epidemiol* 1991; 20: 892-9.

26. Lauterbach MD, Raz S, Sander CJ. Neonatal hypoxic risk in preterm birth infants: the influence of sex and severity of respiratory distress on cognitive recovery. *Neuropsychology* 2001; 15: 411-20.

27. Sacco RL, Boden-Albala B, Gan R, *et al*. Stroke incidence among white, black, and hispanic residents of an urban community: The Northern Manhattan Stroke Study. *Am J Epidemiol* 1998; 147: 259-68.

28. Viscoli CM, Brass LM, Kernan WN, Sarrel PM, Suissa S, Horwitz RI. A clinical trial of estrogen-replacement therapy after ischemic stroke. *N Engl J Med* 2001; 345: 1243-9.

29. Anderson GL, Limacher M, Assaf AR *et al*; Women's Health Initiative Steering Committee. Effects of conjugated equine estrogen in postmenopausal women with hysterectomy: the Women's Health Initiative randomized controlled trial. *JAMA* 2004; 291: 1701-12.

30. Bath PM, Gray LJ. Association between hormone replacement therapy and subsequent stroke: a meta-analysis. *BMJ* 2005; 330: 342.

31. Rossouw, JE, Prentice, RL, Manson, JE, *et al*. Postmenopausal hormone therapy and risk of cardiovascular disease by age and years since menopause. *JAMA* 2007; 297: 1465-77.

32. Grady D, Herrington D, Bittner V, *et al*; HERS Research Group. Cardiovascular disease outcomes during 6.8 years of hormone therapy: Heart and Estrogen/progestin Replacement Study follow-up (HERS II). *JAMA* 2002; 288: 49-57.

33. Grady D, Yaffe K, Kristof M, Lin F, Richards C, Barrett-Connor E. Effect of postmenopausal hormone therapy on cognitive function: the Heart and Estrogen/progestin Replacement Study. *Am J Med* 2002; 113(7): 543-8.

34. Vickers MR, MacLennan AH, Lawton B, *et al*; WISDOM group. Main morbidities recorded in the Women's International Study of long Duration Oestrogen after Menopause (WISDOM): a randomized controlled trial of hormone replacement therapy in postmenopausal women. *BMJ* 2007; 335: 239.

35. Harman S, Brinton E, Cedars M, *et al*. KEEPS: The Kronos Early Estrogen Prevention Study. *Climacteric* 2005; 8: 3-12.

36. Sare GM, Gray LJ, Bath PM. Association between hormone replacement therapy and subsequent arterial and venous vascular events: a meta-analysis. *Eur Heart J* 2008; 29: 2031-41.

37. Friedl KE. Effects of anabolic steroids on physical health. In: *Anabolic Steroids in Sports and Exercise.* Yesalis CE, Ed. Champaign, IL, USA: Human Kinetics Publishers, 2003: 107-50.

38. Akhter J, Hyder S, Ahmed M. Cerebrovascular accident associated with anabolic steroid use in a young man. *Neurology* 1994; 44: 2405-6.

39. Palfi S, Ungurean A, Vecsei L. Basilar artery occlusion associated with anabolic steroid abuse in a 17-year-old bodybuilder. *Eur Neurol* 1987; 37: 190-1.

40. Lisiewicz J, Fijalkowski P, Sankowski J. Ischemic cerebral stroke and anabolic steroids. *Neurol Neurochir Pol* 1999; 32: 137-9.

41. Nagelberg SB, Laue L, Loriaux DL, Liu L, Sherins RJ. Cerebrovascular accident associated with testosterone therapy in a 21-year-old hypogonadal man. *N Engl J Med* 1986; 314: 649-50.

42. Maron BJ, Shirani J, Poliac LC, Mathenge R, Roberts WC, Mueller FO. Sudden death in young competitive athletes. Clinical, demographic, and pathological profiles. *JAMA* 1996; 276: 199-204.

43. Haddad RM, Kennedy CC, Caples SM, *et al*. Testosterone and cardiovascular risk in men: a systematic review and meta-analysis of randomized placebo-controlled trials. *Mayo Clin Proc* 2007; 82: 29-39.

44. Jeppesen LL, Jorgensen HS, Nakayama H, Raaschou HO, Skyhoj T, Winther K. Decreased serum testosterone in men with acute ischemic stroke. *Arterioscler Thromb Vasc Biol* 1996; 16: 749-54.

45. Elwan O, Abdallah M, Issa I, Taher Y, el-Tamawy M. Hormonal changes in cerebral infarction in the young and elderly. *J Neurol Sci* 1990; 98: 235-43.

46. Dash RJ, Sethi BK, Nalini K, Singh S. Circulating testosterone in pure motor stroke. *Funct Neurol* 1991; 6: 29-34.

47. O'Leary DH, Polak JF, Kronmal RA, Manolio TA, Burke GL, Wolfson Jr SK. Carotid-artery intima and media thickness as a risk factor for myocardial infarction and stroke in older adults. Cardiovascular Health Study Collaborative Research Group. *N Engl J Med* 1999; 340: 14-22.

48. Yeap BB, Hyde Z, Almeida OP, *et al*. Lower testosterone levels predict incident stroke and transient ischemic attack in older men. *J Clin Endocrinol Metab* 2009; 94: 2353-9.

49. Norman PE, Flicker L, Almeida OP, *et al*. Cohort Profile: The Health In Men Study (HIMS). *Int J Epidemiol* 2009; 38: 48-52.

50. Herson PS, Koerner IP, Hurn PD. Sex, sex steroids, and brain injury. *Semin Reprod Med* 2009; 27: 229-39.

51. Vagnerova K, Koerner IP, Hurn PD. Gender and the injured brain. *Anesth Analg* 2008; 107: 201-14.

52. Petitti DB. Clinical practice. Combination estrogen-progestin oral contraceptives. *N Engl J Med* 2003; 349: 1443.

53. Douketis JD, Ginsberg JS, Holbrook A, *et al*. A reevaluation of the risk for venous thromboembolism with the use of oral contraceptives and hormone replacement therapy. *Arch Intern Med* 1997; 157: 1522.

54. Gillum LA, Mamidipudi SK, Johnston SC. Ischemic stroke risk with oral contraceptives: a meta-analysis. *JAMA* 2000; 284: 72-8.

55. Chan WS, Ray J, Wai EK, *et al*. Risk of stroke in women exposed to low-dose oral contraceptives: a critical evaluation of the evidence. *Arch Intern Med* 2004; 164: 741-7.

56. Acute myocardial infarction and combined oral contraceptives: results of an international multicentre case-control study. WHO Collaborative Study of Cardiovascular Disease and Steroid Hormone Contraception. *Lancet* 1997; 349: 1202-9.

57. Heinemann LA, Lewis MA, Thorogood M, *et al*. Case-control study of oral contraceptives and risk of thromboembolic stroke: results from international study on oral contraceptives and health of young women. *Br Med J* 1997; 315: 1502.

58. Bousser MG, Conard J, Kittner S, *et al*. Recommendations on the risk of ischaemic stroke associated with use of combined oral contraceptives and hormone replacement therapy in women with migraine. The International Headache Society Task Force on Combined Oral Contraceptives & Hormone Replacement Therapy. *Cephalalgia* 2000; 20: 155-6.

59. Haemorrhagic stroke, overall stroke risk, and combined oral contraceptives: results of an international, multicentre, case-control study. WHO Collaborative Study of Cardiovascular Disease and Steroid Hormone Contraception. *Lancet* 1996; 348: 505-10.

60. Schwartz SM, Siscovick DS, Longstreth WT Jr, *et al.* Use of low-dose oral contraceptives and stroke in young women. *Ann Intern Med* 1997; 127: 596-603.

61. Siritho S, Thrift AG, McNeil JJ, *et al.* Risk of ischemic stroke among users of the oral contraceptive pill: the Melbourne Risk Factor Study (MERFS) Group. *Stroke* 2003; 34: 1575-80.

62. Kemmeren JM, Tanis BC, van den Bosch MA, *et al.* Risk of Arterial Thrombosis in Relation to Oral Contraceptives (RATIO) study: oral contraceptives and the risk of ischemic stroke. *Stroke* 2002; 33: 1202-8.

63. Chakhtoura Z, Canonico M, Gompel A, Thalabard JC, Scarabin PY, Plu-Bureau G. Progestogen-only contraceptives and the risk of stroke: a meta-analysis. *Stroke* 2009; 40: 1059-62.

64. Rasmussen B. Migraine and tension-type headache in a general population: precipitating factors, female hormones, sleep pattern and relation to lifestyle. *Pain* 1993; 53: 65-72.

65. Aegidius K, Zwart JA, Hagen K, *et al.* Oral contraceptives and increased headache prevalence: the Head-HUNT Study. *Neurology* 2006; 66: 349-53.

66. Etminan M, Takkouche B, Isorna FC, Samii A. Risk of ischaemic stroke in people with migraine: systematic review and meta-analysis of observational studies. *BMJ* 2005; 330: 63.

67. Bousser MG, Conard J, Kittner S, *et al.* Recommendations on the risk of ischaemic stroke associated with use of combined oral contraceptives and hormone replacement therapy in women with migraine. The International Headache Society Task Force on Combined Oral Contraceptives & Hormone Replacement Therapy. *Cephalalgia* 2000; 20: 155-6.

68. MacClellan LR, Giles W, Cole J, *et al.* Probable migraine with visual aura and risk of ischemic stroke: the stroke prevention in young women study. *Stroke* 2007; 38: 2438-45.

69. Chasan-Taber L, Stampfer MJ. Epidemiology of oral contraceptives and cardiovascular disease. *Ann Intern Med* 1998; 128: 467-77.

70. Porter JB, Hunter JR, Jick H, Stergachis A. Oral contraceptives and nonfatal vascular disease. *Obstet Gynecol* 1985; 66: 1-4.

71. Vandenbroucke JP, Rosing J, Bloemenkamp KW, *et al.* Medical progress: oral contraceptives and the risk of venous thrombosis. *N Engl J Med* 2001; 344: 1527-35.

72. Gomes MP, Deitcher SR. Risk of venous thromboembolic disease associated with hormonal contraceptives and hormone replacement therapy: a clinical review. *Arch Intern Med* 2004; 64: 1965.

73. Spitzer WO, Lewis MA, Heinemann LAJ, *et al.* Third generation oral contraceptives and risk of venous thromboembolic disorders: an international case-control study. *BMJ* 1996; 312: 83.

74. Effect of different progestagens in low oestrogen oral contraceptives on venous thromboembolic disease. World Health Organization Collaborative Study of Cardiovascular Disease and Steroid Hormone Contraception. *Lancet* 1995; 346: 1582-8.

75. Jick H, Jick SS, Gurewich V, *et al.* Risk of idiopathic cardiovascular death and non-fatal venous thromboembolism in women using oral contraceptives with differing progestagen components. *Lancet* 1995; 346: 1589-93.

76. Jick SS, Kaye JA, Russmann S, Jick H. Risk of nonfatal venous thromboembolism with oral contraceptives containing norgestimate or desogestrel compared with oral contraceptives containing levonorgestrel. *Contraception* 2006; 73: 566-70.

77. Gerstman BB, Piper JM, Freiman JP, *et al.* Oral contraceptive oestrogen and progestin potencies and the incidence of deep venous thromboembolism. *Int J Epidemiol* 1990; 19: 931-6.

78. Lidegaard Ø, Løkkegaard E, Svendsen AL, Agger C. Hormonal contraception and risk of venous thromboembolism: national follow-up study. *BMJ* 2009; 13: 339.

79. Fuertes-de la Haba A, Curet JO, Pelegrina I, Bangdiwala I. Thrombophlebitis among oral and nonoral contraceptive users. *Obstet Gynecol* 1971; 38: 259-63.

80. Böttiger LE, Boman G, Eklund G, Westerholm B. Oral contraceptives and thromboembolic disease: effects of lowering oestrogen content. *Lancet* 1989; 8178: 1097-101.

81. Helmrich SP, Rosenberg L, Kaufman DW, Strom B, Shapiro S. Venous thromboembolism in relation to oral contraceptive use. *Obstet Gynecol* 1987; 69: 91-5.

82. Thorogood M, Mann J, Murphy M, Vessey M. Risk factors for fatal venous thromboembolism in young women: a case-control study. *Int J Epidemiol* 1992; 21: 48-52.

83. Scarabin PY, Oger E, Plu-Bureau G, on behalf of the EStrogen and THromboEmbolism Risk (ESTHER) Study Group. Differential association of oral and transdermal oestrogen replacement therapy with venous thromboembolism risk. *Lancet* 2003; 362: 428-32.

84. Lidegaard O, Edstroem B, Kreiner S. Oral contraceptives and venous thromboembolism: a five-year national case-control study. *Contraception* 2002; 65: 187-96.

85. Vandenbroucke JP, Koster T, Briet E, *et al.* Increased risk of venous thrombosis in oral-contraceptive users who are carriers of Factor V Leiden mutation. *Lancet* 1994; 344: 1453-7.

86. van Vlijmen EF, Brouwer JL, Veeger NJ, *et al.* Oral contraceptives and the absolute risk of venous thromboembolism in women with single or multiple thrombophilic defects: results from a retrospective family cohort study. *Arch Intern Med* 2007; 167: 282-9.

87. Kemmeren JM, Algra A, Meijers JC, *et al.* Effects of second- and third-generation oral contraceptives and their respective progestagens on the coagulation system in the absence or presence of the Factor V Leiden mutation. *Thromb Haemost* 2002; 87: 199-205.

88. Kemmeren JM, Algra A, Meijers JC, *et al.* Effect of second- and third-generation oral contraceptives on the protein C system in the absence or presence of the Factor V Leiden mutation: a randomized trial. *Blood* 2004; 103: 927-33.

89. Grodstein F, Clarkson TB, Manson JE. Understanding the divergent data on postmenopausal hormone therapy. *N Engl J Med* 2003; 348: 645-50.

90. Clarke SC, Kelleher J, Lloyd-Jones H, Slack M, Schofield PM. A study of hormone replacement therapy in postmenopausal women with ischaemic heart disease: the Papworth HRT Atherosclerosis Study. *Br J Obstet Gynaecol* 2002; 109: 1056-62.

91. Cherry N, Gilmour K, Hannaford P, Heagerty A, Khan MA, Kitchener H, McNamee R, Elstein M, Kay C, Seif M, Buckley H. Oestrogen therapy for prevention of reinfarction in postmenopausal women: a randomised placebo controlled trial. *Lancet* 2002; 360(9350): 2001-8.

92. Hoibraaten E, Qvigstad E, Arnesen H, Larsen S, Wickstrom E, Sandset PM. Increased risk of recurrent venous thromboembolism during hormone replacement therapy - results of the randomized, double-blind, placebo-controlled estrogen in venous thromboembolism trial (EVTET). *Thromb Haemost* 2000; 84(6): 961-7.

93. Gallagher JC, Fowler SE, Detter JR, Sherman SS. Combination treatment with estrogen and calcitriol in the prevention of age-related bone loss. *J Clin Endocrinol Metab* 2001; 86: 3618-28.

94. Hall G, Pripp U, Schenck-Gustafsson K, Landgren BM. Long-term effects of hormone replacement therapy on symptoms of angina pectoris, quality of life and compliance in women with coronary artery disease. *Maturitas* 1998; 28: 235-42.

95. Herrington DM, Reboussin DM, Brosnihan KB, Sharp PC, Shumaker SA, Snyder TE, Furberg CD, Kowalchuk GJ, Stuckey TD, Rogers WJ, Givens DH, Waters D. Effects of estrogen replacement on the progression of coronary-artery atherosclerosis. *New Engl J Med* 2000; 343: 522-9.

96. Hodis HN, Mack WJ, Lobo RA, Shoupe D, Sevanian A, Mahrer PR, Selzer RH, Liu C, Liu C, Azen SP, For the Estrogen in the Prevention of Atherosclerosis Trial Research Group. Estrogen in the Prevention of Atherosclerosis. A randomized, double blind, placebo-controlled trial. *Ann Intern Med* 2001; 135: 939-53.

97. Jirapinyo M, Theppisai U, Manonai J, Suchartwatnachai C, Jorgensen LN. Effect of combined oral estrogen/progestogen preparation (Kliogest) on bone mineral density, plasma lipids and postmenopausal symptoms in HRT-naive Thai women. *Acta Obstet Gynecol Scand* 2003; 82: 857-66.

98. Komulainen M, Kroger H, Tuppurainen MT, Heikkinen AM, Alhava E, Honkanen R, Jurvelin J, Saarikoski S. Prevention of femoral and lumbar bone loss with hormone replacement therapy and vitamin D3 in early postmenopausal women: a population-based 5-year randomized trial. *J Clin Endocrinol Metab* 1999; 84: 546-52.

99. Marmorston J. Effect of estrogen treatment in cerebrovascular diseases. *Cerebral Vascular Diseases* 1965: 214-20.

100. Mosekilde L, Beck-Nielsen H, Sorensen OH, Nielsen SP, Charles P, Vestergaard P, Hermann AP, Gram J, Hansen TB, Abrahamsen B, Ebbesen EN, Stilgren L, Jensen LB, Brot C, Hansen B, Tofteng CL, Eiken P, Kolthoff N. Hormonal replacement therapy reduces forearm fracture incidence in recent postmenopausal women - results of the Danish osteoporosis prevention study. *Maturitas* 2000; 36: 181-93.

101. The writing group for the PEPI Trial. Effects of estrogen or estrogen/progestin regimens on heart disease risk factors in postmenopausal women. The postmenopausal estrogen/progestin interventions (PEPI) trial. *JAMA* 1995; 18: 199-208.

102. Angerer P, Stork S, Kothny W, Schmitt P, von Schacky C. Effects of oral postmenopausal hormone replacement on progression of atherosclerosis. A randomized controlled trial. *Arterioscler Thromb Vasc Biol* 2001; 21: 262-8.

103. Recker RR, Davies KM, Dowd RM, Heaney RP. The effect of low-dose continuous estrogen and progesterone therapy with calcium and vitamin D on bone in elderly women. A randomized, controlled trial. *Ann Intern Med* 1999; 130: 897-904.

104. Waters DD, Alderman EL, Hsia J, Howard BV, Cobb FR, Rogers WJ, Ouyang P, Thompson P, Tardif JC, Higginson L, Bittner V, Steffes M, Gordon DJ, Proschan M, Younes N, Verter JI. Effects of hormone replacement therapy and antioxident vitamin supplements on coronary atherosclerosis in postmenopausal women. A randomized controlled trial. *JAMA* 2002; 288: 2432-40.

105. Viscoli CM, Brass LM, Kernan WN, Sarrel PM, Horwitz RI, 1757. Estrogen after ischemic stroke: effect of estrogen replacement on risk of recurrent stroke and death in the Women's Estrogen for Stroke Trial (WEST). *Stroke* 2001; 32: 329.

106. Collins P, Flather M, Lees B, Mister R, Proudler AJ, Stevenson JC, WHISP Pilot Investigators. Randomized trial of effects of continuous combined HRT on markers of lipids and coagulation in women with acute coronary syndromes: WHISP pilot study. *Eur Heart J* 2006; 27: 2046-53.

107. Mant J, Painter R, Vessey M. Risk of myocardial infarction, angina and stroke in users of oral contraceptives: an updated analysis of a cohort study. *Br J Obstet Gynaecol* 1998; 105: 890-6.

108. Royal College of General Practitioners' Oral Contraception Study. Incidence of arterial disease among oral contraceptive users. *J R Coll Gen Pract* 1983; 33: 75-82.

109. Ramcharan S, Pellegrin FA, Ray RM, Hsu JP. The Walnut Creek Contraceptive Drug Study: A prospective Study of the Side Effects of Oral Contraceptives, Volume III, an Interim Report: A Comparison of Disease Occurrence Leading to Hospitalization or Death in Users and Nonusers of Oral Contraceptives. Bethesda, Md: National Institutes of Health, 1981. Center for Population Research Monographs, NIH publication No. 81-564.

110. Vessey MP, Doll R. Investigation of relation between use of oral contraceptives and thromboembolic disease. *Br Med J* 1969; 2: 651-7.

111. Sartwell PE, Masi AT, Arthes FG, *et al*. Thromboembolism and oral contraceptives: an epidemiologic case-control study. *Am J Epidemiol* 1969; 90: 365-80.

112. Hannaford PC, Croft PR, Kay CR. Oral contraception and stroke: evidence from the Royal College of General Practitioners' Oral Contraception Study. *Stroke* 1994; 25: 935-42.

113. Collaborative Group for the Study of Stroke in Young Women. Oral contraception and increased risk of cerebral ischemia or thrombosis. *N Engl J Med* 1973; 288: 871-8.

114. Collaborative Group for the Study of Stroke in Young Women. Oral contraceptives and stroke in young women. *JAMA* 1975; 231: 718-22.

115. Mettinger KL, Soderstrom CE, Neiman J. Stroke before 55 years of age at Karolinska Hospital 1973-77: a study of 399 well-defined cases. *Acta Neurol Scand* 1984; 70: 415-22.

116. Carolei A, Marini C, De Matteis G, for the Italian National Research Council Study Group on Stroke in the Young. History of migraine and risk of cerebral ischaemia in young adults. *Lancet* 1996; 347: 1503-6.

117. Marini C, Carolei A, Roberts RS, *et al*, for the National Research Council Study Group. Focal cerebral ischemia in young adults. *Neuroepidemiology* 1993; 12: 70-81.

118. Lidegaard O. Oral contraception and risk of acerebral thromboembolic attack. *BMJ* 1993; 306: 956-63.

119. Haapaniemi H, Hillbom M, Juvela S. Lifestyle-associated risk factors for acute brain infarction among persons of working age. *Stroke* 1997; 28: 26-30.

120. Thorogood M, Mann J, Murphy M, Vessey M. Fatal stroke and use of oral contraceptives. *Am J Epidemiol* 1992; 136: 35-45.

121. World Health Organization Collaborative Study of Cardiovascular Disease and Steroid Hormone Contraception. Ischaemic stroke and combined oral contraceptives. *Lancet* 1996; 348: 498-505.

122. Poulter NR, Chang CL, Farley TM, *et al*, for the WHO Collaborative Study of Cardiovascular Disease and Steroid Hormone Contraception. Effect on stroke of different progestagens in low oestrogen dose oral contraceptives. *Lancet* 1999; 354: 301-2.

123. Chang CL, Donaghy M, Poulter N, for the WHO Collaborative Study of Cardiovascular Disease and Steroid Hormone Contraception. Migraine and stroke in young women. *BMJ* 1999; 318: 13-8.

124. Petitti DB, Sidney S, Bernstein A, *et al*. Stroke in users of low-dose oral contraceptives. *N Engl J Med* 1996; 335: 8-15.

125. Schwartz SM, Petitti DB, Siscovick DS, *et al*. Stroke and use of low-dose oral contraceptives in young women. *Stroke* 1998; 29: 2277-84.

126. Heinemann LA, Lewis MA, Spitzer WO, *et al*, for the Transnational Research Group on Oral Contraceptives and the Health of Young Women. Thromboembolic stroke in young women. *Contraception* 1998; 57: 29-37.

127. Lidegaard O. Smoking and use of oral contraceptives. *Am J Obstet Gynecol* 1999; 180: S357-363.

128. Lidegaard O, Edstrom B, Kreiner S. Oral contraceptives and venous thromboembolism: a case control study. *Contraception* 1998; 57: 291-301.

129. Cardiovascular disease and use of oral contraceptives. WHO Collaborative Study. *Bull World Health Organ* 1989; 67: 417-23.

130. Beaumont V, Malinow MR, Sexton G, Wilson D, Lemort N, Upson B, *et al*. Hyperhomocyst(e)inemia, anti-estrogen antibodies and other risk factors for thrombosis in women on oral contraceptives. *Atherosclerosis* 1992; 94: 147-52.

131. Hirvonen E, Idanpaan-Heikkila J. Cardiovascular death among women under 40 years of age using low-estrogen oral contraceptives and intrauterine devices in Finland from 1975 to 1984. *Am J Obstet Gynecol* 1990; 163(1 Pt 2): 281-4.

132. Porter JB, Jick H, Walker AM. Mortality among oral contraceptive users. *Obstet Gynecol* 1987; 70: 29-32.

133. Gerstman BB, Piper JM, Tomita DK, Ferguson WJ, Stadel BV, Lundin FE. Oral contraceptive estrogen dose and the risk of deep venous thromboembolitic disease. *Am J Epidemiol* 1991; 133: 32-7.

Chapter 14

The management of cerebrovascular complications in cardiac procedures

Sara Hocker MD, Fellow, Division of Critical Care Neurology
Mayo Clinic, Rochester, Minnesota, USA

José Biller MD FACP FAAN FAHA, Professor and Chairman
Department of Neurology, Loyola University Chicago
Stritch School of Medicine
Maywood, Illinois, USA

Introduction

Cerebrovascular complications of cardiac procedures are common in comparison with general, non-cardiac surgery. The incidence of stroke complicating cardiac surgery ranges from 1.4-9.8%, depending on the type and timing of the procedure [1-9]. More strokes occur after urgent surgery than after elective surgery [6]. Peri-operative strokes result in a prolonged hospital stay and increased rates of disability, discharge to long-term care facilities, and death after surgery [8].

Mechanisms of brain injury include global ischemia secondary to hypotension or hypoxia, focal brain ischemia secondary to hypoperfusion in the border zones (watershed territories), ischemic stroke secondary to embolization of thrombi, atherosclerotic plaque, fat or air, and less commonly, intracranial hemorrhage. The majority of strokes in patients undergoing cardiac surgery are not related to hypoperfusion, but rather are due to embolism. Hypotension induced by anesthesia does not seem to adversely affect cerebral perfusion or increase the risk of peri-operative stroke due to hypoperfusion in patients with carotid artery stenosis [7, 10, 11] **(IIb/B)**.

While the majority of cerebrovascular complications of cardiac procedures are ischemic in nature, hemorrhagic complications do occur secondary to coagulopathy, antithrombotic medications, elevated blood pressure or rupture of an intracranial aneurysm. Ischemic complications of cardiac procedures account for at upward of 85% of periprocedural strokes, the majority of which are embolic [7, 12-14]. In this chapter we will focus on the most common cerebrovascular complications of specific cardiac procedures.

Because of the procedural nature of these studies and the obvious difficulties of blinding either patients or clinicians, level I evidence in the management of post-procedural strokes is limited. This chapter will review evidence, where available, to minimize and manage cerebrovascular complications of cardiac procedures. Management of peri-operative strokes, when they do occur, should follow guidelines for the management of non-peri-operative strokes, except in regards to treatment of acute ischemic stroke. In patients who have recently undergone major surgery, treatment with intravenous recombinant tissue plasminogen activator (rt-PA) is contraindicated (Ia/A). Evidence for treatment with intra-arterial administration of rt-PA and endovascular mechanical clot disruption is limited to case series or case reports (III/B).

Coronary artery bypass grafting

Coronary artery bypass grafting (CABG) is the most common surgical procedure performed in the United States. The incidence of symptomatic stroke after CABG varies from 0.8-5.2% [15]. Using highly sensitive diffusion-weighted MRI increases the incidence of cerebral infarctions to 18%. However, about two thirds of these infarcts are asymptomatic [16]. The clinical picture of post-CABG cerebrovascular events varies, and it depends on the location, number, and extent of lesions affecting the brain. In a study of strokes after CABG, embolic strokes accounted for 62.1%, followed by multiple etiologies (10.1%), hypoperfusion (8.8%), lacunar (3.1%), thrombotic (1%), and hemorrhage (1%). Nearly 14% of strokes after CABG were of unknown etiology. Nearly 45% (105 of 235) of the embolic, and 56% (18 of 32) of hypoperfusion-related strokes occurred within the first postoperative day, and an additional 20% occurred by day 2 [17]. Early embolism typically results from manipulations of the heart and aorta or release of particulate matter from the cardiopulmonary-bypass pump [4, 6, 8]. Less commonly, strokes can occur several days postoperatively and then tend to be related to cardiac arrhythmias such as atrial fibrillation, myocardial infarction or coagulopathy [4].

Risk factors for peri-operative stroke among patients undergoing CABG include advanced age, non-elective surgery, female gender, low ejection fraction (EF), atherosclerotic vascular disease, diabetes mellitus, and impaired renal function [18]. Among patients with a low ejection fraction, the risk of stroke may be lower with coronary angioplasty than with CABG [19] (III/B). Atheromatous aorta and carotid artery disease are known to be predictors for stroke after CABG. A study from Japan suggested that prophylactic cerebrovascular interventions and the selective use of aorta no-touch, off-pump coronary artery bypass (OPCAB) significantly reduces the incidence of peri-operative stroke [20, 21]. A 'no-touch' technique avoids manipulations of the ascending aorta and is advised whenever feasible in patients with aortic arch disease. Because OPCAB avoids both aortic cannulation and cardiopulmonary bypass, neurological complications would be expected to be less. However, three randomized controlled trials (RCTs) [22-24] have not firmly established a significant change in neurological outcomes between OPCAB patients and conventional CABG patients. Currently, there is insufficient evidence of a difference in neurological outcomes for patients undergoing OPCAB compared with those undergoing conventional CABG [25] (Ia/A).

The optimal level of blood pressure during surgery is debatable. In one study, the incidence of cardiac and neurologic complications, including stroke, was significantly lower when the mean systemic arterial pressure was 80-100mm Hg during CABG, as compared with 50 - 60mm Hg. This suggests that a higher mean systemic arterial pressure during CABG is safe and may improve outcomes [26]. Charlson *et al* reported that prolonged changes of more than 20mm Hg or 20% in relation to pre-operative levels result in peri-operative complications [27]. Matching intra-operative and early postoperative blood pressure to the patient's pre-operative range may reduce the risks of peri-operative stroke and death [28] **(Ib/A)**. While the management of the patient's temperature during surgery may also influence outcomes, a Cochrane review from 2001 could find no definite advantage of hypothermia over normothermia in the incidence of clinical events **(Ia/A)**. Hypothermia was associated with a reduced stroke rate, but this is off-set by a trend towards an increase in non-stroke-related peri-operative mortality and myocardial damage [29].

The reader may refer to previous chapters in this book for evidence regarding the management of acute periprocedural strokes, as it will be similar to that of non-periprocedural

Table 1. ACC/AHA guidelines for coronary artery bypass graft surgery.	
◆ In patients having recent anterior MI, pre-operative screening with echocardiography may be considered to detect left ventricular (LV) thrombus, because the technical approach and timing of surgery may be altered.	IIb/C
◆ Carotid endarterectomy is probably recommended before CABG or concomitant to CABG in patients with a symptomatic carotid artery stenosis or in asymptomatic patients with a unilateral or bilateral internal carotid artery stenosis of >80%.	IIa/C
◆ Carotid screening is probably indicated in the following subsets: age >65 years, left main coronary artery stenosis, peripheral vascular disease, history of smoking, history of transient ischemic attack (TIA) or stroke, or carotid bruit on examination.	IIa/C
◆ If clinical circumstances permit, clopidogrel should be withheld for 5 days before the performance of CABG surgery.	I/B
◆ Significant atherosclerosis of the ascending aorta mandates a surgical approach that will minimize the possibility of arteriosclerotic emboli.	I/C
◆ Long-term (3-6 months) anticoagulation is probably indicated for the patient with a recent antero-apical infarct and persistent wall-motion abnormality after coronary bypass.	IIa/C
◆ In post-CABG atrial fibrillation that is recurrent or persists more than 24 hours, warfarin anticoagulation for 4 weeks is probably indicated.	IIa/C

strokes. Because CABG falls under the category of major surgery, intravenous thrombolysis for acute ischemic stroke is contraindicated in these patients. Table 1 lists guidelines for CABG published by the American College of Cardiology/American Heart Association (ACC/AHA) which pertain to stroke [30].

Given that postoperative arrhythmias including postoperative atrial fibrillation are common and can occur following any cardiac surgery or procedure, they will be discussed further in a separate section.

Valvular heart disease

Stroke is the most common neurologic complication of cardiac valvular surgeries. The incidence of stroke is dependent on multiple variables including whether the valve is repaired or replaced, whether open heart surgery, balloon valvuloplasty, or transcatheter placement is used, whether the prosthetic valve is mechanical or bioprosthetic, whether the valve is in the mitral or aortic position, whether concomitant procedures (e.g. left atrial appendage closure, CABG, etc.) are performed, and whether adequate anticoagulation is used. While these variables make it difficult to compare stroke statistics between studies, some generalizations about the epidemiology of stroke after cardiac valve surgery are clear. Stroke is more common with mitral valve (0.3-5%) [31-35] than with aortic valve surgeries (0.2-4.4%) [32, 35-37], and this is thought to be due to an increased likelihood of atrial fibrillation, left atrial enlargement and possible endocardial damage from rheumatic mitral valve disease [38]. Isolated cardiac valve surgery has a lower incidence of stroke than double- or triple-valve surgery or when isolated cardiac valve surgery is combined with CABG, repair of other cardiac abnormalities, or carotid endarterectomy [6, 8, 39, 40]. Intra-operative strokes are commonly due to hypoperfusion or emboli, whereas strokes in the postoperative period are primarily due to emboli from valve thrombosis, left atrial thrombi secondary to atrial fibrillation, and infective endocarditis (IE). Both mechanical and bioprosthetic valves are associated with valve thrombosis. In actuality, in patients with adequate anticoagulation, the rate of stroke is considered equal between bioprosthetic and mechanical valves [41, 42].

Atrial fibrillation is the most significant risk factor for delayed stroke after mitral valve replacement [43]. Postoperative arrhythmias are discussed in a separate section of this chapter.

The development of infective endocarditis after prosthetic valve surgery is a major complication with significant morbidity and a mortality rate of 50%. Stroke is one of the major predictors of mortality with this condition. The neurological manifestations of infective endocarditis are usually consistent with ischemic stroke. Rarely, patients with endocarditis may be found to have intracerebral hemorrhage, subarachnoid hemorrhage, cerebral abscess, or mycotic aneurysms. Prosthetic valve endocarditis accounts for 7-25% of cases of infective endocarditis [44] and the incidence of prosthetic valve endocarditis is reported to be 1-3% during the postoperative period. The incidence of neurologic complications is 20-40% in all cases of infective endocarditis [45, 46]. Mechanical heart valves are probably at higher risk for infection than are bioprostheses during the first 3 months after surgery, but the rates of infection are similar at 5 years [44, 47-49]. The cumulative risk of prosthetic valve endocarditis is approximately 1% at 12 months and 2-3% at 60 months [44, 50, 51].

The use of anticoagulation in cardiac surgery patients is a debated topic. In general, patients with mechanical heart valves receive long-term anticoagulation, while patients with bioprosthetic heart valves receive a 3-month course of warfarin (target INR 2.5), and then only antiplatelet therapy, such as aspirin. The appropriate use and recommendations regarding anticoagulant therapy in patients with bioprosthetic and mechanical valve replacements are reviewed elsewhere in this book.

Invasive electrophysiological procedures for cardiac arrhythmias

The cerebrovascular complications that can occur with invasive electrophysiological studies include TIA and stroke. The incidence of these events is extremely low. Table 2 lists mechanisms of stroke associated with invasive electrophysiologic procedures [52-54]. A complete discussion of these procedures is beyond the scope of this chapter.

As atrial fibrillation is the most common cardiac arrhythmia, associated with significant morbidity including thromboembolism, radiofrequency catheter ablation for patients with symptomatic atrial fibrillation refractory to antiarrhythmic drugs will be discussed here. While ablation may reduce the occurrence of future stroke in patients with atrial fibrillation **(Ia/A)**, periprocedural stroke and TIA do occur with a reported incidence of 0.4-2.1% [55-59]. Predictors of periprocedural stroke with atrial fibrillation ablation are not fully understood. Scherr and colleagues conducted a review of 721 cases in which ten periprocedural ischemic strokes occurred (1.4%) and concluded that a CHADS 2 score > or = to 2 [60] and history of stroke are independent predictors of stroke after atrial fibrillation ablation [61]. It is unknown which, if any, of the stroke mechanisms listed in Table 2 are predominant. Typically, patients undergo transesophageal echocardiography and anticoagulation prior to the procedure and intraprocedural anticoagulation to minimize the risk of periprocedural stroke **(IIa/B)**.

Table 2. Mechanisms of stroke during invasive electrophysiologic procedures.

◆ Thromboembolism from:

    o   catheter and sheaths
    o   left atrial appendage
    o   damage to cardiac endothelium
    o   mechanical disruption of LV thrombus or aneurysm

◆ Air embolism during trans-septal catheterization

◆ Direct embolism during radiofrequency energy delivery

◆ Hypoxic-anoxic injury secondary to hypoperfusion from anesthetic complications

---

Cardiac catheterization and percutaneous coronary intervention

In the United States, about 1.5 million cardiac catheterization procedures are performed per year. Over 1 million coronary intervention procedures such as balloon angioplasty and stent placement are performed annually in the United States. Although stroke is a very rare complication of these procedures, it can have devastating consequences and is known to increase both in-hospital and 1-year mortality [62]. Clinically relevant cerebrovascular events complicate diagnostic cardiac catheterization and percutaneous coronary intervention (PCI) in 0.1-0.44% of adult patients [62-71]. A study of approximately 6500 patients who underwent invasive cardiac procedures such as left heart catheterization, balloon angioplasty, and valvuloplasty described an overall 0.4% incidence of neurologic complications. Asymptomatic cerebral infarction is described in 15% of patients as detected by diffusion-weighted MRI in a study that included diagnostic and interventional cardiac catheterization [72].

The etiologies of cerebrovascular complications from cardiac catheterization and PCI are numerous and include thromboembolism, atherosclerosis, air embolism, vessel trauma, vasospasm, systemic hypoxia or hypotension, and bleeding secondary to pharmacotherapy. Stroke with cardiac catheterization may occur during the procedure, immediately after the procedure while the femoral artery sheath is still intact or up to 36 hours after the procedure [66, 71].

Stroke in association with cardiac catheterization is approximately evenly split between the carotid circulation and the vertebrobasilar circulation, with some studies reporting a carotid circulation predominance [73] and others reporting a vertebrobasilar circulation predominance [63, 66, 74]. Evidence from several studies has suggested that vertebrobasilar circulation strokes are more common with the brachial artery approach and carotid circulation events are more common with the femoral artery approach [64, 75-77] (III/B).

The risk factors for stroke with cardiac catheterization and PCI are similar and are detailed in Table 3 below (III/B). Cerebral microemboli are predominantly detected during catheter advancement, catheter flushing, contrast injection, and ventriculography [78] (III/B). There is also a significant correlation between the number of microemboli and the volume of contrast used [78]. It is unclear whether transradial catheterization is superior to femoral catheterization in terms of lesser incidence of stroke. In one study, stroke was significantly associated with the severity of coronary artery disease and the duration of the procedure [69] (III/B). In patients undergoing percutaneous interventions, stiff, large-bore guiding catheters are used which theoretically can be more traumatic to the aorta than diagnostic catheters, which are more flexible and have smaller lumens and tapered tips [71] (III/B).

When stroke occurs during or following cardiac catheterization or PCI, urgent cerebral imaging should be obtained to confirm an ischemic cause, as the use of anticoagulation and several antiplatelet drugs increases the risk of intracerebral hemorrhage. Therapy should be instituted according to guidelines for standard acute stroke management, including the consideration of thrombolytic therapy [73, 79-82] (III/B).

Table 3. Risk factors for cerebrovascular complications with cardiac catheterization and PCI.

Patient-related

- Age over 60
- Worsening New York Heart Association functional class
- Lower ejection fraction
- Greater risk with three-vessel or left main disease
- Left ventricular hypertrophy
- Over 50% stenosis of any coronary artery
- Female gender
- Peripheral vascular disease
- Atheromas or extensive plaques of the aorta, especially mobile ones, on transesophageal echocardiogram
- Hypertension
- Diabetes mellitus
- Renal insufficiency
- Prior stroke

Procedure-related

- Longer fluoroscopic time (duration of the procedure)
- Use of large-caliber catheters
- Introduction of air emboli from catheter, sheath, or line during contrast or saline injection
- Introduction of microemboli during catheter advancement, catheter flushing, contrast injection, and ventriculography
- Large volume of contrast
- Multiple catheter manipulation

Because stroke is an uncommon complication of both diagnostic cardiac catheterization and PCI, evidence guiding prevention and management is limited. Table 4 contains guidelines for cardiac catheterization procedures which pertain to stroke.

Table 4. ACC/AHA guidelines for cardiac catheterization and PCI which pertain to stroke.

• In STEMI patients with a prior history of stroke and TIA for whom primary PCI is planned, prasugrel is not recommended as part of a dual-antiplatelet therapy regimen [83].	III/C
• The addition of aspirin to clopidogrel increases the risk of hemorrhage. Combination therapy of aspirin and clopidogrel is not routinely recommended for ischemic stroke or TIA patients unless they have a specific indication for this therapy (i.e. coronary stent or acute coronary syndrome) [84].	III/A

Aortic surgery

The incidence of stroke following open surgery for thoracic aortic disease has been reported at 6-11% [85]. Khoynezhad and colleagues reported on 153 patients from 1998 to 2005, who underwent 184 thoracic endovascular aortic repairs (TEVARs), eight of which were complicated by cerebral ischemia [86]. A similar incidence (3.1%) of stroke following endovascular treatment of thoracic aortic disease was calculated from data taken from the European Collaborators on Stent/Graft Techniques for Aortic Aneurysm Repair (EUROSTAR) Registry published in 2007 [87]. A prospective study by Gutsche and colleagues found a higher incidence of 5.8% [88]. Risk factors for cerebral ischemia in these patients included obesity, significant intra-operative blood loss, evidence of peripheral vascular thrombosis, severe atheromatous disease involving the aortic arch, longer duration of intervention and female gender [87, 88]. Manipulation of the aorta has resulted in embolization of neo-endothelium to the vertebral artery and cerebellar infarction, as was reported in the case of a patient undergoing redilation of an aortic stent [89]. Several similar neurologic syndromes with progressive supranuclear palsy (PSP)-like clinical manifestations have been described as occurring after surgery on the ascending aorta with or without aortic valve replacement [90-92]. These patients had lesions in variable locations including the cerebellum, pons and both cerebral hemispheres. Most of these patients had a history of aortic dissections or bicuspid aortic valve. The mechanism of these lesions is not yet well understood. The incidence of spinal cord ischemia resulting in paraparesis or paraplegia following endovascular procedures of the thoracic aorta has been reported to be from 2.5-3.8% [85, 86]. This is contrasted with reported rates of paraplegia following open surgery for thoracic aortic disease of 3-19% [85]. A recent meta-analysis of open versus endovascular repair for ruptured descending thoracic aortic aneurysms which included 224 patients showed a 30-day occurrence rate of stroke (10.2% vs 4.1%; OR 2.67; p=.117) and paraplegia (5.5% vs 3.1%; OR 1.83; p=.405), failing to reach statistical significance [93]. Risk factors for spinal cord ischemia include aneurysm as an underlying pathology, the use of an iliac conduit, and coverage of the hypogastric artery [86]. In the EUROSTAR Registry, spinal cord ischemia was associated with left subclavian artery covering without revascularization, renal failure, open abdominal aorta surgery at the same time, and use of three or more stent grafts [87]. Overstenting of the left subclavian artery with or without revascularization is controversial, although studies have indicated the need for surgical revascularization when there is a flow-limiting stenosis of the right vertebral artery, occlusion of an internal carotid artery, or when the left vertebral artery is dominant [87, 94, 95].

The reader may refer to other chapters in this book for evidence regarding management of acute peri-procedural strokes as it will be similar to that of non-periprocedural strokes. Because open surgery for thoracic aortic disease falls under the category of major surgery, thrombolysis is contraindicated in these patients (Ia/A).

Table 5 lists guidelines for thoracic aortic disease published by the American College of Cardiology/American Heart Association (ACC/AHA) which pertain to cerebrovascular and spinal cord ischemia [96].

Table 5. ACC/AHA guidelines for thoracic aortic disease.	

♦ Motor or somatosensory evoked potential monitoring can be useful when the data will help to guide therapy. It is reasonable to base the decision to use neurophysiologic monitoring on individual patient needs, institutional resources, the urgency of the procedure, and the surgical and perfusion techniques to be employed in the open or endovascular thoracic aortic repair. IIa/B

♦ A brain protection strategy to prevent stroke and preserve cognitive function should be a key element of the surgical, anesthetic, and perfusion techniques used to accomplish repairs of the ascending aorta and transverse aortic arch. I/B

♦ Deep hypothermic circulatory arrest, selective antegrade brain perfusion, and retrograde brain perfusion are techniques that alone or in combination are reasonable to minimize brain injury during surgical repairs of the ascending aorta and transverse aortic arch. Institutional experience is an important factor in selecting these techniques. IIa/B

♦ Peri-operative brain hyperthermia is not recommended in repairs of the ascending aortic and transverse aortic arch as it is probably injurious to the brain. III/B

♦ Cerebrospinal fluid drainage is recommended as a spinal cord protective strategy in open and endovascular thoracic aortic repair for patients at high risk of spinal cord ischemic injury. I/B

♦ Spinal cord perfusion pressure optimization using techniques, such as proximal aortic pressure maintenance and distal aortic perfusion, is reasonable as an integral part of the surgical, anesthetic, and perfusion strategy in open and endovascular thoracic aortic repair patients at high risk of spinal cord ischemic injury. Institutional experience is an important factor in selecting these techniques. IIa/B

♦ Moderate systemic hypothermia is reasonable for protection of the spinal cord during open repairs of the descending thoracic aorta. IIa/B

♦ Adjunctive techniques to increase the tolerance of the spinal cord to impaired perfusion may be considered during open and endovascular thoracic aortic repair for patients at high risk of spinal cord injury. These include distal perfusion, epidural irrigation with hypothermic solutions, high-dose systemic glucocorticoids, osmotic diuresis with mannitol, intrathecal papaverine, and cellular metabolic suppression with anesthetic agents. IIb/B

♦ Neurophysiological monitoring of the spinal cord (somatosensory evoked potentials or motor evoked potentials) may be considered as a strategy to detect spinal cord ischemia and to guide reimplantation of intercostal arteries and/or hemodynamic optimization to prevent or treat spinal cord ischemia. IIb/B

Congenital heart disease

Congenital heart diseases (CHD) represent a diverse group of rare disorders. A detailed review of specific cardiac defects and procedures are beyond the scope of this chapter. Stroke accounts for 20% of the non-cardiac causes of death in this population [97]. Age, duration of bypass, and re-operation may be associated with stroke risk [98]. As with adults undergoing surgery on the aortic arch, spinal cord ischemia can occur. Children with coarctation of the aorta have a 7% incidence of intracranial aneurysms, predisposing them to intracerebral hemorrhage or subarachnoid hemorrhages. Other described cerebrovascular complications of surgery for pediatric CHD include intracranial hemorrhages, arterial ischemic strokes, cerebral venous gas embolism [99], venous thrombosis, spinal cord ischemia, and hypoxic-ischemic injury. Predisposing factors are multifactorial and include pre-operative brain malformations, peri-operative hypoxemia and low cardiac output states, sequelae of cardiopulmonary bypass, deep hypothermic circulatory arrest, and postoperative arrhythmias [100]. It should also be noted that children with CHD undergoing surgery may have underlying genetic abnormalities (e.g. genetic polymorphisms mediating an inflammatory response to cardiopulmonary bypass) or acquired abnormalities (e.g. hemoglobinopathies, coagulation disturbances) that predispose them to thrombosis [101]. Invasive diagnostic tests such as cardiac catheterization and other procedures predispose these children to thrombosis and stroke [101]. As previously noted, neurologic complications occur in 0.24% of diagnostic catheterizations in children [102]. Stroke accounts for greater than half of the neurologic complications. However, two thirds of these children have no neurologic sequelae on long-term follow-up [102]. The risk of complications increases with interventional procedures during the catheterization, with prolonged duration of the procedure and with the presence of a right-to-left shunt [102]. Since the advent of neonatal repair of complex lesions in the 1970s, an estimated 85% of patients with CHD survive into adult life. Because true surgical cures of CHD are infrequent, almost all patients who have undergone surgery are left with some form of sequelae, many of which predispose to infective endocarditis [44, 97, 103-108]. The ACC/AHA recommend that adults with congenital heart disease (ACHD) are managed by regional ACHD centers (IV/C). The interested reader may refer to the ACC/AHA guidelines for the management of ACHD [109] for further recommendations regarding the management of these patients including recommendations for infective endocarditis.

Cardiac transplantation

Cardiac transplantation is a widely accepted procedure for the treatment of end-stage heart failure. While awaiting cardiac transplantation, patients may require treatment with a left ventricular assist device (LVAD) that have been shown to improve survival rates and quality of life in patients with advanced heart failure when compared to medical therapy alone [110]. Treatment with a LVAD reduces the risk of stroke when compared with medical therapy alone [111] (Ib/A). Furthermore, treatment with a continuous-flow LVAD significantly improved the probability of survival free from stroke at 2 years as compared with a pulsatile device [112] (Ib/A). Despite major advances since the early days of cardiac transplantation, there is still a 4% risk of death from all neurologic causes and a need to reduce neurologic morbidity associated with the procedure [113]. Cerebrovascular events occurring in the immediate post-transplantation period are similar to those seen after valvular or coronary revascularization surgery. However, the overall incidence of complications is higher than with elective CABG or elective valve replacement surgery [114]. Ischemic stroke occurs in 2-14% of patients in clinical series of patients undergoing cardiac transplantation [115-120]. However, autopsy series have documented as high as a 50% rate of cerebrovascular events in post-transplantation patients [115, 121, 122]. Etiologies of stroke in the peri-operative period include cardioembolism of fibrin and platelet microthrombi, embolization of atherosclerotic debris during cross-clamping and cannulation of the aorta, air embolism during cardiectomy, and embolization of material from infective endocarditis from the donor patient [117, 119, 120, 123]. Most heart transplant recipients are anticoagulated pre-operatively, reversed before surgery, reanticoagulated during bypass, and then reversed again. The wide variation in coagulation function during this process poses a risk of cerebral infarction of hemorrhage at the extremes of the spectrum. Strokes are the cause of early death (0-30 days) after transplantation in 6.7% of patients [124], while stroke occurring later may be related to diagnostic procedures including cardiac catheterizations and right heart biopsy, acute rejection, and atrial arrhythmias [120]. Intracranial hemorrhage has been reported in 5% of early transplant recipients [116] and may be related to systemic anticoagulation, disseminated intravascular coagulation, relative cerebral hyperperfusion in the presence of impaired cerebral autoregulation and angioinvasive opportunistic infections, such as aspergillosis, candidal meningoencephalitis, and herpes simplex encephalitis [120, 125].

The reader may refer to other chapters in this book for evidence regarding management of acute periprocedural strokes as it will be similar to that of non-periprocedural strokes. Cardiac transplantation is a major surgery; thus, intravenous thrombolysis for acute ischemic stroke is contraindicated in these patients **(Ia/A)**.

Closure of patent foramen ovale / atrial septal aneurysm

Clinicians sometimes consider anticoagulation or patent foramen ovale (PFO) closure in patients who are found to have a large PFO and atrial septal aneurysm (ASA) during the evaluation of cryptogenic TIA or ischemic stroke. A study of 35 patients who had PFO closure after stroke compared the number of cerebral infarctions proven by MRI before and after closure [126]. The rate of new microembolic lesions was 8.6%, whereas the rate of microembolic closure-related events with neurologic deficit was 2.8%. Surgical options for PFO closure include open thoracotomy foraminal closure, minimally invasive surgery, and percutaneous closure techniques. Cerebrovascular complications of percutaneous PFO closure can include air embolism or thromboembolism, atrial fibrillation, infective endocarditis or delayed cardioembolic stroke due to infective endocarditis or thrombus formation around the device.

Intracardiac tumors

Primary cardiac tumors are rare, with a reported prevalence of 0.001-0.03% at autopsy series. Cardiac myxomas account for 40-50% of primary cardiac tumors, typically arising from left-sided cardiac structures, predominantly the left atrium [127, 128]. Atrial myxomas can result in stroke due to embolism of myxomatous material or thrombus. Intracerebral or subarachnoid hemorrhage can occur as can delayed complications from tumor recurrence with embolization, progressive vascular stenosis, aneurysm formation and rupture, or parenchymal metastasis [129, 130]. Late neurologic sequelae after resection are rare and may occur without recurrence of the myxoma. Aneurysms may enlarge or appear for the first time after tumor resection [131]. In a series of 38 patients who had surgical resection of a cardiac myxoma, 7.9% developed postoperative neurologic complications including TIAs and stroke [132]. While recurrence of myxoma after resection is rare (2-3%) [133, 134], it has been associated with recurrent cerebral infarctions and cerebral fusiform aneurysms [135].

Definitive treatment for primary and secondary stroke prevention is surgical resection of the tumor. Resection of primary cardiac tumors can be complicated by stroke; however, operative risk is generally low [136-138] (III/B).

Postoperative arrhythmias

Atrial fibrillation occurs in 30-50% of patients following cardiac surgery. Onset is typically between the second and fourth postoperative days [4, 6, 12, 14, 18, 139, 140]. Postoperative arrhythmias are associated with an increased incidence of postoperative stroke [6, 8, 12, 14]. Electrolyte levels and fluid volume should be optimized, and the patient must be closely monitored for signs of heart failure and arrhythmias during the postoperative period. A 2004 Cochrane review looking at treatment of postoperative atrial fibrillation concluded that prophylactic administration of amiodarone and β-blockers, beginning 5 days prior to cardiac surgery may reduce the incidence of postoperative atrial fibrillation and stroke [141] (Ia/A). Patients with pre-existing atrial fibrillation who are receiving anti-arrhythmic or rate-controlling agents, should be continued on these agents throughout the peri-operative period (Ia/A). New onset postoperative atrial fibrillation often resolves spontaneously after 4-6 weeks. No RCTs have specifically addressed the use of anticoagulation in these patients. The American College of Chest Physicians recommends consideration of heparin therapy for high-risk patients (i.e. those with a history of stroke or TIA) in whom atrial fibrillation develops after surgery and the continuation of anticoagulation therapy for 30 days after the return of a normal sinus rhythm [142] (IV/C). Occlusion of the left atrial appendage (LAA) has been considered to be a potential alternative to warfarin in patients with atrial fibrillation who have contraindications to anticoagulation; however, currently, the evidence is insufficient to support LAA occlusion.

Table 6 lists the guidelines for post-cardiac surgery atrial fibrillation published by the American College of Cardiology/American Heart Association (ACC/AHA).

Table 6. ACC/AHA guidelines for post-cardiac surgery atrial fibrillation.	
◆ Patients with pre-existing atrial fibrillation who are receiving anti-arrhythmic or rate-controlling agents, should be continued on these agents throughout the peri-operative period.	I/C
◆ Unless contraindicated, an oral β-blocker is recommended to prevent postoperative AF for patients undergoing cardiac surgery.	I/A
◆ An AV nodal blocking agent is recommended for rate control in patients who develop postoperative AF.	I/B
◆ Pre-operative amiodarone reduces the incidence of AF in patients undergoing cardiac surgery and represents appropriate prophylactic therapy for patients at high risk for postoperative AF.	IIa/A
◆ It is reasonable to restore sinus rhythm by pharmacologic cardioversion with ibutilide or direct-current cardioversion in patients who develop postoperative atrial fibrillation, as advised for non-surgical patients.	IIa/B
◆ It is reasonable to administer anti-arrhythmic medications in an attempt to maintain sinus rhythm in patients with recurrent or refractory postoperative atrial fibrillation.	IIa/B
◆ Antithrombotic medication is reasonable in patients who develop postoperative AF.	IIa/B
◆ Prophylactic administration of sotalol may be considered for patients at risk of developing atrial fibrillation after cardiac surgery.	IIb/B

Conclusions

In patients who have recently undergone major cardiac surgeries or procedures, treatment with intravenous rt-PA is clearly contraindicated due to an increased risk of bleeding. Evidence for intra-arterial (IA) administration of rt-PA is limited to case series which suggest that the use of IA rt-PA within 6 hours of onset of a peri-operative stroke is relatively safe [143, 144] **(III/B)**. Chalela and colleagues reported on a case series of 36 patients who recieved IA rt-PA for peri-operative stroke, 80% of whom had complete recanalization, and 38% had no symptoms or slight disability at discharge. While 25% of these patients suffered ICH after administration of IA rt-PA, only 8% had worsening of symptoms. The mortality rate in this series was similar to that reported in non-surgical patients who have received IA rt-PA [144]. Data are even more limited for the use of mechanical thrombectomy or embolectomy in patients with peri-operative stroke.

Several principles in the reduction of peri-procedural stroke apply to cardiac surgery in general and were not discussed above. These include: minimization of the duration of surgery whenever possible, avoidance of intra-operative and postoperative hyperglycemia [145, 146], and the prevention and treatment of inflammation and infections during the pre-operative and postoperative periods, as both pre-operative and postoperative high leukocyte counts have been correlated with the development of postoperative atrial fibrillation and stroke [147, 148]. Pre-operative administration of statins, regardless of the patient's lipid profile, has been shown to reduce peri-operative stroke in cardiac surgery [149] **(Ib/A)**. Antiplatelet therapy such as aspirin reduces the incidence of postoperative stroke without increasing the incidence of bleeding complications [150, 151] **(Ia/A)**.

Discontinuation of warfarin or antiplatelet agents in anticipation of surgery increases the risk of peri-operative stroke [152, 153], with the highest risk occurring in patients with coronary artery disease [152] **(IIa/B)**. In patients requiring long-term warfarin therapy, the highest rates of thromboembolic events occur when warfarin is discontinued without administration of IV heparin as bridging therapy (0.6%), in contrast to those who receive IV heparin as bridge therapy (0%) [154]. Thus, bridge therapy with heparin and early postoperative resumption of anticoagulation are recommended in patients at high risk for thromboembolism, such as those with a history of systemic embolism or atrial fibrillation and those with mechanical valves [155].

Randomized, controlled clinical trials are also needed to identify the best preventive and management strategies for peri-operative stroke.

Key points	Evidence level
◆ In patients who have recently undergone major surgery, treatment with intravenous recombinant tissue plasminogen activator (rt-PA) is contraindicated.	Ia/A
◆ Evidence for treatment with intra-arterial administration of rt-PA and endovascular mechanical clot disruption is limited to case series or case reports.	III/B
◆ Matching intra-operative and early postoperative blood pressure to the patient's pre-operative range may reduce the risks of peri-operative stroke and death.	Ib/A
◆ Pre-operative administration of statins, regardless of the patient's lipid profile, has been shown to reduce peri-operative stroke in cardiac surgery.	Ib/A
◆ Antiplatelet therapy such as aspirin reduces the incidence of postoperative stroke without increasing the incidence of bleeding complications.	Ia/A
◆ Discontinuation of warfarin or antiplatelet agents in anticipation of surgery increases the risk of peri-operative stroke, with the highest risk occurring in patients with coronary artery disease.	IIa/B

References

1. Gardner TJ, Horneffer PJ, Manolio TA, *et al*. Stroke following coronary artery bypass grafting: a ten-year study. *Ann Thorac Surg* 1985; 40(6): 574-81.

2. Redmond JM, Greene PS, Goldsborough MA, *et al*. Neurologic injury in cardiac surgical patients with a history of stroke. *Ann Thorac Surg* 1996; 61(1): 42-7.

3. Roach GW, Kanchuger M, Mangano CM, *et al*. Adverse cerebral outcomes after coronary bypass surgery. Multicenter Study of Perioperative Ischemia Research Group and the Ischemia Research and Education Foundation Investigators. *N Engl J Med* 1996; 335(225): 1857-63.

4. Hogue CW Jr, Murphy SF, Schechtman KB, Dávila-Román VG. Risk factors for early or delayed stroke after cardiac surgery. *Circulation* 1999; 100(6): 642-7.

5. Salazar JD, Wityk RJ, Grega MA, *et al*. Stroke after cardiac surgery: short- and long-term outcomes. *Ann Thor Surg* 2001; 72(4): 1195-201.

6. Bucerius J, Gummert JF, Borger MA, *et al*. Stroke after cardiac surgery: a risk factor analysis of 16,184 consecutive adult patients. *Ann Thorac Surg* 2003; 75: 472-8.

7. Likosky DS, Caplan LR, Weintraub RM, *et al*. Intraoperative and postoperative variables associated with strokes following cardiac surgery. *Heart Surg Forum* 2004; 7: E271-6.

8. McKhann GM, Grega MA, Borowicz LM Jr, Baumgartner WA, Selnes OA. Stroke and encephalopathy after cardiac surgery: an update. *Stroke* 2006; 37: 562-71.

9. Hamon M, Baron JC, Viader F, Hamon M. Periprocedural stroke and cardiac catheterization. *Circulation* 2008; 118(6): 678-83.

10. Paramo JA, Rifon J, Llorens R, Casares J, Paloma MJ, Rocha E. Intra- and postoperative fibrinolysis in patients undergoing cardiopulmonary bypass surgery. *Haemostasis* 1991; 21: 58-64.

11. Naylor AR, Mehta Z, Rothwell PM, Bell PR. Carotid artery disease and stroke during coronary artery bypass: a critical review of the literature. *Eur J Vasc Endovasc Surg* 2002; 23: 283-94.

12. Limburg M, Wijdicks EF, Li H. Ischemic stroke after surgical procedures: clinical features, neuroimaging, and risk factors. *Neurology* 1998; 50: 895-901.

13. Brooker RF, Brown WR, Moody DM, *et al*. Cardiotomy suction: a major source of brain lipid emboli during cardiopulmonary bypass. *Ann Thorac Surg* 1998; 65: 1651-5.

14. Restrepo L, Wityk RJ, Grega MA, *et al*. Diffusion- and perfusion-weighted magnetic resonance imaging of the brain before and after coronary artery bypass grafting surgery. *Stroke* 2002; 33: 2909-15.

15. Stamou SC. Stroke and encephalopathy after cardiac surgery: the search for the holy grail. *Stroke* 2006; 37(2): 284-5.

16. Floyd TF, Shah PN, Price CC, *et al*. Clinically silent cerebral ischemic events after cardiac surgery: their incidence, regional vascular occurrence, and procedural dependence. *Ann Thorac Surg* 2006; 81(6): 2160-6.

17. Likosky DS, Marrin CA, Caplan LR, *et al*. Determination of etiologic mechanisms of strokes secondary to coronary artery bypass graft surgery. *Stroke* 2003; 34: 2830-4.

18. van Wermeskerken GK, Lardenoye JW, Hill SE, *et al*. Intraoperative physiologic variables and outcome in cardiac surgery: Part II. Neurologic outcome. *Ann Thorac Surg* 2000; 69: 1077-83.

19. O'Keefe JH Jr, Allan JJ, McCallister BD, *et al*. Angioplasty versus bypass surgery for multivessel coronary artery disease with left ventricular ejection fraction < or = 40%. *Am J Cardiol* 1993; 71: 897-901.

20. Sharony R, Grossi EA, Saunders PC, *et al*. Propensity case-matched analysis of off-pump coronary artery bypass grafting in patients with atheromatous aortic disease. *J Thorac Cardiovasc Surg* 2004; 127: 406-13.

21. Nakamura M, Okamoto F, Nakanishi K, *et al*. Does intensive management of cerebral hemodynamics and atheromatous aorta reduce stroke after coronary artery surgery? *Ann Thorac Surg* 2008; 85(2): 513-9.

22. Diegeler A, Hirsch R, Schneider F, *et al*. Neuromonitoring and neurocognitive outcome in off-pump versus conventional coronary bypass operation. *Ann Thorac Surg* 2000; 69: 1162-6.

23. Lloyd CT, Ascione R, Underwood MJ, Gardner F, Black A, Angelini GD. Serum S-100 protein release and neuropsychologic outcome during coronary revascularization on the beating heart: a prospective randomized study. *J Thorac Cardiovasc Surg* 2000; 119: 148-54.

24. van Dijk D, Jansen EW, Hijman R, *et al*, for the Octopus Study Group. Cognitive outcome after off-pump and on-pump coronary artery bypass graft surgery: a randomized trial. *JAMA* 2002; 287: 1405-12.

25. Iglesias I, Murkin JM. Beating heart surgery or conventional CABG: are neurologic outcomes different? *Semin Thorac Cardiovasc Surg* 2001; 13: 158-69.

26. Gold JP, Charlson ME, Williams-Russo P, *et al*. Improvement of outcomes after coronary artery bypass: a randomized trial comparing intraoperative high versus low mean arterial pressure. *J Thorac Cardiovasc Surg* 1995; 110: 1302-11.

27. Charlson ME, MacKenzie CR, Gold JP, Ales KL, Topkins M, Shires GT. Intraoperative blood pressure: what patterns identify patients at risk for postoperative complications? *Ann Surg* 1990; 212: 567-80.

28. Gold JP, Torres KE, Maldarelli W, Zhuravlev I, Condit D, Wasnick J. Improving outcomes in coronary surgery: the impact of echo-directed aortic cannulation and perioperative hemodynamic management in 500 patients. *Ann Thorac Surg* 2004; 78: 1579-85.

29. Rees K, Beranek-Stanley M, Burke M, Ebrahim S. Hypothermia to reduce neurological damage following coronary artery bypass surgery. *Cochrane Database Syst Rev* 2001; 1: CD002138.

30. Eagle KA, Guyton RA, Davidoff R, Edwards FH, Ewy GA, Gardner TJ, Hart JC, Herrmann HC, Hillis LD, Hutter AM Jr, Lytle BW, Marlow RA, Nugent WC, Orszulak TA, Antman EM, Smith SC Jr, Alpert JS, Anderson JL, Faxon DP, Fuster V, Gibbons RJ, Gregoratos G, Halperin JL, Hiratzka LF, Hunt SA, Jacobs AK, Ornato JP; American College of Cardiology/American Heart Association Task Force on Practice Guidelines Committee to Update the 1999 Guidelines for Coronary Artery Bypass Graft Surgery; American Society for Thoracic Surgery; Society of Thoracic Surgeons. ACC/AHA 2004 guideline update for coronary artery bypass graft surgery: summary article. A Report of the American College of Cardiology/American Heart Association Task Force on Practice Guidelines (Committee to Update the 1999 Guidelines for Coronary Artery Bypass Graft Surgery). *J Am Coll Cardiol* 2004; 44(5): e213-310. Erratum in: *J Am Coll Cardiol* 2005; 45(8): 1377.

31. Drobinski G, Montalescot G, Evans J, Nivet M, Thomas D, Grosgogeat Y. Systemic embolism as a complication of percutaneous mitral valvuloplasty. *Cathet Cardiovasc Diagn* 1992; 25(4): 327-30.

32. Horstkotte D, Scharf RE, Schultheiss HP. Intracardiac thrombosis: patient-related and device-related factors. *J Heart Valve Dis* 1995; 4(2): 114-20.

33. Goldsmith I, Lip GY, Kaukuntla H, Patel RL. Hospital morbidity and mortality and changes in quality of life following mitral valve surgery in the elderly. *J Heart Valve Dis* 1999; 8(6): 702-7.

34. Thourani VS, Weintraub WS, Guyton R A, *et al*. Outcomes and long-term survival for patients undergoing mitral valve repair versus replacement: effect of age and concomitant coronary artery bypass grafting. *Circulation* 2003; 108(3): 298-304.

35. Ruel M, Masters RG, Rubens FD, *et al*. Late incidence and determinants of stroke after aortic and mitral valve replacement. *Ann Thorac Surg* 2004; 78(1): 77-83.

36. Akins CW. Results with mechanical cardiac valvular prostheses. *Ann Thorac Surg* 1995; 60(6): 1836-44.

37. Kvidal P, Bergström R, Malm T, Ståhle E. Long-term follow-up of morbidity and mortality after aortic valve replacement with a mechanical valve prosthesis. *Eur Heart J* 2000; 21(13): 1099-111.

38. Caswell J, O'Brien B, Schneck M. Risk of stroke following valve replacement surgery. *Sem Cerebrovasc Dis Stroke* 2003; 3: 214-8.

39. Wolman RL, Nussmeier NA, Aggarwal A, *et al*. Cerebral injury after cardiac surgery: identification of a group at extraordinary risk. Multicenter Study of Perioperative Ischemia Research Group (McSPI) and the Ischemia Research Education Foundation (IREF) Investigators. *Stroke* 1999; 30(3): 514-22.

40. Fleck JD, O'Donnell JA, Biller J. Cardiac evaluation of patient with carotid artery stenosis and treatment strategies for coexisting disease. In: *Carotid Artery Surgery*. Loftus CM, Kresowik TF, Eds. New York, USA: Thieme, 2000: 121-9.

41. Bloomfield P, Wheatley DJ, Prescott RJ, Miller HC. Twelve-year comparison of a Bjork-Shiley mechanical heart valve with porcine bioprostheses. *N Engl J Med* 1991; 324(9): 573-9.

42. Hammermeister KE, Sethi GK, Henderson WG, Oprian C, Kim T, Rahimtoola S. A comparison of outcomes in men 11 years after heart-valve replacement with a mechanical valve or bioprosthesis. Veteran Affairs Cooperative Study on Valvular Heart Disease. *N Engl J Med* 1993; 328(18): 1289-96.

43. Bando K, Kobayashi J, Hirata M, *et al*. Early and late stroke after mitral valve replacement with a mechanical prosthesis: risk factor analysis of a 24-year experience. *J Thorac Cardiovasc Surg* 2003; 126(2): 358-64.

44. Mylonakis E, Calderwood SB. Infective endocarditis in adults. *N Engl J Med* 2001; 345: 1318-30.

45. Eishi K, Kawazoe K, Kuriyama Y, Kitoh Y, Kawashima Y, Omae T. Surgical management of infective endocarditis associated with cerebral complications. Multi-center retrospective study in Japan. *J Thorac Cardiovasc Surg* 1995; 110(6): 1745-55.

46. Heiro M, Nikoskelainen J, Engblom E, Kotilainen E, Marttila R, Kotilainen P. Neurologic manifestations of infective endocarditis: a 17-year experience in a teaching hospital in Finland. *Arch Intern Med* 2000; 160(18): 2781-7.

47. Ivert TS, Dismukes WE, Cobbs CG, Blackstone EH, Kirklin JW, Bergdahl LA. Prosthetic valve endocarditis. *Circulation* 1984; 69(2): 223-32.

48. Calderwood SB, Swinski LA, Waternaux CM, Karchmer AW, Buckley MJ. Risk factors for the development of prosthetic valve endocarditis. *Circulation* 1985; 72(1): 31-7.

49. Arvay A, Lengyel M. Incidence and risk factors of prosthetic valve endocarditis. *Eur J Cardiothorac Surg* 1988; 2(5): 340-6.

50. Agnihotri AK, McGiffin DC, Galbraith AJ, O'Brien MF. The prevalence of infective endocarditis after aortic valve replacement. *J Thorac Cardiovasc Surg* 1995; 110(6): 1708-20.

51. Vlessis AA, Hovaguimian H, Jaggers J, Ahmad A, Starr A. Infective endocarditis: ten-year review of medical and surgical therapy. *Ann Thorac Surg* 1996; 61(4): 1217-22.

52. Jayachandran JV. Cerebrovascular complications of invasive electrophysiologic procedures. *Sem Cerebrovasc Dis Stroke* 2003; 3(4): 225-7.

53. Hinkle DA, Raizen DM, McGarvey ML, Liu GT. Cerebral air embolism complicating cardiac ablation procedures. *Neurology* 2001; 56(6): 792-4.

54. Sonmez B, Demirsoy E, Yagan N, Unal M, Arbatli H, Sener D, Baran T, Ilkova F. A fatal complication due to radiofrequency ablation for atrial fibrillation: atrio-esophageal fistula. *Ann Thorac Surg* 2003; 76(1): 281-3.

55. Calkins H, Brugada J, Packer DL, Cappato R, Chen SA, Crijns HJ, Damiano RJ Jr, Davies DW, Haines DE, Haissaguerre M, Iesaka Y, Jackman W, Jais P, Kottkamp H, Kuck KH, Lindsay BD, Marchlinski FE, McCarthy PM, Mont JL, Morady F, Nademanee K, Natale A, Pappone C, Prystowsky E, Raviele A, Ruskin JN, Shemin RJ: HRS/EHRA/ECAS Expert Consensus Statement on Catheter and Surgical Ablation of Atrial Fibrillation: Recommendations for Personnel, Policy, Procedures and Follow-up. A Report of the Heart Rhythm Society (HRS) Task Force on Catheter and Surgical Ablation of Atrial Fibrillation. *Heart Rhythm* 2007; 4: 816-61.

56. Natale A, Raviele A, Arentz T, Calkins H, Chen SA, Haïssaguerre M, Hindricks G, Ho Y, Kuck KH, Marchlinski F, Napolitano C, Packer D, Pappone C, Prystowsky EN, Schilling R, Shah D, Themistoclakis S, Verma A. Venice Chart International Consensus Document on Atrial Fibrillation Ablation. *J Cardiovasc Electrophysiol* 2007; 18: 560-80.

57. Pappone C, Rosanio S, Augello G, Gallus G, Vicedomini G, Mazzone P, Gulletta S, Gugliotta F, Pappone A, Santinelli V, Tortoriello V, Sala S, Zangrillo A, Crescenzi G, Benussi S, Alfieri O. Mortality, morbidity, and quality of life after circumferential pulmonary vein ablation for atrial fibrillation: outcomes from a controlled nonrandomized longterm study. *J Am Coll Cardiol* 2003; 42: 185-97.

58. Oral H, Chugh A, Ozaydin M, Good E, Fortino J, Sankaran S, Reich S, Igic P, Elmouchi D, Tschopp D, Wimmer A, Dey S, Crawford T, Pelosi F Jr, Jongnarangsin K, Bogun F, Morady F. Risk of thromboembolic events after percutaneous left atrial radiofrequency ablation of atrial fibrillation. *Circulation* 2006; 114: 759-65.

59. Cappato R, Calkins H, Chen SA, Davies W, Iesaka Y, Kalman J, Kim YH, Klein G, Packer D, Skanes A. Worldwide survey on the methods, efficacy, and safety of catheter ablation for human atrial fibrillation. *Circulation* 2005; 111: 1100-5.

60. Gage BF, Waterman AD, Shannon W, Boechler M, Rich MW, Radford MJ. Validation of clinical classification schemes for predicting stroke: results from the National Registry of Atrial Fibrillation. *JAMA* 2001; 285(22): 2864-70.

61. Scherr D, Sharma K, Dalal D, Spragg D, Chilukuri K, Cheng A, Dong J, Henrikson CA, Nazarian S, Berger RD, Calkins H, Marine JE. Incidence and predictors of periprocedural cerebrovascular accident in patients undergoing catheter ablation of atrial fibrillation. *J Cardiovasc Electrophysiol* 2009; 20(12): 1357-63.

62. Fuchs S, Stabile E, Kinnaird TD, Mintz GS, Gruberg L, Canos DA, Pinnow EE, Kornowski R, Suddath WO, Satler LW, Pichard AD, Kent KM, Weissman NJ. Stroke complicating percutaneous coronary interventions: incidence, predictors, and prognostic implications. *Circulation* 2002; 106: 86-91.

63. Brown DL, Topol EJ. Stroke complicating percutaneous coronary revascularization. *Am J Cardiol* 1993; 72(15): 1207-9.

64. Lazar JM, Uretsky BF, Denys BG, Reddy PS, Counihan PJ, Ragosta M. Predisposing risk factors and natural history of acute neurologic complications of left-sided cardiac catheterization. *Am J Cardiol* 1995; 75: 1056-60.

65. Jackson JL, Meyer GS, Pettit T. Complications from cardiac catheterization: analysis of a military database. *Mil Med* 2000; 165(4): 298-301.

66. Segal AZ, Abernethy WB, Palacios IF, BeLue R, Rordorf G. Stroke as a complication of cardiac catheterization: risk factors and clinical features. *Neurology* 2001; 56(7): 975-7.

67. Akkerhuis KM, Deckers JW, Lincoff AM, Tcheng JE, Boersma E, Anderson K, Balog C, Califf RM, Topol EJ, Simoons ML. Risk of stroke associated with abciximab among patients undergoing percutaneous coronary intervention. *JAMA* 2001; 286(1): 78-82.

68. Dukkipati S, O'Neill WW, Harjai KJ, Sanders WP, Deo D, Boura JA, Bartholomew BA, Yerkey MW, Sadeghi HM, Kahn JK. Characteristics of cerebrovascular accidents after percutaneous coronary interventions. *J Am Coll Cardiol* 2004; 43: 1161-7.

69. Mack MJ, Brown PP, Kugelmass AD, *et al.* Current status and outcomes of coronary revascularization 1999 to 2002: 148,396 surgical and percutaneous procedures. *Ann Thorac Surg* 2004; 77(3): 761-6; discussion 766-8.

70. Wong SC, Minutello R, Hong MK. Neurological complications following percutaneous coronary interventions: a report from the 2000-2001 New York State Angioplasty Registry. *Am J Cardiol* 2005; 96: 1248-50.

71. Sankaranarayanan R, Msairi A, Davis GK. Stroke complicating cardiac catheterization - a preventable and treatable complication. *J Invasive Cardiol* 2007; 19(1): 40-5.

72. Busing KA, Schulte-Sasse C, Flüchter S, *et al.* Cerebral infarction: incidence and risk factors after diagnostic and interventional cardiac catheterization - prospective evaluation at diffusion-weighted MR imaging. *Radiology* 2005; 235: 177-183.

73. Al-Mubarek N, Vitek JJ, Mousa I, Lyer SS, Mgaieth S, Moses J, Roubin GS. Immediate catheter-based neurovascular rescue for acute stroke complicating coronary procedures. *Am J Cardiol* 2002; 90: 173-6.

74. Cho L. Cerebrovascular complications in interventional cardiology. *Sem Cerebrovasc Dis Stroke* 2003; 3(4): 228-32.

75. Dawson DM, Fischer EG. Neurologic complications of cardiac catheterization. *Neurology* 1977; 27(5): 496-7.

76. Kosmorsky G, Hanson MR, Tomsak RL. Neuro-ophthalmologic complications of cardiac catheterization. *Neurology* 1988; 38(3): 483-5.

77. Keilson GR, Schwartz WJ, Recht LD. The preponderance of posterior circulatory events is independent of the route of cardiac catheterization. *Stroke* 1992; 23(9): 1358-9.

78. Lund C, Nes RB, Ugelstad TP, *et al.* Cerebral emboli during left heart catheterization may cause acute brain injury. *Eur Heart J* 2005; 26(13): 1269-75.

79. Zaidat OO, Slivka AP, Mohammad Y, Graffagnino C, Smith TP, Enterline DS, Christoforidis GA, Alexander MJ, Landis D, Suarez JI. Intra-arterial thrombolytic therapy in pericoronary angiography ischemic stroke. *Stroke* 2005; 36: 1083-4.

80. De Marco F, Antonio Fernandez-Diaz J, Lefèvre T, Balcells J, Araya M, Routledge H, Rosas A, Louvard Y, Dumas P, Morice MC. Management of cerebrovascular accidents during cardiac catheterization: immediate cerebral angiography versus early neuroimaging strategy. *Catheter Cardiovasc Interv* 2007; 70: 560-8.

81. Khatri P, Taylor RA, Palumbo V, Rajajee V, Katz JM, Chalela JA, Geers A, Haymore J, Kolansky DM, Kasner SE. The safety and efficacy of thrombolysis for strokes after cardiac catheterization. *J Am Coll Cardiol* 2008; 51: 906-11.

82. Arnold M, Fischer U, Schroth G, Nedeltchev K, Isenegger J, Remonda L, Windecker S, Brekenfeld C, Mattle HP. Intra-arterial thrombolysis of acute iatrogenic intracranial arterial occlusion attributable to neuroendovascular procedures or coronary angiography. *Stroke* 2008; 39: 1491-5.

83. Kushner FG, Hand M, Smith SC Jr, King SB 3rd, Anderson JL, Antman EM, Bailey SR, Bates ER, Blankenship JC, Casey DE Jr, Green LA, Hochman JS, Jacobs AK, Krumholz HM, Morrison DA, Ornato JP, Pearle DL, Peterson ED, Sloan MA, Whitlow PL, Williams DO. 2009 focused updates: ACC/AHA Guidelines for the Management of Patients with ST-elevation Myocardial Infarction (updating the 2004 guideline and 2007 focused update) and ACC/AHA/SCAI Guidelines on Percutaneous Coronary Intervention (updating the 2005 guideline and 2007 focused update): a report of the American College of Cardiology Foundation/American Heart Association Task Force on Practice Guidelines. *J Am Coll Cardiol* 2009; 54(23): 2205-41. Review. Erratum in: *J Am Coll Cardiol* 2010; 55(6): 612. Dosage error in article text. *J Am Coll Cardiol* 2009; 54(25): 2464.

84. Sacco RL, Adams R, Albers G, *et al.* Guidelines for prevention of stroke in patients with ischemic stroke or transient ischemic attack: a statement for healthcare professionals from the American Heart Association/American Stroke Association Council on Stroke. *Stroke* 2006; 37: 577-617.

85. Morales JP, Taylor PR, Bell RE, *et al.* Neurological complications following endoluminal repair of thoracic aortic disease. *Cardiovasc Intervent Radiol* 2007; 30(5): 833-9.

86. Khoynezhad A, Donayre CE, Bui H, Kopchok GE, Walot I, White RA. Risk factors of neurologic deficit after thoracic aortic endografting. *Ann Thorac Surg* 2007; 83(2): S882-9; discussion S890-2.

87. Buth J, Harris PL, Hobo R, *et al*. Neurologic complications associated with endovascular repair of thoracic aortic pathology: incidence and risk factors. A study from the European Collaborators on Stent/Graft Techniques for Aortic Aneurysm Repair (EUROSTAR) Registry. *J Vasc Surg* 2007; 46(6): 1103-10; discussion 1110-1.

88. Gutsche JT, Cheung AT, McGarvey ML, *et al*. Risk factors for perioperative stroke after thoracic endovascular aortic repair. *Ann Thorac Surg* 2007; 84(4): 1195-200; discussion 1200.

89. Boshoff DE, Eyskens B, Gewillig M. Late redilation of a stent in the aorta crossing the subclavian artery complicated with a cerebellar infarction. *Acta Cardiol* 2007; 62(3): 295-7.

90. Mokri B, Ahlskog JE, Fulgham JR, Matsumoto JY. Syndrome resembling PSP after surgical repair of ascending aorta dissection or aneurysm. *Neurology* 2004; 62: 971-3.

91. Eggers S, Moster ML, Cranmer K. Selective saccadic palsy after cardiac surgery. *Neurology* 2008; 70: 318-20.

92. Yee RD, Purvin VA. Acquired ocular motor apraxia after aortic surgery. *Trans Am Ophthalmol Soc* 2007; 105: 152-9.

93. Jonker FHW, Trimarchi S, Verhagen JM, Moll FL, Sumpio BE, Muhs BE. Meta-analysis of open versus endovascular repair for ruptured descending thoracic aortic aneurysm. *J Vasc Surg* 2010; 51: 1026-32.

94. Tiesenhausen K, Hausegger KA, Oberwalder P, *et al*. Left subclavian artery management in endovascular repair of thoracic aortic aneurysms and aortic dissections. *J Card Surg* 2003; 18: 429-35.

95. Schoder M, Grabenwoger M, Holzenbein T, *et al*. Endovascular repair of the thoracic aorta necessitating anchoring of the stent graft across the arch vessels. *J Thorac Cardiovasc Surg* 2006; 131: 380-7.

96. American Heart Association. Heart Disease and Stroke Statistics: 2007 Update. Dallas: 2007. Hiratzka LF, Bakris GL, Beckman JA, Bersin RM, Carr VF, Casey D Jr, Eagle KA, Hermann LK, Isselbacher EM, Kazerooni EA, Kouchoukos NT, Lytle BW, Milewicz DM, Reich DL, Sen S, Shinn JA, Svensson LG, Williams DM, Jacobs AK, Smith SC Jr, Anderson JL, Adams CD, Buller CE, Creager MA, Ettinger SM, Guyton RA, Halperin JL, Hunt SA, Krumholz HM, Kushner FG, Nishimura R, Page RL, Riegel B, Stevenson WG, Tarkington LG, Yancy CW, Lewin JC, May C, Bradfield L, Stewart MD, Keller S, Barrett EA, Welsh JM, Brown N, Whitman GR; American College of Cardiology Foundation; American Heart Association Task Force on Practice Guidelines; American Association for Thoracic Surgery; American College of Radiology; American Stroke Association; Society of Cardiovascular Anesthesiologists; Society for Cardiovascular Angiography and Interventions; Society of Interventional Radiology; Society of Thoracic Surgeons; Society for Vascular Medicine. 2010 CCF/AHA/AATS/ACR/ASA/SCA/SCAI/SIR/STS/SVM Guidelines for the Diagnosis and Management of Patients with Thoracic Aortic Disease. *J Am Coll Cardiol* 2010; 55(14): e27-129.

97. Child JS, Perloff JK, Kubak B. Infective endocarditis: risks and prophylaxis. In: *Congenital Heart Disease in Adults*. Perloff JK, Child JS, Eds. Philadelphia, USA: W.B. Saunders, 1998: 129-43.

98. Domi T, Edgell DS, McCrindle BW, *et al*. Frequency, predictors, and neurologic outcomes of vaso-occlusive strokes associated with cardiac surgery in children. *Pediatrics* 2008; 122(6): 1292-8.

99. Buompadre MC, Arroyo HA. Accidental cerebral venous gas embolism in a young patient with congenital heart disease. *J Child Neurol* 2008; 23(1): 121-3.

100. Andropoulos DB, Stayer SA, Diaz LK, Ramamoorthy C. Neurological monitoring for congenital heart surgery. *Anesth Analg* 2004; 99(5): 1365-75.

101. Caldwell RL. Stroke and congenital heart disease in infants and children. *Sem Cerebrovasc Dis Stroke* 2003; 3(4): 200-6.

102. Liu XY, Wong V, Leung M. Neurologic complications due to catheterization. *Pediatr Neurol* 2001; 24(4): 270-5.

103. Fowler VG, Durack DT. Infective endocarditis. *Curr Opin Cardiol* 1994; 9: 389-400.

104. Dodo H, Child JS. Infective endocarditis in congenital heart disease. *Cardiol Clin* 1996; 14: 383-92.

105. Dajani AS, Taubert KA, Wilson W, *et al*. Prevention of bacterial endocarditis. Recommendations by the American Heart Association. *Circulation* 1997; 96: 358-66.

106. Ferrieri P, Gewitz MH, Gerber MA, *et al*. Unique features of infective endocarditis in childhood. *Circulation* 2002; 105: 2115-26.

107. Deanfield J, Thaulow E, Warnes C, *et al*. Management of grown up congenital heart disease. *Eur Heart J* 2003; 24: 1035-84.

108. Horstkotte D, Follath F, Gutschik E, *et al*. Guidelines on Prevention, Diagnosis and Treatment of Infective Endocarditis Executive Summary; the Task Force on Infective Endocarditis of the European Society of Cardiology. *Eur Heart J* 2004; 25: 267-76.

109. Warnes CA, Williams RG, Bashore TM, Child JS, Connolly HM, Dearani JA, del Nido P, Fasules JW, Graham TP Jr, Hijazi ZM, Hunt SA, King ME, Landzberg MJ, Miner PD, Radford MJ, Walsh EP, Webb GD, Smith SC Jr, Jacobs AK, Adams CD, Anderson JL, Antman EM, Buller CE, Creager MA, Ettinger SM, Halperin JL, Hunt SA, Krumholz HM, Kushner FG, Lytle BW, Nishimura RA, Page RL, Riegel B, Tarkington LG, Yancy CW; American College of Cardiology; American Heart Association Task Force on Practice Guidelines (Writing Committee to Develop Guidelines on the Management of Adults With Congenital Heart Disease); American Society of Echocardiography; Heart Rhythm Society; International Society for Adult Congenital Heart Disease; Society for Cardiovascular Angiography and Interventions; Society of Thoracic Surgeons. ACC/AHA 2008 Guidelines for the Management of Adults with Congenital Heart Disease: a report of the American College of Cardiology/American Heart Association Task Force on Practice Guidelines (Writing Committee to Develop Guidelines on the Management of Adults With Congenital Heart Disease). Developed in Collaboration With the American Society of Echocardiography, Heart Rhythm Society, International Society for Adult Congenital Heart Disease, Society for Cardiovascular Angiography and Interventions, and Society of Thoracic Surgeons. *J Am Coll Cardiol* 2008; 52(23): e1-121.

110. Dembitsky WP, Tector AJ, Park S, Moskowitz AJ, Gelijns AC, Ronan NS, Piccione W Jr, Holman WL, Furukawa S, Weinberg AD, Heatley G, Poirier VL, Damme L, Long JW. Left ventricular assist device performance with long-term circulatory support: lessons from the REMATCH trial. *Ann Thorac Surg* 2004; 78(6): 2123-9; discussion 2129-30.

111. Lazar RM, Shapiro PA, Jaski BE, Parides MK, Bourge RC, Watson JT, Damme L, Dembitsky W, Hosenpud JD, Gupta L, Tierney A, Kraus T, Naka Y. Neurological events during long-term mechanical circulatory support for heart failure: the Randomized Evaluation of Mechanical Assistance for the Treatment of Congestive Heart Failure (REMATCH) experience. *Circulation* 2004; 109(20): 2423-7.

112. Slaughter MS, Rogers JG, Milano CA, Russell SD, Conte JV, Feldman D, Sun B, Tatooles AJ, Delgado RM 3rd, Long JW, Wozniak TC, Ghumman W, Farrar DJ, Frazier OH; HeartMate II Investigators. Advanced heart failure treated with continuous-flow left ventricular assist device. *N Engl J Med* 2009; 361(23): 2241-51.

113. Bourge RC, Kirklin JK, Thomas K, *et al*. The emergence of co-morbid diseases impacting survival after cardiac transplantation, a ten-year multi-institutional experience. *J Heart Lung Transplant* 2001; 20(2): 167-8.

114. Inoue K, Lüth JU, Pottkämper D, Strauss KM, Minami K, Reichelt W. Incidence and risk factors of perioperative cerebral complications. Heart transplantation compared to coronary artery bypass grafting and valve surgery. *J Cardiovasc Surg* (Torino) 1998; 39(2): 201-8.

115. Hotson JR, Pedley TA. The neurologic complications of cardiac transplantation. *Brain* 1976; 99: 673-94.

116. Andrews BT, Hershon JJ, Calanchini P, Avery GJ 2nd, Hill JD. Neurologic complications of cardiac transplantation. *West J Med* 1990; 153(2): 146-8.

117. Adair JC, Call GK, O'Connell JB, Baringer JR. Cerebrovascular syndromes following cardiac transplantation. *Neurology* 1992; 42(4): 819-23.

118. Jarquin-Valdivia AA, Wijdicks EF, McGregor C. Neurologic complications following heart transplantation in the modern era: decreased incidence, but postoperative stroke remains prevalent. *Transplant Proc* 1999; 31(5): 2161-2.

119. Mayer TO, Biller J, O'Donnell J, Meschia JF, Sokol DK. Contrasting the neurologic complications of cardiac transplantation in adults and children. *J Child Neurol* 2002; 17(3): 195-9.

120. Gill WJ, O'Donnell J. Cerebrovascular complications of cardiac transplantation. *Sem Cerebrovasc Diseases and Stroke* 2003; 3(4): 219-24.

121. Schober R, Herman NM. Neuropathology of cardiac transplantation: survey of 31 cases. *Lancet* 1973; i: 962-7.

122. Montero CG, Martinez AJ. Neuropathology of heart transplantation: 23 cases. *Neurology* 1986; 36: 1149-54.

123. Adair JC, Woodley SL, O'Connell JB, Call GK, Baringer JR. Aseptic meningitis following cardiac transplantation: clinical characteristics and relationship to immunosuppressive regimen. *Neurology* 1991; 41(2 (Pt 1)): 249-52.

124. Taylor DO, Edwards LB, Boucek MM, *et al*. Registry of the International Society for Heart and Lung Transplantation: twenty-fourth official adult heart transplant report - 2007. *J Heart Lung Transplant* 2007; 26(8): 769-81.

125. Sila CA. Spectrum of neurologic events following cardiac transplantation. *Stroke* 1989; 20(11): 1586-9.

126. Dorenbeck U, Simon B, Skowasch D, *et al.* Cerebral embolism with interventional closure of symptomatic patent foramen ovale: an MRI-based study using diffusion-weighted imaging. *Eur J Neurol* 2007; 14(4): 451-4.

127. Khan MA, Khan AA, Waseem M. Surgical experience with cardiac myxomas. *J Ayub Med Coll Abbottabad* 2008; 20(2): 76-9.

128. Velicki L, Nicin S, Mihajlovic B, Kovacevic P, Susak S, Fabri M. Cardiac myxoma: clinical presentation, surgical treatment and outcome. *J BUON* 2010; 15(1): 51-5.

129. Price DL, Harris JL, New PF, Cantu RC. Cardiac myxoma: a clinicopathologic and angiographic study. *Arch Neurol* 1970; 23(6): 558-67.

130. Walker MT, Kilani RK, Toye LR, Bird CR. Central and peripheral fusiform aneurysms six years after left atrial myxoma resection. *J Neurol Neurosurg Psychiatry* 2003; 74(2): 281-2.

131. Roeltgen DP, Weimer GR, Patterson LF. Delayed neurologic complications of left atrial myxoma. *Neurology* 1981; 31(1): 8-13.

132. Scrofani R, Carro C, Villa L, Botta M, Antona C. Cardiac myxoma: surgical results and 15-year clinical follow-up. *Ital Heart J Suppl* 2002; 3(7): 753-8.

133. McCarthy PM, Piehler JM, Schaff HV, *et al.* The significance of multiple, recurrent, and 'complex' cardiac myxomas. *J Thorac Cardiovasc Surg* 1986; 91: 389-96.

134. Bjessmo S, Ivert T. Cardiac myxoma: 40 years' experience in 63 patients. *Ann Thorac Surg* 1997; 63: 697-700.

135. Kvitting JE, Engvall J, Broqvist M, *et al.* Recurrence of myxoma in the left ventricle with concurrent cerebral fusiform aneurysms after previous atrial myxoma surgery. *J Thorac Cardiovasc Surg* 2008; 135(5): 1172-3.

136. Loire R. [Myxoma of the left atrium, clinical outcome of 100 operated patients]. *Arch Mal Coeur Vaiss* 1996; 89(9): 1119-25.

137. Pinede L, Duhaut P, Loire R. Clinical presentation of left atrial cardiac myxoma. A series of 112 consecutive cases. *Medicine* (Baltimore) 2001; 80(3): 159-72.

138. Kuroczynski W, Peivandi AA, Ewald P, Pruefer D, Heinemann M, Vahl CF. Cardiac myxomas: short- and long-term follow-up. *Cardiol J* 2009; 16(5): 447-54.

139. Charlesworth DC, Likosky DS, Marrin CA, *et al.* Development and validation of a prediction model for strokes after coronary artery bypass grafting. *Ann Thorac Surg* 2003; 76: 436-43.

140. Lahtinen J, Biancari F, Salmela E, *et al.* Postoperative atrial fibrillation is a major cause of stroke after on-pump coronary artery bypass surgery. *Ann Thorac Surg* 2004; 77: 1241-4.

141. Crystal E, Garfinkle MS, Connolly SS, Ginger TT, Sleik K, Yusuf SS. Interventions for preventing post-operative atrial fibrillation in patients undergoing heart surgery. *Cochrane Database Syst Rev* 2004; 4: CD003611.

142. Epstein AE, Alexander JC, Gutterman DD, Maisel W, Wharton JM; American College of Chest Physicians. Anticoagulation: American College of Chest Physicians Guidelines for the Prevention and Management of Postoperative Atrial Fibrillation after Cardiac Surgery. *Chest* 2005; 128(2 Suppl): 24S-7.

143. Moazami N, Smedira NG, McCarthy PM, *et al.* Safety and efficacy of intra-arterial thrombolysis for perioperative stroke after cardiac operation. *Ann Thorac Surg* 2001; 72: 1933-7.

144. Chalela JA, Katzan I, Liebeskind DS, *et al.* Safety of intra-arterial thrombolysis in the postoperative period. *Stroke* 2001; 32: 1365-9.

145. Gandhi GY, Nuttall GA, Abel MD, *et al.* Intraoperative hyperglycemia and perioperative outcomes in cardiac surgery patients. *Mayo Clin Proc* 2005; 80: 862-6.

146. Krinsley JS. Effect of an intensive glucose management protocol on the mortality of critically ill adult patients. *Mayo Clin Proc* 2004; 79: 992-1000. [Erratum, *Mayo Clin Proc* 2005; 80: 1101.]

147. Albert AA, Beller CJ, Walter JA, *et al.* Preoperative high leukocyte count: a novel risk factor for stroke after cardiac surgery. *Ann Thorac Surg* 2003; 75: 1550-7.

148. Lamm G, Auer J, Weber T, Berent R, Ng C, Eber B. Postoperative white blood cell count predicts atrial fibrillation after cardiac surgery. *J Cardiothorac Vasc Anesth* 2006; 20: 51-6.

149. Durazzo AE, Machado FS, Ikeoka DT, *et al.* Reduction in cardiovascular events after vascular surgery with atorvastatin: a randomized trial. *J Vasc Surg* 2004; 39: 967-75.

150. Mangano DT. Aspirin and mortality from coronary bypass surgery. *N Engl J Med* 2002; 347: 1309-17.

151. Engelter S, Lyrer P. Antiplatelet therapy for preventing stroke and other vascular events after carotid endarterectomy. *Cochrane Database Syst Rev* 2003; 3: CD001458.

152. Maulaz AB, Bezerra DC, Michel P, Bogousslavsky J. Effect of discontinuing aspirin therapy on the risk of brain ischemic stroke. *Arch Neurol* 2005; 62: 1217-20.

153. Genewein U, Haeberli A, Straub PW, Beer JH. Rebound after cessation of oral anticoagulant therapy: the biochemical evidence. *Br J Haematol* 1996; 92: 479-85.

154. Dunn AS, Turpie AG. Perioperative management of patients receiving oral anticoagulants: a systematic review. *Arch Intern Med* 2003; 163: 901-8.

155. Dunn AS, Wisnivesky J, Ho W, Moore C, McGinn T, Sacks HS. Perioperative management of patients on oral anticoagulants: a decision analysis. *Med Decis Making* 2005; 25: 387-97.

Chapter 15

Central nervous system vascular malformations

A. Jess Schuette MD, Resident, Department of Neurosurgery
Emory University, Atlanta, Georgia, USA

C. Michael Cawley MD, Associate Professor, Department of Neurosurgery,
Emory University, Atlanta, Georgia, USA

Daniel L. Barrow MD, MBNA/Bowman Professor and Chairman
Director, Emory Stroke Center, Department of Neurosurgery
Emory University School of Medicine, Atlanta, Georgia, USA

Introduction

Central nervous system vascular malformations are a diverse group of pathologic entities including arteriovenous malformations (AVMs), dural arteriovenous fistulae, developmental venous anomalies (DVAs), cavernous malformations, and capillary telangiectasias [1]. Combined, these malformations occur in 0.1-4.0% of the general population. AVMs alone are about one seventh as common as aneurysms [2, 3].

These non-neoplastic lesions were first categorized by McCormick in 1966 in the pre-computed tomography era [1, 4]. As imaging techniques have improved, our understanding of the symptomatology, pathophysiology, natural history, and angioarchitecture has improved. Advances in microsurgery have combined with endovascular techniques and stereotactic radiosurgery to augment therapeutic options for managing these lesions [5, 6].

As with most cerebrovascular neurosurgical pathology, there are very few randomized studies and therefore very little level I evidence.

Arteriovenous malformations

AVMs represent the most common central nervous system vascular malformation with autopsy studies showing an incidence of 1.4-4.3% in the general population [7, 8]. The annual incidence of symptomatic AVMs has been estimated to be 1.1 per 100,000 population [8]. Intracerebral hemorrhage is the most common and devastating manifestation with over half of patients presenting in this manner [9]. Other symptoms include seizures, headaches, progressive neurologic deficit and pulsatile tinnitus [2, 10].

Our understanding of the natural history of these lesions remains incomplete. However, natural history studies estimate the risk of hemorrhage to be between 2-4% per year **(III/B)** [2, 10-12]. Early literature estimates the morbidity and mortality of an initial hemorrhage to be between 10-30%; more recent estimates have been lower [13, 14]. There are some data to suggest that there is an increased risk of rehemorrhage in the first year following an initial hemorrhage – estimated between 6-25% [15-17] **(II/B)**. Studies have attempted to evaluate risk factors for hemorrhage in patients with AVMs. Though inconsistent, some risk factors include small AVM size, deep location, ventricular or periventricular location, posterior fossa location, intranidal aneurysms, deep venous drainage, and high feeding arterial pressures [7, 18].

The gold standard for AVM diagnosis remains digital subtraction angiography (DSA) [7]. DSA allows a detailed evaluation of the feeding arteries, nidus venous drainage, and any associated aneurysms. CT scanning is relatively insensitive for diagnosis but may demonstrate calcifications or evidence of past hemorrhages [19]. Magnetic resonance imaging (MRI) provides for the most accurate anatomical localization and size estimation [20].

Treatment options for AVMs have increased as have the quality of those options. When a clinician first evaluates a patient with an AVM, the initial step is to determine if the patient requires any treatment of their AVM. In cases of hemorrhage, this decision may be straightforward. In other cases, where an AVM is discovered incidentally, the decision process may be much more difficult. Currently, between 54-62% of AVMs are discovered prior to rupture [6, 21]. Again, there are no randomized trials to provide guidance in this population though most specialists recommend some form of treatment of low-intermediate grade lesions. Additionally, the question of which AVMs are treatable and untreatable remains a topic of much debate. Once the risks and benefits of treatment are weighed, the decision can be made to proceed with expectant management versus treatment.

Therapeutic options include observation, microsurgical resection, embolization, stereotactic radiosurgery or a combination of these modalities [5]. Only complete obliteration of the AVM, documented by angiography, eliminates the risk of future hemorrhage [22]. Partial treatment does not appear to favorably alter the natural history [7]. The advantage of microsurgical resection is that it provides an immediate and permanent cure [22, 23]. Embolization alone rarely cures an AVM, but is more often used as an adjunct to other therapies to reduce flow and size of the nidus in preparation for surgery or radiosurgery [7, 24]. Occasionally, partial embolization is indicated for obliteration of associated aneurysms or to reduce flow in an AVM presenting with progressive neurological deficit from a cerebrovascular 'steal' phenomenon [7]. Radiosurgery is effective in obliterating some AVMs and is less invasive than microsurgery [25, 26]. Drawbacks of radiosurgery include the long interval to obliteration and the lack of universal effectiveness [22]. Currently, a large prospective randomized trial in the treatment of unruptured AVMs is ongoing (ARUBA) [21, 27, 28]. This trial will randomize patients into a best possible treatment arm and a non-treatment arm. The goal is to determine if invasive or non-invasive therapy will reduce the risk of death or symptomatic stroke.

Treatment options

Microsurgery

Surgical resection of AVMs is most often performed in an elective manner **(III/B)** [7, 22]. Even in cases of emergent operations due to a large hematoma, definitive resection of the AVM may be deferred unless the malformation is superficial and the anatomy is easily visible or if hemostasis can not be achieved [7]. As with all treatment options, pre-operative imaging with both DSA and MRI is helpful to elucidate the angioarchitecture of the lesion and to properly grade the patient so that an estimate of surgical risk can be determined.

Surgery for an intracerebral AVM involves a generous craniotomy over the AVM so that all of the superficial feeding arteries and draining veins are visualized in the exposure. Deeper lesions require thoughtful approaches through corridors that avoid injury to functionally important anatomical regions. Image guidance can be a useful adjunct in these cases. Using the operating microscope, the surgeon works circumferentially around the nidus to progressively coagulate and divide feeding arteries only as they are committed to the AVM. As the AVM is devascularized, the turgor is reduced. Care is taken to preserve a final draining vein to prevent intra-operative hemorrhage. After all feeders are taken, the draining vein is coagulated and divided. Intra-operative DSA is very useful in documenting complete obliteration and reduces the need for re-operation for residual AVM [29].

The most widely used grading system to estimate risk in AVM surgery is the Spetzler-Martin (SM) Grading Scale introduced in 1986 (Table 1) [29]. The scale was tested in a retrospective manner and successfully estimated surgical risk. Later prospective studies

Table 1. Spetzler-Martin AVM grading system.

AVM feature	Points
Size	
<3cm	1
3-6cm	2
>6cm	3
Eloquence of surrounding brain	
Non-eloquent	0
Eloquent	1
Venous drainage	
Superficial only	0
Deep	1

confirmed the scale's applicability [23, 30, 31] (II/B). The scale is based on three characteristics of the AVM: size, venous drainage, and eloquence of surrounding cortex. Scores are summarative, ranging from 1-5 as demonstrated in the table. Favorable outcomes following surgery for SM I lesions have been reported to be 92-100%, while SM V have a 57.1% chance of good outcome. Additionally, experienced surgeons recognize there are additional features of AVMs that influence surgical risk, such as compactness of the nidus. Lawton *et al* further demonstrated the heterogenous nature of grade III AVMs and proposed a modification of the SM grading scale [31].

SM III AVMs are more heterogenous with some being >6cm in non-eloquent cortex, while some are smaller AVMs with deep venous drainage or located in eloquent cortex [32]. For this reason, a modification was proposed for the SM grading system (mSM) [33]. The mSM subdivided grade III as follows: grade IIIA with size >6cm and IIIB involving deep venous drainage or eloquent cortex. In this case study, the authors recommended embolization plus surgery for IIIA and radiosurgery for IIIB (III/B). A second modification divided the class into:

◆ small AVMs (S1, venous drainage 1, eloquence 1);
◆ medium/deep (S2, V1, E0), medium/eloquent (S2, V0, E1); and
◆ large AVM (S3, V0, E0).

A new deficit or death was noted in 2.9% of (S1, V1, E1), 7.1% in (S2, V1, E0), and 14.8% in (S2, V0, E1). There were no large AVMs in the series. The authors recommended microsurgery in small AVMs, and felt that medium/eloquent lesions deserve conservative management (III/B).

In SM I and II patients, surgical extirpation has been shown to have excellent results in 92-100% and 94-95% of patients, respectively (III/B) [30]. Surgical risk is significantly higher in SM IV and V patients and caution must be exercised in the use of surgery alone, or more commonly, a multimodality treatment regimen is required (II/B) [23, 30].

Endovascular

Endovascular techniques have advanced markedly over the last decade due to technological progress and greater experience. With the introduction of new catheters, advanced angiography suites, and improved embolic agents, endovascular surgeons can navigate into smaller vessels and achieve pinpoint embolizations of the nidus of the AVM. Embolization has the lowest cure rate when used alone with complete obliteration rates of 9.9% in some studies [34] (III/B). For this reason, embolization is used primarily as an adjunct to surgical or radiosurgical treatments with the goal of eliminating feeding arteries and reducing nidus size for future treatment [7]. There are reports indicating palliative embolization for relief of epilepsy and vascular steal in a subset of patients [35, 36] (III/B). Outcomes after embolization alone has been shown to have generally low morbidity and mortality (13% and 1%, respectively [24] (III/B).

One randomized controlled study demonstrated no significant differences in pre-operative embolization between N-butyl cyanoacrylate (NBCA) and polyvinyl alcohol (PVA) and a second more recent study demonstrated no significant difference between NBCA and Onyx [37, 38]

(Ib/A). Therefore, the agent used does not appear to affect complication rate or embolization efficacy, when used as a pre-operative adjunct. If embolization is used to reduce nidus size prior to radiosurgery there may be a benefit to the use of more permanent 'glues' to embolize the portion of the AVM that will remain outside the radiosurgical target [39, 40].

There are no prospective studies comparing AVM surgery with or without embolization. The immediate advantage of pre-operative embolization includes reduced surgical time and decreased blood loss. There are multiple level III studies indicating reduced nidal size and low morbidity prior to microsurgical treatment [34, 41, 42].

The goal in preradiosurgical embolization includes reducing the nidus size to less than 3cm, treating associated aneurysms, and reducing venous hypertensive symptoms [34]. In large AVMs, preradiosurgical embolization has been reported to be helpful in some cases [41] (III/B). Alternatively, there is a report of decreased obliteration rates in a retrospective case control study of 47 matched patients when comparing radiosurgery with and without embolization. There was no significant difference in outcomes between the two groups (IIb/B).

Radiation

Stereotactic radiosurgery (SRS) acts on the blood vessels of the malformation causing progressive luminal obstruction [43]. By focusing radiation doses, the surrounding brain receives a smaller dose of radiation. Studies indicate that SRS is most successful in AVMs with maximal diameters less than 3cm and volumes less than 10cm^3 [43, 44]. For this reason, SRS is most commonly used for small AVMs in deep and eloquent brain. The large majority of SRS studies are level III data indicating that SRS is safe and effective in the treatment of specific AVMs [26, 43, 45, 46].

In patients who receive SRS alone, immediate complications are rare. Most morbidity is seen in a delayed fashion corresponding with the time course for treatment [26, 45]. Though imaging findings of radiation injury is present in up to 10% of patients, disabling permanent deficits were present in 2% of patients at 34 months (III/B) [26]. The same group reported that radiation dose and AVM size predicted obliteration. Complication rates were most often related to radiation dosage and AVM volume [45] (III/B). Paired series comparing microsurgery and SRS demonstrated similar cure rates with higher morbidity in surgery but higher rebleed rates in SRS [25].

Developmental venous anomaly

Developmental venous anomalies (DVAs) represent an exaggeration of normal venous structures that drain normal cerebral tissue [47]. Often, DVAs are discovered incidentally after radiographic imaging for unrelated reasons. Due to the fact that these venous structures drain normal cerebral tissues, removal or radiation of DVAs leads to venous infarction of the region drained by the DVA. Though the data come from case series (III/B), conservative management is the treatment of choice for these lesions [48, 49]. More recently, it has been recognized that DVAs are commonly associated with spatially adjacent but anatomically distinct cavernous malformations [50]. It is now well recognized that a 'hemorrhage' in association with a DVA is actually due to an associated cavernous malformation [47, 50, 51]. When resecting the cavernous malformation, extreme care needs to be undertaken to preserve the associated DVA.

Cavernous malformations

Cavernous malformations (CM) are dilated sinusoidal capillaries with a thin endothelial lining [52]. There is no interposed cerebral tissue in the lesion but the permeability of the lining predisposes them to leakage of blood with damage to the surrounding brain. These lesions were initially referred to as angiographically occult vascular malformations as they are generally invisible on cerebral angiography (except for the occasional associated DVAs [4]). Unlike AVMs, CMs have blood flow through them that is low flow and low pressure [53]. Therefore, the risk of hemorrhage is far less than for AVMs and when they bleed, they do so with much less vigor and thus less morbidity and mortality [54, 55]. With the advent of MRI, a greater understanding of CMs has been possible [56, 57]. CMs represent 10-15% of vascular malformations with the incidence ranging from 0.4-0.8% [52]. In general, CMs have an equal prevalence in men and women [58].

Numerous natural history studies have examined the epidemiology and hemorrhage rates of CMs. CMs occur both sporadically and within families. Although previously thought to be congenital, it is now recognized that CMs may also be acquired. For these reasons, prospective studies of natural history are preferred [55, 58-61]. Familial forms of this lesion are well documented, accounting for 6-50% of cases and are more common in Hispanic populations [62, 63]. Patients with familial CMs have multiple lesions in over 50% in cases, whereas sporadic cases are multiple in less than 20% [52, 63].

Prior to MRI, the vast majority of CMs presented with hemorrhage [64]. Many are now discovered incidentally in patients undergoing imaging for unrelated symptoms. Presently, in supratentorial lesions, the most common presenting symptom is seizure [52, 58]. Infratentorial lesions commonly present with neurological deficit or gait disturbances [65]. Deep brainstem and basal ganglia CMs often present with any number of neurologic symptoms including movement disorders, sensory deficits, cranial nerve dysfunction and hydrocephalus, depending on location and degree of hemorrhage [66]. Despite numerous prospective, level IIb studies, quoted hemorrhage rates vary greatly [55, 58-61]. Early retrospective (III/B) studies reported a hemorrhage rate of 0.25% per patient/year and 0.10% per lesion/year [54]. More recent prospective studies report annual hemorrhage rates of 0.7-6% per patient/year [55, 58-61]. Rebleed rates have been reported from 0-22.9% per patient/year [58, 59, 61] (IIb/B).

Surgery

The first report of successful surgery for a CM was in 1904 by Englehart [52]. Since that time, there are numerous series (III/B) promoting the effectiveness of surgical extirpation of

CMs [67-70]. Supratentorial resections in lesions coming to the pial surface result in excellent outcomes in the majority of cases [69, 70]. CMs in deep basal ganglia, brainstem, and spinal cord are more complex surgical problems [66, 71]. In 1991, a level III case series explored results after surgical resection of deep CMs with the indications for surgery being progressive neurologic deficit [71]. In this series, 28% of the patient population suffered severe complications. The highest risk was in patients with basal ganglia, thalamus, and insular CMs. There have been numerous case studies (III/B) reporting results of surgical resection at brainstem and thalamic CMs with 10-14% long-term morbidity rates with modern microsurgical and imaging techniques [65, 72]. Although indications for surgery of brainstem CMs vary, most authorities agree there should be at least one symptomatic hemorrhage prior to surgery for superficial brain stem lesions [72]. Deeper lesions can be reached by utilizing anatomical approaches for 'safe entry zones' [72]. Surgery is generally delayed 2-3 weeks after hemorrhage to allow for liquefaction of the surrounding hematoma [52].

Stereotactic radiosurgery

SRS for cavernous malformations remains a controversial subject. There have been multiple level III case series indicating a reduction in hemorrhage rates, most pronounced after 2 years [73-75]. Other studies have indicated that hemorrhage clustering may account for the observed lower bleed rates after 2 years and that SRS may not be an effective treatment for CMs [66]. A retrospective review of SRS versus surgery in 46 supratentorial patients demonstrated improved seizure-free rates and rebleed rates in surgery patients [76] (IIb/B). As of this time, there is no prospective case-control, cohort or randomized control series (I/A or IIa/B) to support SRS for CMs.

Capillary telangiectasias

Capillary telangiectasias are enlarged normal capillaries with low flow and generally asymptomatic presentation [4, 77]. These lesions are not normally visualized by angiography. With modern MRI techniques such as susceptibility and diffusion-weighted imaging, this lesion is being diagnosed more frequently [78]. They are typically located in the pons and less commonly in the white matter [77]. There are reports of treatment with surgery in the literature, though generally, the appropriate management is observation [77, 79] (III/B).

Dural arteriovenous fistulae

Dural arteriovenous fistulae (dAVF), sometimes also referred to as dural arteriovenous malformations, are direct fistulous A-V connections within the dural leaflets. These lesions can occur throughout the intracranial and spinal dura and are described by their location and venous drainage pattern. In general, the natural history is related to the anatomy of the venous drainage and symptoms are related to location. DAVFs have generated multiple classification systems that relate to anatomical considerations and hemorrhage rate. For simplicity's sake, these lesions are divided into spinal and cranial varieties.

Cranial dAVFs

The majority of cranial dAVFs are idiopathic and believed to be acquired and represent approximately 6% of supratentorial and 35% of infratentorial vascular malformations [80-82]. Symptoms are generally associated with changes in venous flow in the affected sinus [83]. There is no universal classification system for cranial dAVFs, though the most commonly used system was described by Borden *et al* and Cognard *et al* (Table 2) [84]. This system grades dAVFs from I-III depending on venous drainage. Numerous case studies have shown that the presence of leptomeningeal venous drainage is the single most important factor in predicting an aggressive natural history [84-86] (III/B). Therefore, treatment is generally pursued in Borden II and III fistulae, as they are reported to have hemorrhage rates of approximately 8.1% per year [85, 87]. Recently, the absence of hemorrhage or neurological deficit has been associated with a more benign course with a recommendation of a modification of the grading system to include this observation [83, 88, 89]. Often, observation is the best recommendation for patients with no retrograde leptomeningeal drainage (Borden I fistulae) given the benign clinical course [90] (III/B). For patients with non-aggressive fistulae but with intolerable symptoms, palliative therapy may be considered. There remains a 2% risk from observational studies that Borden I fistulae may go on to develop cortical venous drainage and associated aggressive behavior [90].

Table 2. dAVF classification schemes.

Borden		Cognard	
I	Anterograde or retrograde venous drainage into dural venous sinus	I	Anterograde drainage into dural venous sinus
II	Anterograde or retrograde venous drainage into dural venous sinus and retrograde leptomeningeal venous drainage	IIa	Retrograde venous drainage into dural venous sinus
		IIb	Anterograde venous drainage into dural venous sinus and retrograde leptomeningeal venous drainage
		IIa+IIb	Retrograde venous drainage into dural venous sinus and retrograde leptomeningeal venous drainage
III	Retrograde leptomeningeal venous drainage only	III	Retrograde leptomeningeal venous drainage only, no ectasia
		IV	Retrograde leptomeningeal venous drainage only, with ectasia
		V	Spinal venous drainage

Endovascular

Endovascular therapy is generally the first therapeutic option for most patients requiring treatment for intolerable symptoms or presence of leptomeningeal venous drainage. The goal of treatment is obliteration of the fistulous point and immediate cortical venous drainage by either transarterial or transvenous therapy [91-93]. There are many level III case series reporting successful endovascular treatments of cranial dAVFs in the literature [91, 94, 95]. Given the aggressive nature of this disease in patients with leptomeningeal venous drainage, a comparison to natural history is rarely made. Embolic agents may be delivered transarterially or transvenously and cure rates of 60-80% are quoted in the literature [91, 95]. There have been no head to head comparisons between different embolic agents.

Anatomical considerations remain important in treatment selection. High-risk areas for embolization such as ethmoidal artery fistulae may carry a risk of visual loss with treatment [96]. If embolization is unsuccessful or anatomically constrained as in foramen magnum or tentorial dAVFs, microsurgical management should be considered a viable option [81].

Surgery

The primary goal of microsurgery treatment of intracranial dAVFs is correct identification and elimination of the fistulous point or disconnection of the cortical venous drainage [97]. In lesions such as anterior fossa dAVFs where the ophthalmic artery gives ethmoidal feeders to the fistula, surgery is the treatment of choice with good surgical results noted in the literature [96, 98, 99] (III/B). Intra-operative angiography, or more recently, indocyanine green videoangiography can provide accurate intra-operative localization to localize the fistula and verify its obliteration [32, 100].

Radiation

SRS has been shown to be efficatious in the treatment of cranial dAVFs, though obliteration rates vary in the 50-58% range [101, 102]. SRS does appear to be effective in limiting symptoms such as tinnitus and may be a good therapeutic option in patients who suffer severe symptoms of a benign Borden I fistula [102] (III/B). As with all SRS treatments, there is a latency before obliteration that makes this a less appealing option for patients with dural fistulae associated with aggressive natural histories.

Spinal vascular malformations

The most common classification scheme grades lesions as follows: type I malformations are dAVFs, type II are glomus AVMs, type III are juvenile AVMs, and type IV are perimedullary fistulae [103]. Therapeutic options are discussed according to this classification.

Type I spinal dAVF

Type I dAVFs are the most common type of spinal vascular malformations representing 70-80% of spinal vascular malformations [103, 104]. Type I dAVFs lie within the dura at the nerve root sleeve as a fistula between a radicular artery and a medullary vein [105]. These lesions are believed to be acquired and present most commonly in men over the age of 40. Early natural history studies showed that 91% patients with untreated dAVFs are severely disabled at 3 years [106] (III/B).

Endovascular therapy with polyvinyl alcohol (PVA) embolization was associated with unacceptable recurrence rates up to 83% [107] (III/B). More recent series utilizing NBCA and Onyx have shown improved results with success rates of 30-90% [108, 109] (III/B).

Microsurgical ligation of a spinal dAVF requires a laminectomy or hemilaminectomy at the level of the fistula [110]. After opening the dura and identification of the fistula, it is disconnected by clipping or bipolar coagulation and division. Modern surgical series report cure rates of 84-98% [103, 110, 111] (III/B).

Type II intramedullary AVMs

Type II lesions have a distinct intramedullary nidus of vessels fed from the anterior and/or posterior spinal arteries [103]. Unlike type I dAVFs, type II AVMs occur throughout the spinal cord with equal incidence in men and women. They are rare congenital lesions.

There are small case series in the literature for all treatment modalities. Treatment with liquid embolics has been shown to improve symptoms with more recent cure rates near 37.5% [112]. Microsurgurical extirpation typically provides the highest cure rates with or without pre-operative embolization [113, 114] (III/B). Additionally, there are recent reports of successful treatments with radiosurgery in type II lesions showing reduction in AVM size and symptoms [115] (III/B).

Type III diffuse spinal AVMs

Metameric, or juvenile AVMs are large congenital lesions that extend past medullary tissue into the extramedullary space, including bone and skin [103]. These extremely rare lesions are often treated palliatively with embolization, though there are rare reports of cure with multimodality treatment in the literature [116] (III/B).

Type IV perimedullary arteriovenous fistulae

These intradural, extramedullary lesions are direct fistulae from the anterior spinal artery, or, less often, posterior spinal artery to the perimedullary venous system [103]. These fistulae are subclassified based on size and flow characteristics. Smaller type IV (subtype A and B) lesions have classically been treated with microsurgical obliteration with good results as long as ASA branches are preserved [117, 118] (III/B). Cho *et al* compared surgical treatment with endovascular and found that embolization cured five of nine while surgical treatment cured nine of ten [119] (IIb/B). Only embolization was attempted in IVC patients. Giant, multipediculated subtype C lesions have been readily treated with endovascular embolization [120, 121] (III/B).

Conclusions

Central nervous system vascular malformations incorporate many heterogeneous lesions with varied natural histories and treatments. Through improved technology and research, a greater understanding of these entities has been gained. As evidenced by the lack of level I studies, there remains a gap in our knowledge that could improve outcomes and treatment in the future.

Key points	Evidence level
◆ There are very few randomized studies and therefore very little level I evidence involving central nervous system vascular malformations.	
◆ AVM treatment is dependent on SM grading with grade I and II lesions being ideal for surgical excision and higher-grade malformations requiring multimodality treatments.	IIb/B
◆ The appropriate management for DVAs and capillary telangiectasis should be observation.	III/B
◆ Cavernous malformations (CM) are most effectively treated with surgery. Multiple studies show excellent results when the CM comes to the surface. In deep lesions, 'safe entry zones' should be utilized.	III/B
◆ Treatment for cranial dAVFs is dependent on Borden classification. In most cases, endovascular treatment is the first-line therapy.	III/B
◆ Spinal dAVFs are also treated based on classification. Type I can be treated with microsurgery or endovascular means depending on the spinal level of the lesion. Type II and IV lesions are treated most often with open surgery or multimodality regimens. Type III malformations are difficult lesions that can be treated with palliative embolization or multimodality treatment regimens.	III/B

References

1. McCormick WF. The pathology of vascular ('arteriovenous') malformations. *J Neurosurg* 1966; 24(4): 807-16.
2. Wilkins RH. Natural history of intracranial vascular malformations: a review. *Neurosurgery* 1985; 16(3): 421-30.
3. Stein BM, Kader A. (Honored guest lecture) Intracranial arteriovenous malformations. *Clin Neurosurg* 1992; 39: 76-113.
4. McCormick WF, Nofzinger JD. 'Cryptic' vascular malformations of the central nervous system. *J Neurosurg* 1966; 24(5): 865-75.
5. van Beijnum J, Bhattacharya JJ, Counsell CE, Papanastassiou V, Ritchie V, Roberts RC, *et al.* Patterns of brain arteriovenous malformation treatment: prospective, population-based study. *Stroke* 2008; 39(12): 3216-21.

6. Hartmann A, Mast H, Choi JH, Stapf C, Mohr JP. Treatment of arteriovenous malformations of the brain. *Curr Neurol Neurosci Rep* 2007; 7(1): 28-34.

7. Ogilvy CS, Stieg PE, Awad I, Brown RD, Jr., Kondziolka D, Rosenwasser R, *et al*. AHA Scientific Statement: Recommendations for the Management of Intracranial Arteriovenous Malformations: a Statement for Healthcare Professionals from a special writing group of the Stroke Council, American Stroke Association. *Stroke* 2001; 32(6): 1458-71.

8. The Arteriovenous Malformation Study Group. Arteriovenous malformations of the brain in adults. *N Engl J Med* 1999; 340(23): 1812-8.

9. Brown RD, Jr., Wiebers DO, Torner JC, O'Fallon WM. Frequency of intracranial hemorrhage as a presenting symptom and subtype analysis: a population-based study of intracranial vascular malformations in Olmsted Country, Minnesota. *J Neurosurg* 1996; 85(1): 29-32.

10. Brown RD, Jr., Wiebers DO, Forbes G, O'Fallon WM, Piepgras DG, Marsh WR, *et al*. The natural history of unruptured intracranial arteriovenous malformations. *J Neurosurg* 1988; 68(3): 352-7.

11. Fults D, Kelly DL, Jr. Natural history of arteriovenous malformations of the brain: a clinical study. *Neurosurgery* 1984; 15(5): 658-62.

12. Crawford PM, West CR, Chadwick DW, Shaw MD. Arteriovenous malformations of the brain: natural history in unoperated patients. *J Neurol Neurosurg Psychiatry* 1986; 49(1): 1-10.

13. Hartmann A, Mast H, Mohr JP, Koennecke HC, Osipov A, Pile-Spellman J, *et al*. Morbidity of intracranial hemorrhage in patients with cerebral arteriovenous malformation. *Stroke* 1998; 29(5): 931-4.

14. Stapf C, Labovitz DL, Sciacca RR, Mast H, Mohr JP, Sacco RL. Incidence of adult brain arteriovenous malformation hemorrhage in a prospective population-based stroke survey. *Cerebrovasc Dis* 2002; 13(1): 43-6.

15. Forster DM, Steiner L, Hakanson S. Arteriovenous malformations of the brain. A long-term clinical study. *J Neurosurg* 1972; 37(5): 562-70.

16. Mast H, Young WL, Koennecke HC, Sciacca RR, Osipov A, Pile-Spellman J, *et al*. Risk of spontaneous haemorrhage after diagnosis of cerebral arteriovenous malformation. *Lancet* 1997; 350(9084): 1065-8.

17. Kondziolka D, McLaughlin MR, Kestle JR. Simple risk predictions for arteriovenous malformation hemorrhage. *Neurosurgery* 1995; 37(5): 851-5.

18. Miyasaka Y, Yada K, Ohwada T, Kitahara T, Kurata A, Irikura K. An analysis of the venous drainage system as a factor in hemorrhage from arteriovenous malformations. *J Neurosurg* 1992; 76(2): 239-43.

19. Kumar AJ, Fox AJ, Vinuela F, Rosenbaum AE. Revisited old and new CT findings in unruptured larger arteriovenous malformations of the brain. *J Comput Assist Tomogr* 1984; 8(4): 648-55.

20. Kucharczyk W, Lemme-Pleghos L, Uske A, Brant-Zawadzki M, Dooms G, Norman D. Intracranial vascular malformations: MR and CT imaging. *Radiology* 1985; 156(2): 383-9.

21. Fiehler J, Stapf C. ARUBA - beating natural history in unruptured brain AVMs by intervention. *Neuroradiology* 2008; 50(6): 465-7.

22. Starke RM, Komotar RJ, Hwang BY, Fischer LE, Garrett MC, Otten ML, *et al*. Treatment guidelines for cerebral arteriovenous malformation microsurgery. *Br J Neurosurg* 2009; 23(4): 376-86.

23. Davidson AS, Morgan MK. How safe is arteriovenous malformation surgery? A prospective, observational study of surgery as first-line treatment for brain arteriovenous malformations. *Neurosurgery* 2010; 66(3): 498-504; discussion -5.

24. Hartmann A, Pile-Spellman J, Stapf C, Sciacca RR, Faulstich A, Mohr JP, *et al*. Risk of endovascular treatment of brain arteriovenous malformations. *Stroke* 2002; 33(7): 1816-20.

25. Nataf F, Schlienger M, Bayram M, Ghossoub M, George B, Roux FX. Microsurgery or radiosurgery for cerebral arteriovenous malformations? A study of two paired series. *Neurosurgery* 2007; 61(1): 39-49; discussion -50.

26. Flickinger JC, Kondziolka D, Lunsford LD, Pollock BE, Yamamoto M, Gorman DA, *et al*. A multi-institutional analysis of complication outcomes after arteriovenous malformation radiosurgery. *Int J Radiat Oncol Biol Phys* 1999; 44(1): 67-74.

27. Mathiesen T. Arguments against the proposed randomised trial (ARUBA). *Neuroradiology* 2008; 50(6): 469-71.

28. Al-Shahi R, Warlow C. Arteriovenous malformations of the brain: ready to randomise? *J Neurol Neurosurg Psychiatry* 2005; 76(10): 1327-9.

29. Spetzler RF, Martin NA. A proposed grading system for arteriovenous malformations. *J Neurosurg* 1986; 65(4): 476-83.

30. Hamilton MG, Spetzler RF. The prospective application of a grading system for arteriovenous malformations. *Neurosurgery* 1994; 34(1): 2-6; discussion -7.

31. Lawton MT. Spetzler-Martin Grade III arteriovenous malformations: surgical results and a modification of the grading scale. *Neurosurgery* 2003; 52(4): 740-8; discussion 8-9.

32. Barrow DL, Boyer KL, Joseph GJ. Intraoperative angiography in the management of neurovascular disorders. *Neurosurgery* 1992; 30(2): 153-9.

33. de Oliveira E, Tedeschi H, Raso J. Multidisciplinary approach to arteriovenous malformations. *Neurol Med Chir* (Tokyo)1998; 38 Suppl:177-85.

34. Vinuela F, Dion JE, Duckwiler G, Martin NA, Lylyk P, Fox A, *et al.* Combined endovascular embolization and surgery in the management of cerebral arteriovenous malformations: experience with 101 cases. *J Neurosurg* 1991; 75(6): 856-64.

35. Vinuela FV, Debrun GM, Fox AJ, Girvin JP, Peerless SJ. Dominant-hemisphere arteriovenous malformations: therapeutic embolization with isobutyl-2-cyanoacrylate. *AJNR Am J Neuroradiol* 1983; 4(4): 959-66.

36. Fox AJ, Girvin JP, Vinuela F, Drake CG. Rolandic arteriovenous malformations: improvement in limb function by IBC embolization. *AJNR Am J Neuroradiol* 1985; 6(4): 575-82.

37. Loh Y, Duckwiler GR; Onyx Trial Investigators. A prospective, multicenter, randomized trial of the Onyx liquid embolic system and N-butyl cyanoacrylate embolization of cerebral arteriovenous malformations. *J Neurosurg* 2010; 113(4): 733-41.

38. n-BCA Trial Investigators. N-butyl cyanoacrylate embolization of cerebral arteriovenous malformations: results of a prospective, randomized, multi-center trial. *AJNR Am J Neuroradiol* 2002; 23(5): 748-55.

39. Dawson RC, 3rd, Tarr RW, Hecht ST, Jungreis CA, Lunsford LD, Coffey R, *et al.* Treatment of arteriovenous malformations of the brain with combined embolization and stereotactic radiosurgery: results after 1 and 2 years. *AJNR Am J Neuroradiol* 1990; 11(5): 857-64.

40. Dion JE, Mathis JM. Cranial arteriovenous malformations. The role of embolization and stereotactic surgery. *Neurosurg Clin N Am* 1994; 5(3): 459-74.

41. Spetzler RF, Martin NA, Carter LP, Flom RA, Raudzens PA, Wilkinson E. Surgical management of large AVMs by staged embolization and operative excision. *J Neurosurg* 1987; 67(1): 17-28.

42. Purdy PD, Samson D, Batjer HH, Risser RC. Preoperative embolization of cerebral arteriovenous malformations with polyvinyl alcohol particles: experience in 51 adults. *AJNR Am J Neuroradiol* 1990; 11(3): 501-10.

43. Lunsford LD, Kondziolka D, Flickinger JC, Bissonette DJ, Jungreis CA, Maitz AH, *et al.* Stereotactic radiosurgery for arteriovenous malformations of the brain. *J Neurosurg* 1991; 75(4): 512-24.

44. Steiner L, Lindquist C, Adler JR, Torner JC, Alves W, Steiner M. Clinical outcome of radiosurgery for cerebral arteriovenous malformations. *J Neurosurg* 1992; 77(1): 1-8.

45. Flickinger JC, Kondziolka D, Lunsford LD, Kassam A, Phuong LK, Liscak R, *et al.* Development of a model to predict permanent symptomatic postradiosurgery injury for arteriovenous malformation patients. Arteriovenous Malformation Radiosurgery Study Group. *Int J Radiat Oncol Biol Phys* 2000; 46(5): 1143-8.

46. Colombo F, Cavedon C, Casentini L, Francescon P, Causin F, Pinna V. Early results of CyberKnife radiosurgery for arteriovenous malformations. *J Neurosurg* 2009; 111(4): 807-19.

47. Zimmer A, Hagen T, Ahlhelm F, Viera J, Reith W, Schulte-Altedorneburg G. [Developmental venous anomaly (DVA)]. *Radiologe* 2007; 47(10): 868, 70-4.

48. Kondziolka D, Dempsey PK, Lunsford LD. The case for conservative management of venous angiomas. *Can J Neurol Sci* 1991; 18(3): 295-9.

49. Garner TB, Del Curling O, Jr., Kelly DL, Jr., Laster DW. The natural history of intracranial venous angiomas. *J Neurosurg* 1991; 75(5): 715-22.

50. Rigamonti D, Spetzler RF. The association of venous and cavernous malformations. Report of four cases and discussion of the pathophysiological, diagnostic, and therapeutic implications. *Acta Neurochir* (Wien)1988; 92(1-4): 100-5.

51. Abdulrauf SI, Kaynar MY, Awad IA. A comparison of the clinical profile of cavernous malformations with and without associated venous malformations. *Neurosurgery* 1999; 44(1): 41-6; discussion 6-7.

52. Awad I, Barrow D. Cavernous malformations. Park Ridge, Ill: American Association of Neurological Surgeons, 1993.

53. Little JR, Awad IA, Jones SC, Ebrahim ZY. Vascular pressures and cortical blood flow in cavernous angioma of the brain. *J Neurosurg* 1990; 73(4): 555-9.

54. Del Curling O, Jr., Kelly DL, Jr., Elster AD, Craven TE. An analysis of the natural history of cavernous angiomas. *J Neurosurg* 1991; 75(5): 702-8.

55. Robinson JR, Awad IA, Little JR. Natural history of the cavernous angioma. *J Neurosurg* 1991; 75(5): 709-14.

56. Rigamonti D, Drayer BP, Johnson PC, Hadley MN, Zabramski J, Spetzler RF. The MRI appearance of cavernous malformations (angiomas). *J Neurosurg* 1987; 67(4): 518-24.

57. Schorner W, Bradac GB, Treisch J, Bender A, Felix R. Magnetic resonance imaging (MRI) in the diagnosis of cerebral arteriovenous angiomas. *Neuroradiology* 1986; 28(4): 313-8.

58. Moriarity JL, Wetzel M, Clatterbuck RE, Javedan S, Sheppard JM, Hoenig-Rigamonti K, *et al*. The natural history of cavernous malformations: a prospective study of 68 patients. *Neurosurgery* 1999; 44(6): 1166-71; discussion 72-3.

59. Kondziolka D, Lunsford LD, Kestle JR. The natural history of cerebral cavernous malformations. *J Neurosurg* 1995; 83(5): 820-4.

60. Porter PJ, Willinsky RA, Harper W, Wallace MC. Cerebral cavernous malformations: natural history and prognosis after clinical deterioration with or without hemorrhage. *J Neurosurg* 1997; 87(2): 190-7.

61. Aiba T, Tanaka R, Koike T, Kameyama S, Takeda N, Komata T. Natural history of intracranial cavernous malformations. *J Neurosurg* 1995; 83(1): 56-9.

62. Bicknell JM. Familial cavernous angioma of the brain stem dominantly inherited in Hispanics. *Neurosurgery* 1989; 24(1): 102-5.

63. Zabramski JM, Wascher TM, Spetzler RF, Johnson B, Golfinos J, Drayer BP, *et al*. The natural history of familial cavernous malformations: results of an ongoing study. *J Neurosurg* 1994; 80(3): 422-32.

64. Bell BA, Kendall BE, Symon L. Angiographically occult arteriovenous malformations of the brain. *J Neurol Neurosurg Psychiatry* 1978; 41(12): 1057-64.

65. Porter RW, Detwiler PW, Spetzler RF, Lawton MT, Baskin JJ, Derksen PT, *et al*. Cavernous malformations of the brainstem: experience with 100 patients. *J Neurosurg* 1999; 90(1): 50-8.

66. Gross BA, Batjer HH, Awad IA, Bendok BR. Cavernous malformations of the basal ganglia and thalamus. *Neurosurgery* 2009; 65(1): 7-18; discussion -9.

67. Yeh HS, Kashiwagi S, Tew JM, Jr., Berger TS. Surgical management of epilepsy associated with cerebral arteriovenous malformations. *J Neurosurg* 1990; 72(2): 216-23.

68. Batra S, Lin D, Recinos PF, Zhang J, Rigamonti D. Cavernous malformations: natural history, diagnosis and treatment. *Nat Rev Neurol* 2009; 5(12): 659-70.

69. Yamasaki T, Handa H, Yamashita J, Paine JT, Tashiro Y, Uno A, *et al*. Intracranial and orbital cavernous angiomas. A review of 30 cases. *J Neurosurg* 1986; 64(2): 197-208.

70. Vaquero J, Salazar J, Martinez R, Martinez P, Bravo G. Cavernomas of the central nervous system: clinical syndromes, CT scan diagnosis, and prognosis after surgical treatment in 25 cases. *Acta Neurochir* (Wien)1987; 85(1-2): 29-33.

71. Bertalanffy H, Gilsbach JM, Eggert HR, Seeger W. Microsurgery of deep-seated cavernous angiomas: report of 26 cases. *Acta Neurochir* (Wien)1991; 108(3-4): 91-9.

72. Gross BA, Batjer HH, Awad IA, Bendok BR. Brainstem cavernous malformations. *Neurosurgery* 2009; 64(5): E805-18; discussion E18.

73. Lunsford LD, Khan AA, Niranjan A, Kano H, Flickinger JC, Kondziolka D. Stereotactic radiosurgery for symptomatic solitary cerebral cavernous malformations considered high risk for resection. *J Neurosurg* 2010; 113(1): 23-9.

74. Kida Y. Radiosurgery for cavernous malformations in basal ganglia, thalamus and brainstem. *Prog Neurol Surg* 2009; 22: 31-7.

75. Kim DG, Choe WJ, Paek SH, Chung HT, Kim IH, Han DH. Radiosurgery of intracranial cavernous malformations. *Acta Neurochir* (Wien) 2002; 144(9): 869-78; discussion 78.

76. Shih YH, Pan DH. Management of supratentorial cavernous malformations: craniotomy versus gammaknife radiosurgery. *Clin Neurol Neurosurg* 2005; 107(2): 108-12.

77. Sayama CM, Osborn AG, Chin SS, Couldwell WT. Capillary telangiectasias: clinical, radiographic, and histopathological features. *J Neurosurg* 2010; 113(4): 709-14..

78. Castillo M, Morrison T, Shaw JA, Bouldin TW. MR imaging and histologic features of capillary telangiectasia of the basal ganglia. *AJNR Am J Neuroradiol* 2001; 22(8): 1553-5.

79. Lobato RD, Perez C, Rivas JJ, Cordobes F. Clinical, radiological, and pathological spectrum of angiographically occult intracranial vascular malformations. Analysis of 21 cases and review of the literature. *J Neurosurg* 1988; 68(4): 518-31.

80. Wilson M, Enevoldson P, Menezes B. Intracranial dural arterio-venous fistula. *Pract Neurol* 2008; 8(6): 362-9.

81. Steiger HJ, Hanggi D, Schmid-Elsaesser R. Cranial and spinal dural arteriovenous malformations and fistulas: an update. *Acta Neurochir Suppl* 2005; 94: 115-22.

82. Newton TH, Cronqvist S. Involvement of dural arteries in intracranial arteriovenous malformations. *Radiology* 1969; 93(5): 1071-8.

83. Zipfel GJ, Shah MN, Refai D, Dacey RG, Jr., Derdeyn CP. Cranial dural arteriovenous fistulas: modification of angiographic classification scales based on new natural history data. *Neurosurg Focus* 2009; 26(5): E14.

84. Borden JA, Wu JK, Shucart WA. A proposed classification for spinal and cranial dural arteriovenous fistulous malformations and implications for treatment. *J Neurosurg* 1995; 82(2): 166-79.

85. van Dijk JM, terBrugge KG, Willinsky RA, Wallace MC. Clinical course of cranial dural arteriovenous fistulas with long-term persistent cortical venous reflux. *Stroke* 2002; 33(5): 1233-6.

86. Cognard C, Gobin YP, Pierot L, Bailly AL, Houdart E, Casasco A, *et al.* Cerebral dural arteriovenous fistulas: clinical and angiographic correlation with a revised classification of venous drainage. *Radiology* 1995; 194(3): 671-80.

87. Duffau H, Lopes M, Janosevic V, Sichez JP, Faillot T, Capelle L, *et al.* Early rebleeding from intracranial dural arteriovenous fistulas: report of 20 cases and review of the literature. *J Neurosurg* 1999; 90(1): 78-84.

88. Soderman M, Pavic L, Edner G, Holmin S, Andersson T. Natural history of dural arteriovenous shunts. *Stroke* 2008; 39(6): 1735-9.

89. Strom RG, Botros JA, Refai D, Moran CJ, Cross DT, 3rd, Chicoine MR, *et al.* Cranial dural arteriovenous fistulae: asymptomatic cortical venous drainage portends less aggressive clinical course. *Neurosurgery* 2009; 64(2): 241-7; discussion 7-8.

90. Satomi J, van Dijk JM, Terbrugge KG, Willinsky RA, Wallace MC. Benign cranial dural arteriovenous fistulas: outcome of conservative management based on the natural history of the lesion. *J Neurosurg* 2002; 97(4): 767-70.

91. Cognard C, Januel AC, Silva NA, Jr., Tall P. Endovascular treatment of intracranial dural arteriovenous fistulas with cortical venous drainage: new management using Onyx. *AJNR Am J Neuroradiol* 2008; 29(2): 235-41.

92. Stiefel MF, Albuquerque FC, Park MS, Dashti SR, McDougall CG. Endovascular treatment of intracranial dural arteriovenous fistulae using Onyx: a case series. *Neurosurgery* 2009; 65(6 Suppl): 132-9; discussion 9-40.

93. Kirsch M, Liebig T, Kuhne D, Henkes H. Endovascular management of dural arteriovenous fistulas of the transverse and sigmoid sinus in 150 patients. *Neuroradiology* 2009; 51(7): 477-83.

94. Saraf R, Shrivastava M, Siddhartha W, Limaye U. Evolution of endovascular management of intracranial dural arteriovenous fistulas: single center experience. *Neurol India* 2010; 58(1): 62-8.

95. Macdonald JH, Millar JS, Barker CS. Endovascular treatment of cranial dural arteriovenous fistulae: a single-centre, 14-year experience and the impact of Onyx on local practise. *Neuroradiology* 2010; 52(5): 387-95.

96. Lawton MT, Chun J, Wilson CB, Halbach VV. Ethmoidal dural arteriovenous fistulae: an assessment of surgical and endovascular management. *Neurosurgery* 1999; 45(4): 805-10; discussion 10-1.

97. van Dijk JM, TerBrugge KG, Willinsky RA, Wallace MC. Selective disconnection of cortical venous reflux as treatment for cranial dural arteriovenous fistulas. *J Neurosurg* 2004; 101(1): 31-5.

98. Lawton MT, Sanchez-Mejia RO, Pham D, Tan J, Halbach VV. Tentorial dural arteriovenous fistulae: operative strategies and microsurgical results for six types. *Neurosurgery* 2008; 62(3 Suppl 1): 110-24; discussion 24-5.

99. Zhou LF, Chen L, Song DL, Gu YX, Leng B. Tentorial dural arteriovenous fistulas. *Surg Neurol* 2007; 67(5): 472-81; discussion 81-2.

100. Raabe A, Nakaji P, Beck J, Kim LJ, Hsu FP, Kamerman JD, *et al.* Prospective evaluation of surgical microscope-integrated intraoperative near-infrared indocyanine green videoangiography during aneurysm surgery. *J Neurosurg* 2005; 103(6): 982-9.

101. Wu HM, Pan DH, Chung WY, Guo WY, Liu KD, Shiau CY, *et al.* Gamma knife surgery for the management of intracranial dural arteriovenous fistulas. *J Neurosurg* 2006; 105 Suppl: 43-51.

102. Pan DH, Chung WY, Guo WY, Wu HM, Liu KD, Shiau CY, *et al.* Stereotactic radiosurgery for the treatment of dural arteriovenous fistulas involving the transverse-sigmoid sinus. *J Neurosurg* 2002; 96(5): 823-9.

103. Barrow DL, Awad IA. Spinal vascular malformations. Park Ridge, Ill: American Association of Neurological Surgeons, 1999.

104. Narvid J, Hetts SW, Larsen D, Neuhaus J, Singh TP, McSwain H, *et al.* Spinal dural arteriovenous fistulae: clinical features and long-term results. *Neurosurgery* 2008; 62(1): 159-66; discussion 66-7.

105. Aminoff MJ, Barnard RO, Logue V. The pathophysiology of spinal vascular malformations. *J Neurol Sci* 1974; 23(2): 255-63.

106. Aminoff MJ, Logue V. The prognosis of patients with spinal vascular malformations. *Brain* 1974; 97(1): 211-8.

107. Hall WA, Oldfield EH, Doppman JL. Recanalization of spinal arteriovenous malformations following embolization. *J Neurosurg* 1989; 70(5): 714-20.

108. Dehdashti AR, Da Costa LB, terBrugge KG, Willinsky RA, Tymianski M, Wallace MC. Overview of the current role of endovascular and surgical treatment in spinal dural arteriovenous fistulas. *Neurosurg Focus* 2009; 26(1): E8.

109. Medel R, Crowley RW, Dumont AS. Endovascular management of spinal vascular malformations: history and literature review. *Neurosurg Focus* 2009; 26(1): E7.

110. Eskandar EN, Borges LF, Budzik RF, Jr., Putman CM, Ogilvy CS. Spinal dural arteriovenous fistulas: experience with endovascular and surgical therapy. *J Neurosurg* 2002; 96(2 Suppl): 162-7.

111. Steinmetz MP, Chow MM, Krishnaney AA, Andrews-Hinders D, Benzel EC, Masaryk TJ, *et al.* Outcome after the treatment of spinal dural arteriovenous fistulae: a contemporary single-institution series and meta-analysis. *Neurosurgery* 2004; 55(1): 77-87; discussion -8.

112. Corkill RA, Mitsos AP, Molyneux AJ. Embolization of spinal intramedullary arteriovenous malformations using the liquid embolic agent, Onyx: a single-center experience in a series of 17 patients. *J Neurosurg Spine* 2007; 7(5): 478-85.

113. Bostrom A, Krings T, Hans FJ, Schramm J, Thron AK, Gilsbach JM. Spinal glomus-type arteriovenous malformations: microsurgical treatment in 20 cases. *J Neurosurg Spine* 2009; 10(5): 423-9.

114. Tai PA, Tu YK, Liu HM. Surgical treatment of spinal arteriovenous malformations: vascular anatomy and surgical outcome. *J Formos Med Assoc* 2001; 100(6): 389-96.

115. Sinclair J, Chang SD, Gibbs IC, Adler JR, Jr. Multisession CyberKnife radiosurgery for intramedullary spinal cord arteriovenous malformations. *Neurosurgery* 2006; 58(6): 1081-9; discussion -9.

116. Spetzler RF, Zabramski JM, Flom RA. Management of juvenile spinal AVMs by embolization and operative excision. Case report. *J Neurosurg* 1989; 70(4): 628-32.

117. Oldfield EH, Doppman JL. Spinal arteriovenous malformations. *Clin Neurosurg* 1988; 34: 161-83.

118. Kikuchi Y, Miyasaka K. Treatment strategy of spinal arteriovenous malformations based on a simple classification. *J Clin Neurosci* 1998; 5 Suppl: 16-9.

119. Cho KT, Lee DY, Chung CK, Han MH, Kim HJ. Treatment of spinal cord perimedullary arteriovenous fistula: embolization versus surgery. *Neurosurgery* 2005; 56(2): 232-41; discussion -41.

120. Ioannidis I, Sfakianos G, Nasis N, Prodromou P, Andreou A. Successful embolization of a giant perimedullary arteriovenous fistula of the cervical spine in a 6-year-old child. *Childs Nerv Syst* 2007; 23(11): 1327-30.

121. Ricolfi F, Gobin PY, Aymard A, Brunelle F, Gaston A, Merland JJ. Giant perimedullary arteriovenous fistulas of the spine: clinical and radiologic features and endovascular treatment. *AJNR Am J Neuroradiol* 1997; 18(4): 677-87.

Index

abciximab 8, 54, 97, 98

AbESTT-II trial (Abciximab in Emergent Stroke Treatment Trial) 8

ACCESS trial (Acute Candesartan Cilexetil therapy in stroke Survivors Study) 27

ACCORD trial (Action to Control Cardiovascular Risk in Diabetes) 27-9

ACE inhibitors 25, 26, 27, 30, 179, 242

ACE trial (ASA and Carotid Endarterectomy) 53

acetazolamide 214

ACTIVE-W trial (Atrial Fibrillation Clopidogrel Trial with Irbesartan for prevention of Vascular Events – Warfarin) 54, 72

acute coronary syndrome (ACS) 73, 229, 242

adult polycystic kidney disease (APKD) 137

ADVANCE trial (Action in Diabetes and Vascular Disease) 29

AFASAK-1/AFASAK-2 trials (Atrial Fibrillation Aspirin and Anticoagulant Therapy) 72

African Americans 22

age 21-2

    see also elderly patients

alcohol use 34-5

ALLHAT trial (Antihypertensive and Lipid-Lowering Treatment to prevent Heart Trial) 29-30

amiodarone 290, 291

amniotic fluid embolism 243

analgesia 180

ancrod 5

androgens

    in men 261-2, 269

    in postmenopausal women 256

anesthesia 248, 279

aneurysms *see* cerebral aneurysms

angioedema, orolingual 7

angiography

    acute ischemic stroke 91

    AVMs 302, 303

    cerebral aneurysms/SAH 142-3

    cerebral vasospasm 153

    CVT 209

    ICH 185-6

angioplasty

    for acute stroke 95

    for cerebral vasospasm 159

    for intracranial stenosis 116-17

antibiotics 212, 241

anticoagulants 59-61, 78-9

    in acute ischemic stroke/TIA 9, 60, 61-5, 232-3

    bridging therapy 65, 292

    in children 68, 216, 226, 229, 230, 232-3

    in CVT 66, 212-13, 213-14, 216, 243

in pregnancy 216, 243, 244, 245
prophylactic 48-9, 61, 78-9
    in arterial disease 55, 67-8, 116, 226, 230
    in cancer 77
    in cardiac disease 54, 69-76, 229, 245, 283, 290, 292
    in hypercoagulable disorders 76-7
    in ICH 190-1
reversal of effect 60, 186-9
anticonvulsants 190, 215
antidepressants 131
anti-factor Xa 233
antifibrinolytic agents 147-8
antihypertensives
    in ICH 177-8
    in pregnancy 242, 244, 247
    in SAH 147
    in stroke prevention 24-7, 29-30, 244
    thrombolysis and 10
antiphospholipid antibody syndrome (APL) 76-7, 210
antiplatelet agents 45-8, 55-6
    anticoagulants and 61, 74
    in arterial dissection/stenosis 55, 67-8, 230
    in cardiac disease 54, 74-5, 292
    in carotid endarterectomy 52-3
    in carotid stenting 54
    in children 226, 230, 231
    combination therapy 49-52, 53, 54
    in pregnancy 242, 244
    thrombolysis and 46, 97
antithrombotic therapy *see* anticoagulants; antiplatelet agents
aortic atherosclerosis 68, 280
aortic surgery 286-7
arrhythmia, cardiac
    in pregnancy 243
    see also atrial fibrillation
arteriovenous malformations (AVMs) 137, 248, 301-5, 311
ARUBA trial (A Randomized clinical trial of Unruptured Brain AVMs) 302
aSAH *see* subarachnoid hemorrhage, aneurysmal
aspirin 45-6
    in arterial dissection/stenosis 55, 67-8, 230
    in atrial fibrillation 54
    in cardiac disease 74-5
    in carotid endarterectomy 52-3
    in children 226, 230, 231
    with/compared to clopidogrel 49-52, 53, 54
    with dipyridamole 49, 50-1
    non-responsiveness 46-7
    in pregnancy 244
ATACH trial (Antihypertensive Treatment of Acute Cerebral Hemorrhage) 178
atorvastatin 31, 33

atrial fibrillation
  anticoagulation 54, 70-3, 75-6
  after cardiac surgery 282, 290-1
  radiofrequency catheter ablation 283
AVMs (arteriovenous malformations) 137, 248, 301-5, 311

BAATAF trial (Boston Area Anticoagulation Trial for Atrial Fibrillation) 72
BAFTA trial (Birmingham Atrial Fibrillation Treatment of the Aged) 72
balloon angioplasty
  for acute ischemic stroke 95
  for cerebral vasospasm 159
  for intracranial stenosis 116-17
Baltimore-Washington Cooperative Young Stroke Study 222
barbiturates, coma induction 183
BASICS registry (Basilar Artery International Cooperation Study) 6, 98
basilar artery 6, 98-9
bed position, in ICH 180
bed rest, in SAH 147
benzodiazepines 190
beta-blockers 179, 242, 290
blood pressure
  during CABG 280-1
  hypotension 279
  in ICH 176-8, 247
  in SAH 147
  thrombolysis and 9-10
  see also antihypertensives; hypertension
blood transfusions 223-4
body mass index (BMI) 35
body temperature
  in acute ischemic stroke 128
  cardiac surgery and 281
  in ICH 183-4, 189-90
  thrombolysis and 11
bone marrow transplantation 225
BRASIL trial (Bleeding Risk Analysis in Stroke Imaging before Thrombolysis) 11
British Aneurysm Nimodipine Trial 155

CABG (coronary artery bypass grafting) 280-2
CAD (cervical artery dissection) 8-9
CAFA trial (Canadian Atrial Fibrillation Anticoagulation) 72
calcium channel blockers
  for cerebral vasospasm 155-6, 160, 243
  in ICH 178, 179
  in pregnancy 247
cancer
  anticoagulation 77
  cardiac 70, 229, 290
  intracranial choriocarcinoma 247
candesartan (ACCESS trial) 27
capillary telangiectasias 307

cardiomyopathy 73, 229
    peripartum 242
cardiovascular causes of stroke 69-70, 279-80, 291-2
    anticoagulation and 54, 69-76, 229, 245, 283, 290, 292
    aortic procedures 286-7
    atrial fibrillation 54, 70-3, 75-6, 282, 283, 290-1
    CABG 280-2
    catheterization 284-5
    in children 227-9, 288
    congenital malformations 74-5, 229, 242, 288, 289
    heart transplantation 288-9
    in pregnancy 241-2, 243-4, 245
    radiofrequency catheter ablation 283
    tumor resection 290
    valvular disease 73-4, 75, 228, 241, 244, 282-3
CARE trial (Cholesterol and Recurrent Events) 31
carers 131
CARESS trial (Clopidogrel and Aspirin for Reduction of Emboli in Symptomatic carotid Stenosis) 52
carotid artery
    cavernous fistulae in pregnancy 248
    dissection in children 229-30
    endarterectomy (CEA) 107, 117, 118
        compared with CAS-P 115-16
        CT scan results and 108-9
        emergency 113-14
        plus antiplatelet agents 52-3
        in stable disease 109-13, 115-16
    stents (CAS) 54, 97-8, 115-16, 117
    thrombolysis 97, 114
CAST trial (Chinese Acute Stroke Trial) 46
catheterization, cardiac 284-5
cavernous malformations (CMs) 306-7, 311
    carotid cavernous fistulae in pregnancy 248
CCAD (cervicocephalic arterial dissection) 229-30
CDVST (cerebral dural venous sinus thrombosis) 243
CEA see carotid artery, endarterectomy
cerebellar hemorrhage 192
cerebellar infarction 131-2
cerebral aneurysms
    epidemiology 135-6
    imaging 142-3
    natural history 137-40, 161
    pathology 136
    in pregnancy 247
    risk factors 136-7, 161
    treatment 138
    see also subarachnoid hemorrhage, aneurysmal
cerebral dural venous sinus thrombosis (CDVST) 243
cerebral edema 123, 132-3
    antiedematous drugs 124, 131, 182
    diagnosis 128

hemicraniectomy 99, 124-31, 133
hypothermia 128
cerebral spinal fluid (CSF) 141
cerebral vasospasm
in PPCA 243
in SAH 148, 152-60, 162-3
cerebral venous thrombosis (CVT) 217
in children 213, 216
diagnosis 206-7, 216
epidemiology 205
management 66, 212-16, 217
prognosis 205, 210-11
risk factors 206, 209-10
in women taking OCs 267
cervical artery dissection (CAD) 8-9
cervicocephalic arterial dissection (CCAD) 229-30
CHADS2 score 70
CHARISMA trial (Clopidogrel for High Atherothrombotic Risk and Ischemic Stabilization, Management and Avoidance) 50, 51
children
anticoagulants 68, 216, 226, 229, 230, 232-3
antiplatelet agents 226, 230, 231
CVT 213, 216
ischemic stroke 68, 221-2
cardiac disease 227-9, 288
CCAD 229-30
management 231-5
moyamoya disease 225-7
sickle cell disease 222-5
chlorthalidone 30
cholesterol 10-11, 30-3
choriocarcinoma 247
cilexetil (ACCESS trial) 27
cilostazol 47
citicoline 12
CLAIR trial (Clopidogrel plus Aspirin for Infarction Reduction) 52
clazosentan 157
Clear IVH trial (Clot Lysis: Evaluating Accelerated Resolution of Intraventricular Hemorrhage) 195
clinical evaluation/presentation
acute ischemic stroke 89-90, 128
cerebral vasospasm 143
CVT 205
moyamoya disease 225
SAH 140-1
clopidogrel 47-8, 49-52, 53, 54, 231
CMs see cavernous malformations
coagulation factors in ICH 184-5, 189
coagulopathies 23
ICH and 186-9
see also hypercoagulable disorders

coils, endovascular, in SAH 150-2, 162, 247

coma, induced 183

compression stockings 190

computed tomography (CT)

    acute ischemic stroke 90-1, 124, 128

    CEA and 108-9

    CVT 206-7

    hemicraniectomy 129

    SAH 141

computed tomography angiography (CTA)

    cerebral aneurysms/SAH 142-3

    ICH (spot sign) 185-6

    ischemic stroke 91

congenital heart disease 74-5, 229, 242, 288, 289

cooling *see* hypothermia

coronary artery bypass grafting (CABG) 280-2

corticosteroids 214

coumarins *see* warfarin

craniectomy, suboccipital 131-2

    see also hemicraniectomy

cranioplasty 130

craniotomy 191-2, 303

crescendo TIAs 113-14

CREST trial (Carotid Revascularization Endarterectomy versus Stenting Trial) 115

CSPS trial (Cilostazol Stroke Prevention Study) 47

CT *see* computed tomography

CTA *see* computed tomography angiography

CVT *see* cerebral venous thrombosis

cytochrome P450 (CYP) variants 48

D-dimer test 209

dabigatran 49, 75

dAVFs (dural arteriovenous fistulae) 307-10, 311

DECIMAL trial (DEcompressive Craniectomy in MALignant middle cerebral artery infarcts) 99, 125-8

deep venous thrombosis (DVT) 65, 130, 190-1

depression 131

desmoteplase 5

desogestrel 266

DESTINY trial (DEcompressive Surgery for the Treatment of malignant INfarction of the middle cerebral arterY) 99, 125-8

developmental venous anomalies (DVAs) 305-6, 311

diabetes mellitus 27-30

diagnosis

    acute ischemic stroke 90-1

    AVMs 302

    CVT 206-7, 216

    SAH/cerebral aneurysm 140-3, 153-4, 161

    see also imaging

diet 35

digital subtraction angiography (DSA) 302, 303

dipyridamole 49, 50-1
direct thrombin inhibitors 48-9, 75
Doppler ultrasound, transcranial 154, 223
drospirenone 267
dural arteriovenous fistulae (dAVFs) 307-10, 311
dural venous sinus thrombosis 243
DVAs (developmental venous anomalies) 305-6, 311
DVT (deep venous thrombosis) 65, 130, 190-1

EAFT trial (European Atrial Fibrillation Trial) 72
ECASS trials (European Cooperative Acute Stroke Study) 2, 91
        ECASS-3 4-5
eclampsia 247
edema, cerebral *see* cerebral edema
elderly patients
        anticoagulation 70-1
        CVT 210
        decompressive surgery 99
        thrombolysis 5, 8
electroencephalography (EEG) 154
embolectomy 6-7, 93-4, 98, 114-15
embolization
        of AVMs 302, 304-5
        of dAVFs 309, 310
emergency department treatment 113-14, 146, 176
Emergency Management of Stroke Bridging Trial 93
enalapril 179
encephaloduroarteriosynangiosis 225, 226
endocarditis, infective 70, 241, 243, 282-3
endoscopic surgery in ICH 193
endothelin/endothelin receptor antagonists 157
endovascular treatments
        coils 150-2, 162, 247
        embolectomy 6-7, 93-4, 98, 114-15
        embolization 302, 304-5, 309, 310
        stents 54, 95-8, 115-17
epidemiology
        cerebral aneurysms 135-6
        CVT 205
        ICH 175, 186, 302
        SAH 135, 147, 247
        stroke 19, 89, 107
                after cardiovascular surgery 279, 280, 282, 284, 286, 289
                in children 222, 225, 229
                in pregnancy/puerperium 239
        vascular malformations 301, 306
        see also risk factors
epilepsy *see* seizures
eprosartan (MOSES trial) 27
esmolol 179
ESPRIT trial (European/Australasian Stroke Prevention in Reversible Ischemia Trial) 68
estrogens 271

CVT and 216
guidelines on use of OCs 268-9
stroke risk 22, 33, 256, 257-60, 261-4, 269
venous thrombosis risk 264-5, 266-7
ethnicity 22
European Carotid Surgery Trial 107-8, 112
evidence levels x, 20
exercise 36-7

Fabry disease 23
Factor V Leiden 76, 267
Factor VII, activated (FVIIa) 184-5, 189
Factor Xa inhibitors 76
FAST trial (Factor VII for Acute Hemorrhagic Stroke Trial) 185
FASTER trial (Fast Assessment of Stroke and Transient ischemic attack to prevent Early Recurrence) 51
fentanyl 180
fever, in ICH 189-90
FFP (fresh frozen plasma) 187, 188
Fisher grading of SAH 145
FISS/FISS-3 trials (Fraxiparine Ischemic Stroke Study) 63, 64
fosphenytoin 190
Framingham Heart Study 21
free radicals 157-8
fresh frozen plasma (FFP) 187, 188

gemfibrozil 33
gender
obesity and 36
as a risk factor 22, 257
genetic risk factors
cerebral aneurysms 137
CVT 210
stroke 23
gestodene 266
glucose levels
in ICH 189
stroke risk in diabetes 27-9
thrombolysis and 11
glycoprotein IIb/IIIa antibodies 8, 54, 97, 98

HAEST trial (Heparin in Acute Embolic Stroke Trial) 63, 64
HAMLET trial (Hemicraniectomy After Middle cerebral artery infarction with Life-threatening Edema Trial) 99, 125-8
headache
in CVT 215
in SAH 140
stroke risk and migraine 264, 268, 269-70
Heart Protection Study (HPS) 31
hemicraniectomy
for acute ischemic stroke 99, 124-31, 132-3

    for CVT 214

hemorrhage, anticoagulation and 60, 62-3, 70-1

hemorrhagic stroke

    cardiac surgery and 279, 289

    in pregnancy 240, 246-7

    statins and 33

    see also intracranial hemorrhage; subarachnoid hemorrhage, aneurysmal

heparin 60

    in acute ischemic stroke/TIA 61-5, 230, 232-3

    as bridging therapy 65, 292

    in CDVST 243

    in children 230, 232-3

    in CVT 66, 212-13

    in DVT 65

    in ICH 190-1

    in pregnancy 243, 244

    see also low-molecular-weight (LMW) heparin

HERS-I/HERS-II trials (Heart and Estrogen/Progestin Replacement Study) 256, 258, 259

HIMS (Health in Men Study) 261-2

Hispanic Americans 22

HMG-CoA reductase inhibitors *see* statins

HOPE trial (Heart Outcomes Prevention Evaluation) 25, 30

hormone replacement therapy (HRT) 271

    stroke risk 22, 255-60, 269

    venous thrombosis risk 264, 267

Hunt and Hess grading of SAH 143

hydralazine 179

hydrocephalus 183

hydroxyurea 224-5

hypercholesterolemia 31-3, 268

hypercoagulable disorders

    anticoagulation 76-7

    venous thrombosis risk 209-10, 213-14, 267, 270

hyperglycemia 11, 189

hypertension

    eclampsia 247

    in ICH 176-7, 247

    as a risk factor 24-7, 29-30

    thrombolysis and 9-10

    see also antihypertensives

hypertensive hypervolemic hemodilution (triple-H) therapy 154-5

hyperthermia 11, 189-90

hypertonic saline 182-3

hyperventilation 180-2, 226

hypoglycemia 11

hypotension 279

hypothermia

    in acute ischemic stroke 128

    cardiac surgery and 281

    in ICH 183-4

ICH *see* intracranial hemorrhage
ICP *see* intracranial pressure
idraparinux 76
imaging
        acute ischemic stroke 90-1, 124, 128
        AVMs 302
        CCAD 229
        CEA and 108-9
        cerebral aneurysms/SAH 141-3
        CVT 206-7, 215, 216
        hemicraniectomy 125, 129
        ICH 185-6
        moyamoya disease 226
immunosuppressive agents 247
IMS trial (Interventional Management of Stroke) 93
intensive care units (ICUs) 176
INTERACT trial (Intensive Blood Pressure Reduction in Acute Cerebral Hemorrhage Trial) 177
internal carotid artery (ICA)
        dissection 229-30
        occlusion 97-8, 114-16
International Cooperative Study on the Timing of Aneurysm Surgery 149
International Normalized Ratio (INR) 59-60, 187, 233
intra-arterial therapy
        thrombolysis 5-7, 92-3, 98, 291
        vasodilators 159-60
intracranial hemorrhage (ICH)
        as a complication of
                cardiac surgery 279, 289
                CEA 109-10
                thrombolysis 2, 4, 8-11
        epidemiology 175, 186
        management 175, 195-7
                of blood pressure 176-8, 247
                of coagulopathy 186-9
                hemostasis 184-6
                immediate 176
                of raised ICP 180-4
                supportive care 189-91
                surgery 183, 191-5, 247-8
        in pregnancy 246-8
        vascular malformations and 302, 306, 308
intracranial pressure (ICP), raised
        in CVT 214
        in ICH 178-84
        see also cerebral edema
intracranial stenosis 55, 67, 116-17
intraventricular hemorrhage 183, 194-5
intubation 176, 180
ISAT trial (International Subarachnoid Aneurysm Trial) 151-2
ischemic stroke 12-14, 99-100, 133
        angioplasty 95

antithrombotic therapy 9, 60, 61-5, 97, 231-3
    in children 221-35
    clinical assessment 89-90
    epidemiology 18, 89, 107, 239
    imaging 90-1, 124, 128
    pathology 123
    in pregnancy 239-46
    stents 95-7, 97-8, 115
    surgery 99, 113-14, 124-33
    thrombolysis *see* thrombolysis
ISCVT trial (International Study on Cerebral Vein and Dural Sinus Thrombosis) 210-11, 213
IST trial (International Stroke Trial) 46, 63, 64
ISUIA study (International Study of Unruptured Intracranial Aneurysms) 137-9

J-MUSIC trial (Japan-Multicenter Stroke Investigators' Collaboration) 92
Joint Study of Extracranial Arterial Occlusion 109

KEEPS trial (Kronos Early Estrogen Prevention Study) 259-60

labetalol 179
left ventricular assist devices 288
levetiracetam 190
levonorgestrel 266, 267
lifestyle 22, 33-7
lipid peroxidation inhibitors 157-8
LIPID trial (Long-term Intervention with Pravastatin in Ischemic Disease) 31
lipids
    guidelines for OC use 268
    post-thrombolysis ICH and 10-11
    as a risk factor 30-3
loss of consciousness 140, 176
low-molecular-weight (LMW) heparin 60
    in acute ischemic stroke/TIA 61-5, 230, 232-3
    as bridging therapy 65
    in cancer patients 77
    in CDVST 243
    in children 230, 232-3
    in CVT 212-13, 216
    in DVT 65
    in pregnancy 216, 243, 244
    see also heparin
lumbar puncture 141, 214
lumbo-peritoneal shunt 214
lysosomal α-galactosidase A 23

magnesium 156
magnetic resonance angiography (MRA) 143
magnetic resonance imaging (MRI)
    acute ischemic stroke 91
    cerebral vasospasm 154
    CVT 207-8, 215

ICH risk after thrombolysis 9-10

SAH 142

malignant MCA infarction *see* middle cerebral artery (MCA) infarction

mannitol 124, 131, 182

MAST-I trial (Multicenter Acute Stroke Trial) 46

MATCH trial (Management of Atherothrombosis with Clopidogrel and High-risk patients) 49-50, 51

MCA *see* middle cerebral artery

mechanical embolectomy 6-7, 93-4, 98, 114-15

medroxyprogesterone acetate 255-6

men

       androgens 261-2, 269

       obesity 36

       stroke risk 22

meningismus 140

Merci Retriever®/MERCI trial 6-7, 93, 98, 114-15

mestranol 267

microbleeds 11

MicroLysUS™ infusion catheter 95

microsurgery

       for AVMs 303-4

       for CMs 306-7

       for dAVFs 309, 310

       for SAH 151-2, 162, 248

       see also stereotactic surgery

middle cerebral artery (MCA) infarction 123-4, 132-3

       antiedema drugs 124

       diagnosis 128

       hemicraniectomy 99, 124-31

       hypothermia 128

       rehabilitation 131

       thrombolysis 5

middle cerebral artery (MCA) vasospasm 153

migraine 264, 268, 269-70

MISTIE trial (Minimally-Invasive surgery plus rt-PA for Intracerebral Hemorrhage Evacuation) 194

mitral valve 73, 228, 282

mortality

       CVH 205

       ICH 175

       SAH 139-40, 147

       stroke 89, 239

MOSES trial (Morbidity and Mortality after Stroke, Eprosartan Compared with Nitrendipine for Secondary Prevention) 27

moyamoya disease 225-7

MRA (magnetic resonance angiography) 143

MRI *see* magnetic resonance imaging

Multi-MERCI trial 6-7, 93, 98

myocardial infarction 73, 229

myxoma 70, 229, 290

NASCET trial (North American Symptomatic Carotid Endarterectomy Trial) 107-8, 110, 112
NBCA (N-butyl cyanoacrylate) embolic agent 304, 310
neonates
       CVT 216
       ischemic stroke 233
NEUROLINK™ stent 116
neuroprotection studies 12
neutropenia 48
niacin 33
nicardipine 156, 178, 179
nimodipine 155-6, 243, 247
NINDS rt-PA Stroke Study (National Institute of Neurological Disorders and Stroke) 2, 46, 89, 91-2
nitrendipine (MOSES trial) 27
nitrite infusions 158
nitroprusside 179
nitrous oxide (NO) 158
Nurses' Health Study 257

obesity 35-6
OCs see oral contraceptives
ocular hemorrhage 141
off-pump coronary artery bypass (OPCAB) 280
Ogilvy and Carter grading of SAH 145-6
ONTARGET trial (Ongoing Telmisartan Alone and in Combination with Ramipril Global Endpoint Trial) 27
Onyx embolic agent 304, 310
opioids 180
optic nerve compression 215
oral contraceptives (OCs) 271
       CVT and 216
       guidelines on use 268-9
       stroke risk 33, 262-4, 269
          and migraine 264, 269-70
       venous thrombosis risk 264-7, 270
osmotic therapy 124, 131, 182-3
ovarian hyperstimulation syndrome (OHS) 243

pain relief 180
papaverine 159-60
patent foramen ovale (PFO) 74-5, 229, 242, 289
pediatrics see children
pentobarbital 183
Penumbra system™ 94
percutaneous coronary intervention 284-5
perindopril (PROGRESS trial) 26
peripartum cardiomyopathy (PPCM) 242
PFO (patent foramen ovale) 74-5, 229, 242, 289
physical activity 36-7
pioglitazone 29
platelet function assays 46-7

polycystic kidney disease (APKD) 137
polyvinyl alcohol (PVA) embolic agent 304, 310
posterior circulation stroke 6, 7, 98-9
postpartum cerebral angiopathy (PPCA) 243
prasugrel 48
pravastatin 31, 159
pregnancy 248-9
       contraindicated drugs 216, 242, 244, 247
       CVT 216
       hemorrhagic stroke 240, 246-8
       ischemic stroke
              causes and risk factors 239-43
              management 242, 244, 249
              primary prevention 243-4
              secondary prevention 244-6
PROACT I and II trials (Prolyse in Acute Cerebral Thromboembolism) 5, 92, 93
PROACTIVE trial (Prospective Pioglitazone Clinical Trial in Macrovascular Events) 29
PRoFESS trial (Prevention Regimen for Effectively avoiding Secondary Strokes) 27, 50-1
progestogens
       stroke risk 255-6, 257-60, 264
       venous thrombosis risk 266, 267, 270
PROGRESS trial (Perindopril Protection Against Recurrent Stroke Study) 26
propofol 180
prosthetic valves 73-4, 241
       infective endocarditis 70, 241, 243, 282-3
protamine sulfate 60
prothrombin complex concentrates 188-9
prothrombotic conditions *see* hypercoagulable disorders
prourokinase (PROACT trials) 5, 92, 93
pulmonary embolism 190-1, 265
pyrexia, in ICH 189-90

radiosurgery
       for AVMs 302, 305
       for CMs 307
       for dAVFs 309
raloxifene 260
ramipril 25, 27, 30
Rankin scale 90, 126
RAPID trial (Rapid Anticoagulation to Prevent Ischemic Damage) 63
RE-LY trial (Randomized Evaluation of Long-Term Anticoagulant Therapy) 49
RECANALISE trial 7
rehabilitation, after hemicraniectomy 131
retinal hemorrhage 141
Reye's syndrome 231
rhabdomyoma, cardiac 229
risk factors 38
       age 21-2
       androgens in men 261-2, 269
       in cardiac procedures 280, 282, 284, 286, 288
       in children 222-30, 288

cholesterol levels 30-3
for CVT 206, 209-10
diabetes 27-30
gender 22, 257
genetic 23, 137, 210
HRT 257-60, 269
hypertension 24-7, 29-30
for ICH 246-7, 302
lifestyle 33-7
oral contraceptives 262-4, 269-70, 271
in pregnancy 239-43, 246-7
for SAH/cerebral aneurysms 136-7, 161
rosiglitazone 29
rt-PA (recombinant tissue plasminogen activator)
anterior circulation strokes 91-3
blood pressure and 9-10
after cardiac surgery 291
carotid artery occlusion 97, 114
cervical artery dissection 8-9
in children 233-4
complications 2, 4, 7, 11
hyperglycemia 11
hyperthermia 11
after ICH 194, 195
in older patients 5, 8
posterior circulation strokes 6, 7, 98-9
in pregnancy 244
time window of intravenous therapy 1-4, 8, 92, 97

SAH *see* subarachnoid hemorrhage, aneurysmal
SAINT I/II trials 12
saline, hypertonic 182-3
Scandinavian Simvastatin Survival Study (4S) 31
sedation 180
seizures
in CVT 215
in ICH 190
in SAH 141
SHEP trial (Systolic Hypertension in the Elderly Program) 25
shunts, in CVT 214
SICHPA trial (Stereotactic Treatment of Intracerebral Hematoma by means of a Plasminogen Activator) 193-4
sickle cell disease (SCD) 222-5
simvastatin 31, 159
sinking skin flap syndrome 129-30
SITS-ISTR registry (Safe Implementation of Thrombolysis in Stroke) 4
SITS-MOST study 2
smoking 33-4
SPAF trials (Stroke Prevention Atrial Fibrillation) 72
SPARCL trial (Stroke Prevention by Aggressive Reduction in Cholesterol Levels) 10, 31, 33
Spetzler-Martin (SM) Grading Scale (for AVMs) 303-4

SPINAF trial (Stroke Prevention in non-Rheumatic Atrial Fibrillation) 72
spinal cord ischemia 286, 287
spinal vascular malformations 309-10, 311
SPIRIT trial (Stroke Prevention in Reversible Ischemia) 68
SPS3 trial (Secondary Prevention of Small Subcortical Strokes) 27
SSYLVIA trial (Stenting of Symptomatic Atherosclerotic Lesions in the Vertebral or Intracranial Arteries) 116
statins 10-11, 31-3, 159, 292
stents 54, 95-8, 115-17
stereotactic surgery
      ICH aspiration 193-4
      radiosurgery
            for AVMs 302, 305
            for CMs 307
            for dAVFs 309
STICH trials (International Surgical Trial in Intracerebral Hemorrhage) 191-2
STOP trials (Stroke Prevention Trial in Sickle Cell Anemia) 223-4
STOP-IT trial (Spot Sign for Predicting and Treating ICH Growth) 185
streptokinase 5
stroke on awakening 7-8
stroke centers 20
stroke in evolution 113-14
subarachnoid hemorrhage, aneurysmal (aSAH) 160-3
      cerebral vasospasm 148, 152-60, 162-3
      diagnosis 140-3, 153-4, 161
      epidemiology 135, 147, 247
      etiology 136
      grading 143-6, 162
      management
            cerebral vasospasm 154-60, 162-3
            in the ED 146
            microsurgery and coiling 149-52, 162, 247-8
            prevention of rehemorrhage 147-8, 162
      natural history 139-40, 161
      in pregnancy 247-8
      risk factors 136-7, 161
subclavian artery 286
surgery
      for acute ischemic stroke 99, 124-33
            see also carotid artery, endarterectomy
      for AVMs 302, 303-4, 305
      cardiac, cerebrovascular complications of 279-92
      for CMs 306-7
      for CVT 214
      for dAVFs 309, 310
      for ICH 183, 191-5
      in moyamoya disease 226-7
            SCD-related 225
      for SAH 149-52, 162, 247-8
SWITCH trial (Stroke With Transfusions Changing to Hydroxyurea) 225
Syst-Eur trial (Systolic Hypertension in Europe) 25